# CLINICAL SKILLS MANUAL
## FOR MATERNITY AND PEDIATRIC NURSING

### Fifth Edition

**Ruth C. McGillis Bindler, RNC, PhD**
*Professor Emeritus*
*Washington State University*
*College of Nursing*
*Spokane, Washington*

**Jane W. Ball, RN, DrPH, CPNP**
*Consultant, American College of Surgeons*
*Gaithersburg, Maryland*

**Marcia L. London, RN, MSN, APRN, CNS, NNP-BC-E**
*Senior Clinical Instructor and Director of Neonatal Nurse Practitioner Program*
*Beth-El College of Nursing and Health Sciences*
*University of Colorado*
*Colorado Springs, Colorado*

**Michele R. Davidson, RN, PhD, CNM, CFN**
*Associate Professor of Nursing and Women's Studies*
*George Mason University College of Health and Human Services*
*School of Nursing*
*Fairfax, Virginia*

**PEARSON**

Boston   Columbus   Indianapolis   New York   San Francisco
Amsterdam   Cape Town   Dubai   London   Madrid   Milan   Munich   Paris   Montréal
Toronto   Delhi   Mexico City   São Paulo   Sydney   Hong Kong   Seoul   Singapore   Taipei   Tokyo

**Publisher:** Julie Levin Alexander
**Publisher's Assistant:** Sarah Henrich
**Executive Editor:** Lisa Rahn
**Editorial Assistant:** Erin Sullivan
**Project Manager:** Maria Reyes
**Program Manager:** Erin Rafferty
**Development Editor:** Mary Cook
**Director, Publishing Operations:** Etain O'Dea
**Team Lead, Program Management:** Melissa Bashe
**Team Lead, Project Management:** Cynthia Zonneveld
**Manufacturing Buyer:** Maura Zaldivar-Garcia
**Art Director:** Mary Siener
**Vice President of Sales & Marketing:** David Gesell
**Vice President, Director of Marketing:** Margaret Waples
**Senior Product Marketing Manager:** Phoenix Harvey
**Field Marketing Manager:** Debi Doyle
**Marketing Specialist:** Michael Sirinides
**Media Project Manager:** Lisa Rinaldi
**Full-Service Vendor:** Cenveo® Publisher Services
**Printer/Binder:** RR Donnelley/Kendallville
**Cover Printer:** Lehigh-Phoenix Color/Hagerstown
**Cover Image:** Getty Images/Hero Images; Getty Images/ERproductions Ltd; Shutterstock/Chaikom

**Notice:** Care has been taken to confirm the accuracy of information presented in this book. The authors, editors, and the publisher, however, cannot accept any responsibility for errors or omissions, or for consequences from application of the information in this book, and make no warranty, express or implied, with respect to its contents.

The authors and publisher have exerted every effort to ensure that drug selections and dosages set forth in this text are in accord with current recommendations and practice at time of publication. However, in view of ongoing research, changes in government regulations, and the constant flow of information relating to drug therapy and drug reactions, the reader is urged to check the package inserts and other drug references of all drugs for any change in indications of dosage and for added warnings and precautions. This is particularly important when the recommended agent is a new and/or infrequently employed drug.

**Library of Congress Cataloging-in-Publication Data**
Names: Bindler, Ruth McGillis, author. | Ball, Jane (Jane W.), author. |
  London, Marcia L., author. | Davidson, Michele R., author.
Title: Clinical skills manual for maternity and pediatric nursing / Ruth C.
  McGillis Bindler, Jane W. Ball, Marcia L. London, Michele R. Davidson.
Other titles: Clinical skills manual for maternal & child nursing care
Description: Fifth edition. | Hoboken, New Jersey : Pearson Education, Inc.,
  [2017] | Preceded by Clinical skills manual for maternal & child nursing
  care / Ruth C. McGillis Bindler . . . [et al.]. 4th ed. c2014. | Includes
  bibliographical references and index.
Identifiers: LCCN 2016000881 | ISBN 9780134257006 (alk. paper) | ISBN 0134257006 (alk. paper)
Subjects: | MESH: Maternal-Child Nursing--methods | Pediatric Nursing—methods
Classification: LCC RG951 | NLM WY 157.3 | DDC 618.92/00231—dc23
LC record available at http://lccn.loc.gov/2016000881

10  9  8  7  6  5  4  3  2  1

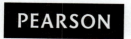

ISBN-13: 978-0-13-425700-6
ISBN-10:    0-13-425700-6

# Contents

## ■ Chapter 13

# Intravenous Access    123

## ■ Chapter 14

# Neurologic Assessment and Care    136

## ■ Chapter 15

# Cardiorespiratory Care    141

# Preface

Performance of skills in a safe and competent manner is an essential component of nursing interventions. This clinical skills manual is designed to assist you in planning and performing nursing skills. It is an independent skills procedure manual and is portable so that it can be carried to clinical settings and referred to quickly when you need to perform a skill. As a text companion, it helps you to translate theoretical concepts into performance while you care for health clients in a variety of settings.

Nurses caring for childbearing women often use skills that are specialized to prenatal care, birth, and the postnatal period, thereby providing maternity nursing care. Skills can be challenging to perform on children because of their differing levels of growth and development, lack of ability to communicate or understand information about procedures, and some differences from techniques used with adults. Therefore, this maternity and pediatric clinical skills manual is intended to enable practitioners to assist in and safely carry out skills commonly performed on childbearing women, newborns, and children. We recognize that students now often learn skill performance in a combination of simulation and actual clinical experiences. This book allows for the student to verify correct procedures prior to performing those skills in the clinical setting.

Skills are grouped into chapters that reflect types of intervention. The following chapters are included:

- Protective methods
- Women's health and prenatal care
- Intrapartum
- Postpartum
- Newborn
- Informed consent for children
- Physical assessment of newborns and children
- Pain assessment and management
- Positioning and restraining therapies
- Transporting the child
- Specimen collection
- Administration of medication and irrigation
- Intravenous access for newborns and children
- Neurologic assessment and care of newborns and children
- Cardiorespiratory care of newborns and children
- Nutrition skills for newborns and children
- Elimination skills for newborns and children
- Skin and musculoskeletal care

Each skill begins with a short description, followed by the preparation needed, equipment and supplies required, and the procedure itself. Rationales are inserted within the skill presentations to explain the reason for certain preparations and actions. Be sure to read the introduction to this manual, which lists general guidelines that must be applied whenever performing skills.

The skills are presented concisely to emphasize essential information. This manual builds on the basic skills content in nursing programs; it does not seek to replace a nursing foundations course. Rather, it is designed to emphasize childbearing and pediatric variations and the essential information needed to perform the most vital skills with childbearing women, newborns, children, and youth. Several approaches are used to assist the student in understanding and carrying out the skills. Photographs provide a visual image of equipment and technique. Boxes and tables highlight important safety issues, growth and development considerations, family teaching, and clinical tips.

The clinical skills manual ends with appendices that provide information on growth grids and calculation of body surface area for medication administration.

**NOTE:** Students and nurses should always consult their agency's procedure manual or other references for more detailed and specific information when needed.

## Acknowledgments

This clinical skills manual has become a reality through the dedication and hard work of many individuals. Our thanks go to Julie Levin Alexander, our publisher. Julie is committed to excellence and creativity. She is the driving force behind the exciting changes occurring at Pearson Health Science and is truly a creative futurist in publishing. Mary Cook, our development editor, was attuned to detail, organized the components of this edition, and coordinated all aspects of the project. We are grateful for her skill, dedication, and guidance.

Many of the photographs were taken by George Dodson and Roy Ramsey; both of these talented individuals are sensitive to issues related to children and families in clinical settings and are creative and proficient in capturing the images of family members and nurses.

We also want to thank the following reviewers for the honest and valuable feedback that they provided for this revision:

Karen Hessler, PhD, FNP-C
*Associate Professor*
*University of Northern Colorado*
*Greeley, Colorado*

Meredith Lahl, MSN, PCNS-BC,
PPCNP-BC, CPON
*Senior Director of Advanced Practice Nursing*
*Cleveland Clinic*
*Cleveland, Ohio*

Sharon Rappold, MSN, RN, BC
*Wharton County Junior College*
*Wharton, Texas*

Maria Burkhalter Ronquillo, MS, RNC-OB, C-EFM
*Samuel Merritt University*
*San Mateo, California*

JoAnne Silbert-Flagg, DNP, PNP, IBCLC
*Assistant Professor*
*Johns Hopkins University*
*Baltimore, Maryland*

Maureen P. Tippen, RN, C, MS
*Clinical Assistant Professor*
*University of Michigan*
*Flint, Michigan*

Ruth C. Bindler
Jane W. Ball
Marcia L. London
Michele R. Davidson

# Introduction

## General Guidelines

Two major concerns the nurse should keep in mind when performing procedures are safety and comfort. The nurse ensures that correct procedures are followed so that the childbearing woman or the child being cared for is kept free from harm. Approaches should be used to promote understanding and comfort for both the client and family members. Nurses play a vital role in skill performance that enhances the effectiveness of preventive measures, diagnosis, and treatment in many settings.

Childbearing women may need procedures with which they are not familiar, and potentially at a time that is also stressful. Clear explanations for the woman, the presence of support persons, reassurance, and explanations during the procedure are helpful.

Nurses often perform procedures on children in homes, clinics, and hospitals. These procedures, although similar to those performed on adults, differ in several ways. Nurses must therefore be knowledgeable about skills commonly performed in child health settings, as well as understand variations in preparation, equipment, and techniques needed to perform skills on children. The nurse also integrates knowledge of health promotion and disease prevention by performing screening in children.

Children are taken to a treatment room or to another room in the clinic or hospital for potentially painful or frightening procedures. The child's room and the playroom are thus kept as "safe" areas in which painful procedures are not performed. If parents wish to be present, they can be helped to support the child. When possible, it is best to have other personnel immobilize the child or assist with the procedure so that the child does not view the parent as being the cause of the discomfort. The child and family should receive support after the procedure as needed.

When a clinical skill is to be performed, general guidelines for performing the procedure include the following:

- Check the medical order or prescription to verify the procedure.
- Review the procedure as needed. Consult the agency's policy and procedure manual as needed.
- Identify the individual by two types of identification, such as name band, medication record, verbal statement, or other means.
- Verify that the consent is signed if needed.
- Greet the childbearing woman or child receiving care and the family members.
- Give developmentally and culturally appropriate explanations and instructions about the specific plan to the childbearing woman or child and family. Arrange for translators to perform the explanation if needed.
- Verify understanding and ask if there are questions about the procedure.
- Inquire if the parent wishes to be present when the skill is to be performed on a child. Ask the childbearing woman if she wants someone with her. Clarify the roles of any family member present, such as immobilizing a limb or offering comfort measures.
- Perform hand hygiene.
- Prepare necessary equipment and supplies.
- Don clean or sterile gloves as needed.
- Perform the procedure.
- Clean the area as needed.
- Document the performance of the procedure, results, and responses of the client and family.

Nursing skills provide a unique opportunity to provide a high level of care for childbearing women, children, parents, and families, and to communicate in a sensitive and effective manner. We hope that this skills manual assists you in providing safe and comprehensive care for childbearing women, infants, children, and adolescents.

# Chapter 1
# Protective Methods

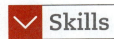 **Skills**

## Infection Control Methods

Special methods are used to provide infection control. There are two levels of precautions: standard and transmission-based. Consult the Centers for Disease Control and Prevention (CDC) and the Healthcare Infection Control Practices Advisory Committee for details on infection control (Siegel, Rhinehart, Jackson, et al., 2007).

---

**BOX 1–1  RECOMMENDATIONS AND GUIDELINES FOR PARTICULAR RISKS**

General recommendations as well as specific guidelines for particular risks, such as hand hygiene, catheter-related infection, norovirus, and environmental issues, can be found at http://www.cdc.gov/hicpac /pubs.html. Specific recommendations for managing persons at risk for Ebola virus are available (Centers for Disease Control and Prevention [CDC], 2014a).

---

Prior to client contact, decide what types of personal protective equipment (PPE) are needed:

- *Masks* are needed for protection from pathogens that are shed through respiratory droplets.
- *Gloves* are used to protect the skin from contact with pathogens. They are worn when there is contact with mucous membranes, nonintact skin, body fluids, or blood.
  RATIONALE: *Gloves protect both the client and the healthcare provider from contamination and transferal of infective agents.*
- *Gowns (protective apparel)* are used for protection against contact with pathogens when it is likely that body substances will come in contact with the healthcare provider's clothing. Gowns are changed between contacts with different clients.
- *Protective eyewear,* such as goggles or face shields, is worn if there is a risk of blood or body fluids being splattered. Wear protective eyewear when the eyes, nose, or mouth may be splashed by the client's body substances and when in close proximity to any open skin lesions.

## Standard Precautions

Standard precautions are used in the care of all clients, no matter what their diagnoses, whenever contact with blood, body fluids, secretions, excretions, nonintact skin, mucous membranes, or materials contaminated with these substances might occur. Always have access to protective equipment and add items as needed. The following general guidelines should be used:

1. Conduct hand hygiene before and after client contact; after contact with blood, body fluids, or contaminated surfaces (even if gloves are worn); before invasive procedures; and after removing gloves (wearing gloves is not enough to prevent the transmission of pathogens in healthcare settings) (CDC, 2014b; World Health Organization, 2014). Soap and water as well as an array of antiseptic agents are available. The U.S. Food and Drug Administration is currently evaluating antiseptic agents to make further recommendations for health care (U.S. Department of Health and Human Services, 2015).

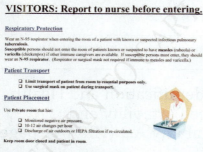

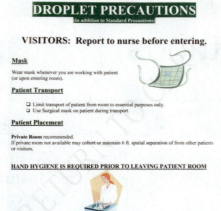

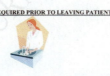

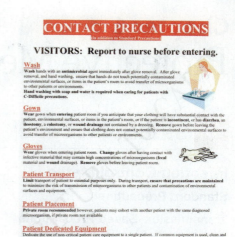

**Figure 1–1** *Isolation signs.*

2. Wear gloves whenever contact with blood, body fluids, secretions, excretions, nonintact skin, or mucous membranes might occur. Change gloves each time they are contaminated with these substances, washing hands before regloving.

3. Wear additional protective equipment such as a gown, mask, and eye shield if body fluid splashes can occur.

4. Wear the protective equipment listed in this chapter to clean up body fluid spills. Discard waste in appropriate body substance waste containers. Clean the area with bleach or another acceptable cleaner. Bag contaminated laundry in secured and labeled bags.

5. Discard needles, scalpels, and lancets in labeled sharps containers without recapping.

6. Place clients who could contaminate the environment with airborne or droplet infection in private rooms.

## Transmission-Based Precautions

In addition to standard precautions, further measures are followed when a client may be infected with a pathogen or communicable disease. The type of precaution taken is indicated by posting the appropriate sign on the person's hospital door (Figure 1–1).

There are three levels of transmission-based precautions:

1. Use *airborne precautions* for diseases transported by the airborne route (see Table 1–1). Health-care providers use high-efficiency particulate air filter respirators (such as a National Institute for Occupational Safety and Health [NIOSH]–certified disposable N95 respirator or personal air-purifying respirator [PAPR] hoods and power packs) for protection. In addition, a negative airflow ventilation system room is needed for tuberculosis. The client in airborne precautions must wear a surgical mask when leaving the room to filter expired air. Label the person's door with a sign instructing visitors to report to the nurses' desk before entering (Figure 1–2).

2. Institute *droplet precautions* for diseases transmitted by the droplet route. A surgical mask is needed when coming within 3 feet of the client. The client wears a mask when leaving the room. The room door can remain open, and special respirators are not required.
   RATIONALE:   *The large particle droplets of these diseases cannot travel over 3 feet.*

3. Use *contact precautions* for diseases that spread by direct contact with the skin or by indirect contact with a contaminated object in the client's environment. Apply gloves to perform all nursing care. Gowns are worn if the healthcare provider's clothing may come in contact with contaminated surfaces or the client. Clients should be placed in a private room or with other clients infected with the same pathogen.
   NOTE:   *A combination of precautions may be needed. For example, for severe acute respiratory syndrome (SARS), a combination of standard, contact, and airborne precautions must be followed.*

| TABLE 1–1 | Examples of Diseases Requiring Transmission-Based Precautions | |
|---|---|---|
| **Airborne** | **Droplet** | **Contact** |
| Measles | *Haemophilus influenzae* type b | Gastrointestinal illness (e.g.) |
| Varicella (chickenpox) | Rubella | *Clostridium difficile* |
| Tuberculosis | Pertussis | *Escherichia coli* |
| | Mumps | Hepatitis A |
| | Pneumonia | Skin infections (e.g.) |
| | Influenza | Scabies |
| | Streptococcal pharyngitis | Impetigo |
| | *Mycoplasma pneumoniae* | Lice |
| | | Genital infections (e.g.) |
| | | Herpes simplex |
| | | Chlamydial |
| | | Syphilis |
| | | Gonorrhea |
| | | General infections (e.g.) |
| | | Conjunctivitis |
| | | Methicillin-resistant *Staphylococcus aureus* (MRSA) |

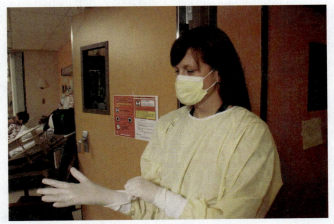

**Figure 1–2** *For clients in contact isolation, gowns, gloves, and masks are worn and the door must be clearly labeled with a sign instructing healthcare providers of equipment needed and telling visitors to stop at the nurses' station before entering.*

## SKILL 1–1 Latex Precautions

Latex sensitivity and allergy are antigen-antibody (IgE) reactions to natural rubber latex products. Precautions are needed to ensure that clients and employees with sensitivity and allergy do not come into contact with latex.

### PREPARATION

1. Reduce and/or eliminate the amount of latex used in agencies by eliminating use of latex gloves where feasible as well as reducing the amount of other latex products used; when latex gloves are used, they should be nonpowdered.

   **RATIONALE:** *The powder in latex gloves contains latex, which is spread into the environment when the gloves are donned.*

2. Identify latex-free materials and supplies in the agency.

3. Be aware of signs of latex sensitivity.

4. Assess all clients for a history of latex allergy or significant risk factors.

5. Be prepared for emergency resuscitation if needed.

### EQUIPMENT AND SUPPLIES

- Latex-free gloves, syringes, and IV ports on IV bags/lines
- Latex-free bellows on ventilator
- Latex-free resuscitator bags
- Stockinette and latex-free tape
- Medications and equipment for treatment of anaphylactic reaction

### PROCEDURE

When clients are identified as being latex sensitive or allergic, prepare the environment before their entry and continue practices as long as they remain:

1. Remove all latex-containing products (e.g., gloves, tourniquets, tape) from the room. If latex products cannot be removed, the items should be located in a closed storage area, such as cabinets and drawers.

2. After removing latex items, thoroughly clean the room/examination area using latex-free (nitrile or vinyl) gloves to remove contaminated latex-containing dust. Do not wear latex or rubber gloves to clean the room. When an allergic individual has surgery or another procedure, the room should be properly prepared and the case should be the first of the day.

3. Mattresses/examination tables may contain latex and should be covered completely with a nonlatex protective cover.

4. Stock rooms with latex-free materials and latex-free gloves.

5. Place a latex precaution sign on the client's door/examination area.

6. Place all monitoring devices and cords/tubes (oximeter, blood pressure, electrocardiograph wires, ports on intravenous tubing) in stockinette, and tape with nonlatex tape to prevent direct skin contact. Items sterilized in ethylene oxide must be rinsed before use. Residual ethylene oxide can cause an allergic response in a latex-allergic client.

7. Use stopcocks rather than latex ports to inject drugs.

8. Label the client's medical record, medication form, and identification bands with allergy alerts. Alert other nurses to the allergy during verbal reports between shifts.

9. Document measures taken.

10. Report promptly and document any signs of sensitivity or allergy.

11. Teach clients and families about latex allergy and how to avoid latex products.

---

**CLINICAL TIP**

Always use nonlatex gloves and supplies when your client has an allergy or sensitivity to latex. See your textbook for information on latex allergy. From 8% to 12% of healthcare workers are sensitive to latex, and the high exposure to latex products in the workplace is a causative factor. Know the sources of latex in the clinical agency where you work, and choose nonlatex alternatives when possible to decrease your exposure and resultant risk for developing latex sensitivity (National Institute for Occupational Safety and Health [NIOSH], 2014).

12. Instruct the family about foods that commonly cause allergies in those with latex allergy, and avoid feeding such foods to the client. These foods include bananas, avocados, kiwis, plums, peaches, cherries, apricots, figs, papayas, tomatoes, potatoes, and chestnuts.

## SKILL 1–2  Visitor Identification and Health Insurance Portability and Accountability Act (HIPAA)

Nurses must reliably identify clients, family members, and other healthcare professionals, and at the same time protect the privacy of clients. The Health Insurance Portability and Accountability Act of 1996 (HIPAA) identifies protected health information (PHI) by establishing standards for the exchange of health information, security standards, and privacy standards. As technology has increased, ensuring the safety of health information has become even more critical. Nurses should apply current guidelines; they often work on interdisciplinary teams within agencies to ensure establishment and integration of security plans (Office of the National Coordinator for Health Information Technology, 2015). PHI identifies an individual or could reasonably be used to identify an individual. It includes the following information about the client:

- Name
- Mental or physical condition
- Diagnosis
- Birth, admission, discharge dates
- Social Security number
- Insurance or payment information
- Address
- Relatives
- Telephone and fax numbers
- Certification/license numbers
- Vehicle identifiers such as license plate and serial numbers
- Device identifiers and serial numbers
- E-mail address, Web universal resource locator (URL), Internet protocol (IP) address
- Medical record, account, and health plan numbers
- Biometric readings such as fingerprints
- Full-face photographic images and any comparable images

An organization/agency may not use or disclose protected health information except as permitted or required by the HIPAA Privacy Rule. Depending on the situation, a client may or may not need to authorize the use of PHI. A client does not need to authorize the use or disclosure of PHI in relation to treatment, payment for care, and healthcare operations.

### PREPARATION

1. Be knowledgeable about HIPAA regulations.
2. Review agency policies about client confidentiality.
3. Review agency safeguards to assist in protection of client information.
4. Identify the HIPAA officer/technology safety office at your agency of employment.
5. Assess the client and family's developmental, cognitive, and cultural abilities to understand protected personal health information.
6. Ensure families have received information about their HIPAA rights.
7. Discuss your professional responsibility to ensure information is being shared only with the legally eligible family or care providers.
8. Explain that you will be clarifying the relationship to the client of all visitors and sharing only appropriate information.
9. Ask the family to identify any anticipated privacy concerns with potential visitors.

### EQUIPMENT AND SUPPLIES

- Client and family name tags, bracelets, or identification badges to be worn while in the agency
- Employee name tag with job position
- Agency description of HIPAA regulations

**PROCEDURE**

1. Apply identification bracelets immediately upon a person's entry to the healthcare facility.

2. Identify all healthcare providers and visitors and define their relationships to the client. Verify the identity of a child's parent/guardian for healthcare decisions. If there are family members who are not legally permitted access or decision-making authority for a minor child, note this on the chart.

3. Never allow a client to be taken off a unit without written permission of the physician and clear identification of the persons involved.

4. Teach the client and family about HIPAA regulations. Secure the appropriate signatures on HIPAA forms or determine that they were obtained from the admissions department per agency protocol; maintain in the client's record.

5. Share PHI and treatment information only with the permission of the client or legal guardian unless it is for ongoing care, payment for treatment, or healthcare operations.

6. Speak in a moderate tone to prevent conversations from being overheard. Lower your voice appropriately in multiple-bed client rooms, hallways, elevators, and other public places.

7. Do not transmit PHI over nonsecure Internet connections.

8. Secure client medical records away from public view. Chart in a secure area; use computer screens that time-out quickly when left unattended; and post client lists or nurse assignments only in staff areas, away from view of the public.

9. Discuss client care in private areas.

10. For pediatric clients, direct visitors and other relatives to the parents/guardians for information about the child, the treatments, and the child's condition.

11. Do not unnecessarily discuss client conditions with colleagues who are not involved in the care.

12. Consult with the agency designee or HIPAA officer when problems or concerns arise.

## SKILL 1–3  Time Out

A universal protocol has been developed to help prevent wrong anatomic sites, procedures, or persons in surgical and other healthcare procedures (Joint Commission, 2015a). The "time out" protocol stops care and ensures that the correct site and the correct procedure are about to be performed on the correct client.

**PREPARATION**

1. Ensure that the agency approach to the time-out protocol is standardized. Designate the person who is responsible for calling a time out.

2. Train all members of the team in the time-out protocol.

**EQUIPMENT AND SUPPLIES**

- All equipment needed for the scheduled procedure
- A planned method of documenting the time out

**PROCEDURE**

1. Verify the client, procedure, and site before beginning. Include client and/or family member in verification whenever possible.

2. Verify that all required test results matching the client's identity are present, and that equipment for the procedure is at hand. Document this process.

3. Mark the procedure site using agency protocol. Involve the client in this process if possible.

4. Call a time out immediately before performing the procedure to verify procedure, site, and client with the entire team. Every team member must communicate the accuracy of and agreement with the plan. Every team member has the responsibility to speak out if there is a question about the procedure, site, or client identity.

5. If a second procedure is planned, the universal protocol must be repeated.

# Chapter 2
# Women's Health and Prenatal Care

## ⌄ Skills

## Breast Self-Examination (BSE)

Monthly breast self-examination (BSE) is a good self-care method for detecting any abnormalities in either breast, especially findings that might indicate breast cancer. A woman who knows the texture and feel of her own breasts is far more likely to detect changes that develop. Thus it is important for a woman to develop the habit of doing BSE as early as possible, preferably as an adolescent. Women at high risk for breast cancer should especially be encouraged to be attentive to the importance of early detection through routine BSE.

In the course of a routine physical examination or during an initial visit to her healthcare provider, the woman should be taught the BSE technique and its importance as a monthly practice. The effectiveness of BSE is determined by the woman's ability to perform the procedure correctly.

---

### SKILL 2–1 Teaching Breast Self-Examination

**PREPARATION**

1. Explain the purpose of BSE.
2. Identify the common risk factors for breast cancer and determine whether the woman has any of them.
3. Create a warm, supportive atmosphere by attitude and communication style—both verbal and nonverbal—and focus on open discussion.

   RATIONALE: *Understanding the purpose and value of BSE can often motivate women to incorporate the practice into their personal routines. A discussion of breast cancer may bring forth many emotions in the woman, including grief for previous cancer-related losses.*

4. Specify the best time to complete the examination.

RATIONALE: *Timing varies according to the phase of a woman's life. Women who are menstruating are advised to perform the BSE about 1 week after each menstrual period when the breasts are not tender or swollen. After menopause, women should perform BSE on the same day each month. They are advised to pick a date that is easy to remember (e.g., birthday).*

## EQUIPMENT AND SUPPLIES

- Private room
- Drape or patient gown
- Mirror
- Examining table, couch, or bed
- Pillow
- Written materials, including American Cancer Society monthly reminder shower card

## PROCEDURE

1. Describe and demonstrate the correct procedure for BSE.

   - Instruct the woman to inspect her breasts by standing or sitting in front of a mirror. She needs to inspect her breasts in three positions: with both arms relaxed at her sides, with both arms stretched straight over her head, and with both hands placed on her hips while leaning forward.

     RATIONALE: *Inspection is done in three positions to detect any changes in size, symmetry, shape, color, thickening, or surface appearance.*

   - Advise the women to look at her breasts individually and in comparison with one another. Note and record the following characteristics for each position.

2. Advise the woman to note the following:

   - Size and symmetry—Breasts may vary but variations should remain constant during rest or movement. Note abnormal contours.

   - Shape and direction of breasts—Breasts should be rounded or pendulous with some variation between breasts. Breasts should be pointing slightly laterally.

     RATIONALE: *Abnormal contours or changes in size or direction may indicate an underlying mass.*

   - Color, thickening, edema, and venous patterns—Check for signs of redness or inflammation. A blue hue with a marked venous pattern that is focused or one-sided may indicate an area of increased blood supply. Symmetric venous patterns are normal. Skin edema looks like thickened skin with enlarged pores ("orange peel" skin).

     RATIONALE: *A marked venous pattern may indicate an increased blood supply associated with a tumor, and skin edema may indicate blocked lymphatic drainage due to a tumor.*

   - Surface of the breasts—Note skin dimpling, puckering, or retraction (pulling) when the hands are pressed together or against the hips. Check for rashes. Striae (stretch marks) red at onset and pale with age are normal.

   - Nipples—Long-standing nipple inversion is normal, but an inverted nipple previously capable of erection is suspicious. Note any deviations, flattening, or broadening of the nipples. Note ulcerations or nipple discharge.

     RATIONALE: *Skin dimpling, pulling, and retraction may indicate an underlying tumor mass. Nipple discharge may be normal if the woman is breastfeeding but may also suggest malignancy.*

3. After she inspects her breasts, instruct her to palpate them as follows:

   - Lie down. Place one hand behind your head. With the other hand, fingers flattened, gently feel your breast. Press lightly (Figure 2–1).

   - Figure 2–2 shows you how to check each breast. Begin with the outer portion of the breast and follow the arrows, moving in an up and down pattern starting from the underarm and progressing toward the sternum. Be sure to cover all the tissue, going up to the collar bone and down until you feel the ribs. Feel gently but firmly for a lump or area of thickening. Help her to identify her "normal lumps" (e.g., mammary ridge, ribs, nodularity in the upper outer quadrants). Remember to feel all areas of the

> **CLINICAL TIP**
>
> While the woman is palpating her breasts, take her hand and help her identify "normal lumps" such as the mammary ridge, ribs, and nodularity in the upper outer quadrants. If a breast model is available, have the woman palpate it and identify the lumps.

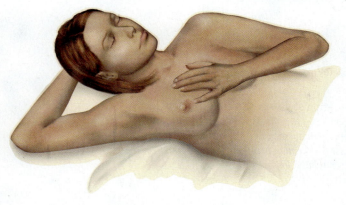

**Figure 2–1** *With one hand behind your head, flatten your fingers and press lightly on your breast, feeling gently for a lump or thickening.*

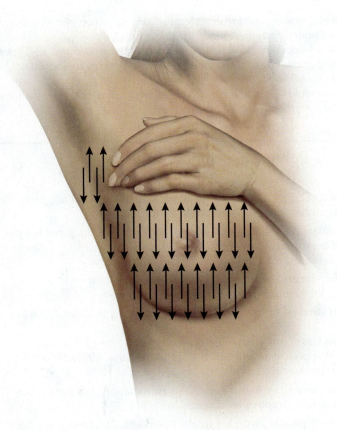

**Figure 2–2**  *Check each breast in an up-and-down pattern, feeling all parts of the breast.*

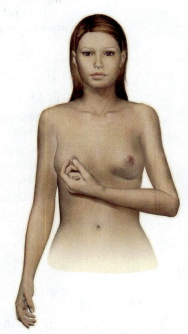

**Figure 2–3**  *Squeeze your nipple between your thumb and forefinger; look for any clear or bloody discharge.*

breast, including the "tail" of tissue near the armpit. (Note: Some women prefer to use a lateral technique, moving the fingers back and forward across the breast.)

- Repeat the process on the other breast.
- Sit up and repeat the palpation with your hand behind your head.
  **RATIONALE:** *Palpation, done monthly, helps the woman learn the feel of her breasts and enables her to recognize any changes.*

4. Instruct her to end the palpation of each breast by squeezing the nipple between her thumb and index finger. She should note any discharge—clear or bloody (Figure 2–3).

5. Determine whether the client has any questions about her findings during this examination. If she has questions, palpate the area and attempt to identify whether it is normal.

6. Provide information on the warning signs of breast cancer and what she should do if she identifies any of these signs during BSE.

7. Provide her with a reminder symbol for monthly BSE and to be specific based on whether she is premenopausal, pregnant, postmenopausal, or postmenopausal receiving hormone therapy. The American Cancer Society provides such items to hang in the shower, place on the refrigerator or mirror, and so forth.

# Pelvic Examination

Women are advised to have their first screening pelvic examination and Papanicolaou (Pap) smear when they reach the age of 21. The American College of Obstetricians & Gynecologists (ACOG) recommends Pap smears every 3 years for women ages 21 to 29. Women over the age of 30 should be screened with a Pap smear and cotesting for human papillomavirus (HPV). Women between the ages of 30 and 65 with negative test results can then be screened every 5 years with both types of testing. If HPV testing is not available, Pap smear frequency should be every 3 years for this age group. Cervical cancer screening should be discontinued in women older than 65 if they have no history of cervical intraepithelial neoplasia (CIN) 2, CIN 3, adenocarcinoma in situ, or cervical cancer. Women over the age of 65 who have also had either three consecutive negative Pap test results or two consecutive negative cotest results within the previous 10 years, with the most recent test performed within the past 5 years, may also discontinue testing. Women who have undergone a total hysterectomy with removal of both the uterus and cervix do not need to continue Pap smears but should continue to have an annual pelvic examination to assess for other abnormalities. The pelvic examination enables the healthcare provider to assess a variety of factors about the woman's vagina, uterus, ovaries, and lower abdominal area. It is often performed after the Pap smear but may also be done without a Pap smear for diagnostic purposes.

Women should be advised to avoid douching, intercourse, female hygiene products, and spermicidal agents immediately before a specimen is obtained for a Pap smear. Specimens should not be obtained during menstruation or when visible cervicitis exists.

Nurse practitioners, certified nurse-midwives, and physicians all perform pelvic examinations. Nurses assist the practitioner and the woman during the examination.

## SKILL 2–2 Assisting With a Pelvic Examination

### PREPARATION

1. Ensure that the room is sufficiently warm by checking the room temperature and adjusting the thermostat if necessary. If overhead heat lamps are available, turn them on.

2. Explain the procedure to the woman. If she has never had a pelvic examination, show her the equipment to be used as part of the explanation.
   RATIONALE: *Explaining the procedure helps reduce anxiety and increase cooperation.*

3. Ask the woman to empty her bladder and to remove clothing below the waist.
   RATIONALE: *An empty bladder promotes comfort during the internal examination.*

4. Have padding on the stirrups. If stirrups are not padded, the woman may prefer to leave her shoes on during the procedure.
   RATIONALE: *Stirrups are usually padded to ease the pressure of the feet against the metal and to decrease the discomfort associated with the touch of the cold stirrups. If they are not padded, however, wearing shoes accomplishes the same purpose.*

5. Give the woman a disposable drape or sheet to use during the examination. Ask her to sit at the end of the examining table with the drape opened across her lap.

6. Position the woman in the lithotomy position with her thighs flexed and adducted. Place her feet in the stirrups. Her buttocks should extend slightly beyond the edge of the examining table.

7. Drape the woman with the sheet, leaving a flap so that the perineum can be exposed.
   RATIONALE: *This position provides the exposure necessary to conduct the examination effectively. The drape helps preserve the woman's sense of dignity and privacy.*

### EQUIPMENT AND SUPPLIES

- Vaginal specula of various sizes, warmed with water or on a heating pad prior to insertion
- Sterile gloves for the examiner
- Water-soluble lubricant
- Materials for Pap smear or liquid-based Pap test method and cultures
- Good light source
  NOTE: *Lubricant may alter the results of tests and cultures and is not used during the speculum examination. Its use is reserved for the bimanual examination.*

### PROCEDURE

1. The examiner dons gloves for the procedure. Explain each part of the procedure as the healthcare provider performs it.

2. Let the woman know that the examiner begins with an inspection of the external genitalia. The speculum is then inserted to allow visualization of the cervix and vaginal walls and to obtain specimens for testing. After the speculum is withdrawn, the examiner performs a bimanual examination of the internal organs using the fingers of one hand inserted in the woman's vagina while the other hand presses over the woman's uterus and ovaries. The final step of the procedure is generally a rectal examination.

3. Ask the woman to breathe slowly and regularly and to use any method she finds effective in helping her to remain relaxed.

4. Let her know when the examiner is ready to insert the speculum and ask her to bear down.
   RATIONALE: *Relaxation helps decrease muscle tension. Bearing down helps open the vaginal orifice and relaxes the perineal muscles.*

5. After the speculum is withdrawn, lubricate the examiner's fingers prior to the bimanual examination.
   RATIONALE: *Lubrication decreases friction and eases insertion of the examiner's fingers.*

### CLINICAL TIP

Women with a history of sexual abuse may have a difficult time during pelvic examinations. The nurse can provide support by explaining the procedure and cuing the woman into what steps the examiner is about to perform. The nurse can also encourage the woman to take slow deep breaths during the examination.

6. After the examiner has completed the examination and moved away from the woman, move to the end of the examination table and face the woman. Cover her with the drape. Apply gentle pressure to her knees and encourage her to move toward the head of the table. Assist her to remove her feet from the stirrups, then offer your hand to her and assist her to sit up.

   RATIONALE: *Assistance is important because the lithotomy position is an awkward one and many women, but especially those women who are pregnant, obese, or older, may find it difficult to get out of the stirrups.*

7. Provide her with tissues to wipe the lubricant from her vagina and perineum.

   RATIONALE: *Vaginal secretions and lubricant may be discharged from the vagina when the woman sits upright.*

8. Provide the woman with privacy while she dresses. Be sure that she is not dizzy and that she is standing or sitting safely before leaving the room.

   RATIONALE: *Lying supine may cause postural hypotension.*

# Deep Tendon Reflexes and Clonus

Preeclampsia, the most common hypertensive disorder in pregnancy, affects all major systems of the body. Central nervous system (CNS) changes associated with preeclampsia are hyperreflexia, headache, and seizures. Deep tendon reflexes (DTRs) are evaluated regularly to detect hyperreflexia, which occurs with CNS irritability. DTRs are also assessed when treatment for preeclampsia is begun because the medications used, which are designed to decrease CNS irritability, depress the deep tendon reflexes.

Clonus should be assessed by vigorously dorsiflexing the woman's foot while her knee is held in a flexed position. Normally, no clonus is present. If it is present, it is measured as 1 to 4 beats, or sustained, and is recorded as such.

## SKILL 2–3 Assessing Deep Tendon Reflexes and Clonus

### PREPARATION

1. Explain the procedure, the indications for its use, and the information that will be obtained.

2. Check the patellar reflex and one other such as the biceps, triceps, or brachioradialis.

   RATIONALE: *DTRs are assessed to gain information about CNS irritability secondary to preeclampsia and to assess the effects of magnesium sulfate if the woman is receiving it.*

> **CLINICAL TIP**
>
> If a percussion hammer is not available, you may use the side of your hand, side of your stethoscope, or tips of your index and middle fingers to elicit DTRs.

### EQUIPMENT AND SUPPLIES

- Percussion hammer

### PROCEDURE

1. Elicit reflexes.

   - *Patellar reflex.* Position the woman with her legs hanging over the edge of the bed (feet should not be touching the floor). (See Figure 2–4.) Briskly strike the patellar tendon, which is located just below the patella. Normal response is extension or a thrusting forward of the foot.

     RATIONALE: *In an inpatient setting, the patellar reflex is often assessed while the woman lies supine. Flex her knees slightly and support them.*

   - *Biceps reflex.* Flex the woman's arm 45 degrees at the elbow and place your thumb on the biceps tendon. Allow your fingers to hold the biceps muscle. Strike your thumb in a slightly downward motion and assess the response. Normal response is flexion of the arm.

   - *Triceps reflex.* Flex the woman's arm up to 90 degrees and allow her hand to hang against the side of her body. Using the percussion hammer, strike the triceps tendon just above the elbow. Normal response is contraction of the muscle, which causes extension of the arm.

   - *Brachioradialis reflex.* Flex the woman's arm slightly and lay it on your forearm with her hand slightly pronated. Using the percussion hammer, strike the brachioradialis tendon, which is found about 1 to 2 inches above the wrist. Normal response is pronation of the forearm and flexion of the elbow.

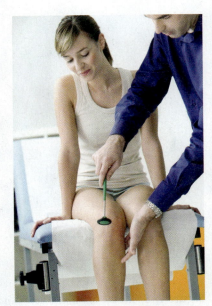

**Figure 2–4** *Correct sitting position for eliciting the patellar reflex.*
Source: © BSIP SA / Alamy.

RATIONALE: *The correct position causes the muscle to be slightly stretched. Then when the tendon is stretched, with a tap the muscle should contract. Correct positioning and technique are essential to elicit the reflex.*

2.  Grade reflexes. Reflexes are graded on a scale of 0 to 4+, as follows:

    4+ Hyperactive; very brisk, jerky, or clonic response; abnormal

    3+ Brisker than average; may not be abnormal

    2+ Average response; normal

    1+ Diminished response; low normal

    No response; abnormal

    RATIONALE: *Normally reflexes are 1+ or 2+. With CNS irritation, hyperreflexia may be present; with high magnesium levels, reflexes may be diminished or absent.*

3.  Assess for clonus. With the woman's knee flexed and the leg supported, vigorously dorsiflex the foot, maintain the dorsiflexion momentarily, and then release. With a normal response, the foot returns to its normal position of plantar flexion. Clonus is present if the foot "jerks" or taps against the examiner's hand. If so, record the number of taps or beats of clonus.

    RATIONALE: *Clonus occurs with more pronounced hyperreflexia and indicates CNS irritability.*

4.  Report and record findings. For example: DTRs 2+, no clonus or DTRs 4+, 2 beats clonus.

## Rh Alloimmunization

Rh alloimmunization occurs when an Rh-negative woman is exposed to Rh-positive blood. During pregnancy, this most commonly occurs when an Rh-negative woman carries an Rh-positive fetus. The woman develops antibodies to the Rh-positive blood. These antibodies can attack the fetal red blood cells, causing severe anemia. Rh immune globulin causes passive immunity to occur and "tricks" the mother's body into believing that it is not necessary to develop antibodies. Consequently, immunization is indicated any time there is a potential for maternal exposure to Rh-positive blood. See Figure 2–5.

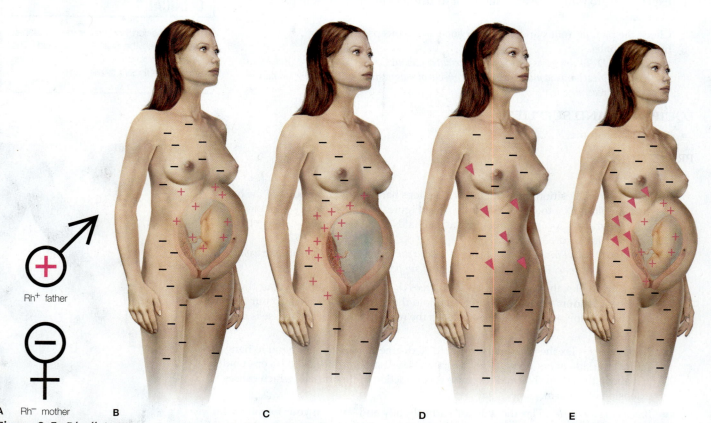

**Figure 2–5** *Rh alloimmunization sequence. **A**, Rh-positive father and Rh-negative mother. **B**, Pregnancy with an Rh-positive fetus. Some Rh-positive blood enters the mother's bloodstream. **C**, As the placenta separates, the mother is further exposed to the Rh-positive blood. **D**, Anti–Rh-positive antibodies (triangles) are formed. **E**, In subsequent pregnancies with an Rh-positive fetus, Rh-positive red blood cells are attacked by the anti–Rh-positive maternal antibodies, causing hemolysis of the red blood cells in the fetus.*

Rh immune globulin is administered to an unsensitized Rh-negative woman following any pregnancy-related event that might result in fetal–maternal bleeding, including miscarriage, abortion (spontaneous or therapeutic), antepartum hemorrhage, mismatched blood transfusion, ectopic pregnancy, evacuation of a molar pregnancy, amniocentesis, chorionic villus sampling, and percutaneous umbilical blood sampling (PUBS). It is also administered prophylactically to all Rh-negative women at about 28 weeks' gestation to decrease possible transplacental bleeding concerns, and again within 72 hours of childbirth if it is indicated because the baby is Rh positive, direct Coombs negative.

## SKILL 2–4  Administration of Rh Immune Globulin (RhoGAM, HypRho-D)

### PREPARATION

1. Confirm that Rh immune globulin is indicated by checking the woman's prenatal or intrapartal record to verify that she is Rh negative. Then confirm that sensitization has not occurred— maternal indirect Coombs negative. During postpartum, confirm that the baby is Rh positive but not sensitized (direct Coombs negative) and that the mother's indirect Coombs is negative. Rh immune globulin is not indicated if the baby is Rh negative.
   RATIONALE: *Rh immune globulin is only indicated for an Rh-negative, unsensitized woman.*

2. Confirm that the woman does not have a history of allergies to immune globulin preparations by checking entries on medication allergies in her chart and by asking her whether she has ever had any allergic reactions to medications, globulins, or blood products.
   RATIONALE: *Rh immune globulin is made from the plasma portion of blood. Allergic reactions are possible.*

3. Explain the purpose and procedure. Have a consent form signed if required by agency policy.
   RATIONALE: *Many agencies require separate consent for the administration of rh immune globulin because it is a blood product. The woman should clearly understand the purpose of the rh immune globulin, its rationale, the administration procedure, and any related risks. Generally, the primary side effects are redness and tenderness at the injection site and allergic responses.*

### EQUIPMENT AND SUPPLIES

- Rh immune globulin, which is obtained from the blood bank or pharmacy according to agency protocol. Lot numbers for the drug and the cross-match should be the same.
- Syringe and intramuscular (IM) needle

### PROCEDURE

1. Confirm the woman's identity and administer one vial of 300 mcg Rh immune globulin IM in the deltoid muscle.
   RATIONALE: *The normal 300-mcg dose provides passive immunity following exposure to 15 mL of transfused red blood cells (RBCs) or 30 mL of fetal blood.*

2. An immune globulin microdose is used after miscarriage, elective abortion, ectopic pregnancy, or molar pregnancy occurring within the first 12 weeks' gestation. During antepartum, the Rh immune globulin is generally given within 3 hours of the event but not longer than 72 hours after the event.

3. If a larger bleed is suspected at birth (as in cases of severe abruptio placentae), additional doses may be administered at one time using multiple sites or at regular intervals as long as all doses are given within 72 hours of childbirth.

4. Provide opportunities for the woman to ask questions and express concerns.
   RATIONALE: *Many women, especially primigravidas, are not aware of the risks for an Rh-positive fetus of a sensitized Rh-negative mother. They need to understand the importance of receiving Rh immune globulin for each pregnancy to ensure continued protection.*

5. Chart according to agency policy. Most agencies chart lot number, route, dose, and patient education.

> **CLINICAL TIP**
>
> In most cases, Rh immune globulin is administered in the deltoid muscle. However, in an extremely thin woman, or in the case of a larger-than-normal dose, consider administering the medication in the ventrogluteal or posterior gluteal site. You may also divide the dose into multiple injections. Both Rhophiac and WinRho-SDF may be administered intravenously.

# Amniocentesis

Amniocentesis is a procedure performed to obtain a sample of amniotic fluid for testing. The amniotic fluid is withdrawn through a needle inserted through the abdominal wall into the uterus. The analysis of amniotic fluid can provide valuable information about fetal status. The nurse assists the healthcare provider during the amniocentesis and supports the woman undergoing the procedure.

## SKILL 2–5  Assisting During Amniocentesis

### PREPARATION

1. Explain the procedure and the indications for it and reassure the woman.
   RATIONALE: *Explanation of the procedure decreases anxiety.*

2. Determine whether an informed consent form has been signed. If not, verify that the woman's healthcare provider has explained the procedure and ask her to sign a consent form.
   RATIONALE: *It is the healthcare provider's responsibility to obtain informed consent. The woman's signature indicates her awareness of the risks and gives her consent to the procedure.*

### EQUIPMENT AND SUPPLIES

Prepare and arrange the following items so they are easily accessible:

- Sterile gloves
- 22-gauge spinal needle with stylet
- 10- and 20-mL syringes
- 1% lidocaine (Xylocaine)
- Povidone-iodine (Betadine)
- Three 10-mL test tubes with tops (amber colored or covered with tape)
  RATIONALE: *Amniotic fluid must be protected from light to prevent the breakdown of bilirubin.*

### PROCEDURE

1. Obtain baseline vital signs, including maternal blood pressure (BP), pulse, respirations, temperature, and fetal heart rate (FHR) before the procedure begins; then monitor BP, pulse, respirations, and FHR every 15 minutes during the procedure.
   RATIONALE: *Baseline information is essential to detect any changes in maternal or fetal status that might be related to the procedure.*

2. Provide gel for the real-time ultrasound and assist with the procedure to assess needle insertion during the procedure as needed.
   RATIONALE: *Amniocentesis is usually performed laterally in the area of fetal small parts, where pockets of amniotic fluid are often seen. Real-time ultrasound will identify fetal parts, locate the placenta, and locate pockets of amniotic fluid.*

3. Cleanse the woman's abdomen with Betadine solution.
   RATIONALE: *Cleansing the abdomen prior to needle insertion helps decrease the risk of infection.*

4. The physician dons sterile gloves, inserts the needle into the identified pocket of fluid (Figure 2–6), and withdraws a sample.

5. Obtain the filled test tubes from the physician. Label the tubes with the woman's correct identification and send to the laboratory with the appropriate laboratory slips. Document that samples have been sent to the laboratory.

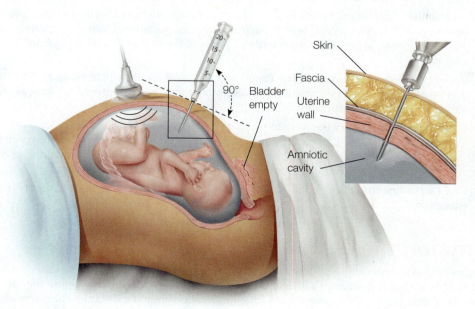

**Figure 2–6**  *Amniocentesis.*

6. Monitor the woman and reassess her vital signs.
   - Determine the woman's BP, pulse, respirations, and the FHR.
   - Palpate the woman's fundus to assess for uterine contractions.
   - Monitor her using an external fetal monitor for 20 to 30 minutes after the amniocentesis.
   - Tilt the woman slightly with a wedge to the left side to counteract any supine hypotension and to increase venous return and cardiac output.

     RATIONALE: *Monitoring maternal and fetal status postprocedure provides information about response to the procedure and helps detect any complications such as inadvertent fetal puncture.*

7. Assess the woman's blood type and determine any need for Rh immune globulin.

8. Administer Rh immune globulin if indicated (see Skill 2–4).

   RATIONALE: *To prevent Rh alloimmunization in an Rh-negative woman, Rh immune globulin is administered prophylactically following amniocentesis.*

9. Instruct the woman to report any of the following changes or symptoms to her primary caregiver:
   - Unusual fetal hyperactivity or, conversely, any lack of fetal movement
   - Vaginal discharge—either clear drainage or bleeding
   - Uterine contractions or abdominal pain
   - Fever or chills

     RATIONALE: *The woman needs to know how to recognize changes or symptoms that require further evaluation.*

10. Encourage the woman to avoid strenuous activity for 24 hours and to increase her fluid intake. Sexual intercourse should be avoided for several days.

    RATIONALE: *A decrease in strenuous maternal activity will decrease uterine irritability and increase uteroplacental circulation. Increased hydration helps replace amniotic fluid through the uteroplacental circulation. Since the procedure is invasive, intercourse should be avoided to avoid infection.*

11. Complete the patient record.
    - Record the type of procedure, the date and time, and the name of the healthcare provider who performed the procedure and the disposition of the specimen.
    - Record the maternal-fetal response such as maternal vital signs, level of discomfort, FHR, and presence of contractions, bleeding, and fluid leakage, if occurred. Discharge instructions given should be documented.

> **CLINICAL TIP**
>
> Have the woman lie on her left side to ensure adequate placental perfusion.

# External Fetal Monitoring

External fetal monitoring is often used to assess fetal well-being during pregnancy. External fetal monitoring (EFM) is used for women with high-risk pregnancies, decreased fetal movement, and, often, during labor. EFM is a low-cost, no-risk intervention that can provide the healthcare team with crucial information for medical decision making.

## SKILL 2–6 External Electronic Fetal Monitoring

### PREPARATION

1. Explain the procedure, the indications for it, and the information that will be obtained.

### EQUIPMENT AND SUPPLIES

- Monitor
- Two elastic monitor belts
- Tocodynamometer ("toco")
- Ultrasound transducer
- Ultrasound gel

### PROCEDURE

1. Have the woman empty her bladder.
2. Turn on the monitor and place the two elastic belts around the woman's abdomen.
3. Place the toco over the uterine fundus off the midline on the area palpated to be most firm during contractions. Secure it with one of the elastic belts.

   RATIONALE: *The uterine fundus is the area of greatest contractility.*

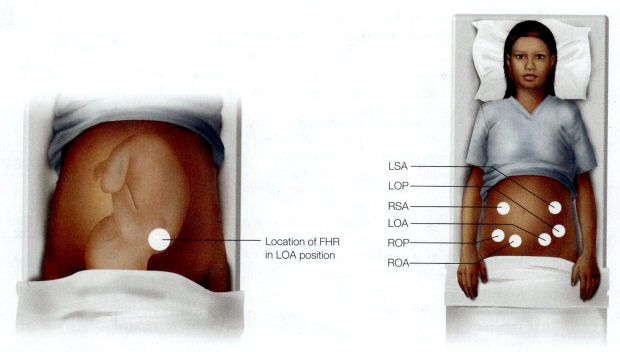

Location of FHR
in LOA position

LSA
LOP
RSA
LOA
ROP
ROA

**Figure 2–7** *Location of the FHR in relation to the more commonly seen fetal positions.*

4. Note the uterine contraction (UC) tracing. The resting tone tracing (i.e., without a UC) should be recording on the 10 or 15 mmHg pressure line. Adjust the line to reflect that reading.
   **RATIONALE:** *If the resting tone is set on the zero line, there often is a constant grinding noise.*

5. Apply the ultrasonic gel to the diaphragm of the ultrasound transducer.
   **RATIONALE:** *Ultrasonic gel is used to maintain contact with the maternal abdomen. The ultrasonic beam is directed toward the fetal heart.*

6. Place the diaphragm on the maternal abdomen in the midline between the umbilicus and the symphysis pubis.

7. Listen for the FHR, which will have a whiplike sound. Move the diaphragm laterally if necessary to obtain a stronger sound (Figure 2–7).

8. When the FHR is located, attach the second elastic belt snugly to the transducer. See Figure 2–8.
   **RATIONALE:** *Firm contact is necessary to maintain a steady tracing.*

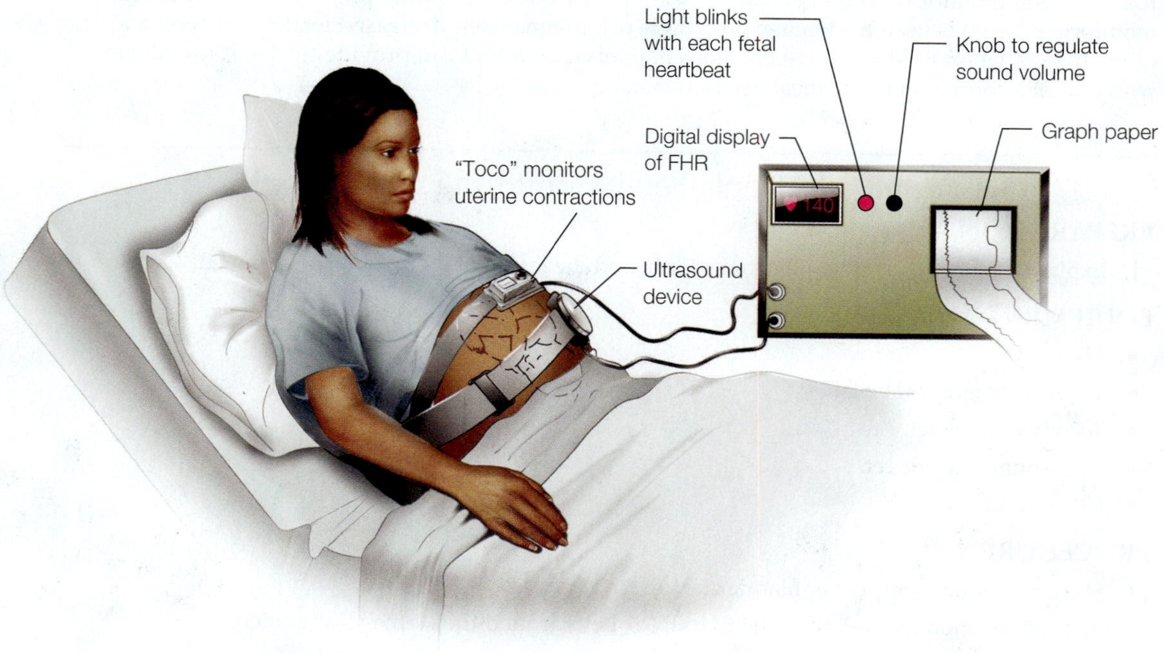

Light blinks
with each fetal
heartbeat

Knob to regulate
sound volume

Digital display
of FHR

Graph paper

"Toco" monitors
uterine contractions

Ultrasound
device

**Figure 2–8** *External electronic fetal monitoring.*

9. Place the following information in the electronic medical record at the onset of electronic fetal monitoring: date, time, gravida, para, membrane status, and name of healthcare provider.

    **NOTE:**    *Each birthing unit may have specific guidelines about additional information to include. Some units may require the mother's identification band to be scanned to confirm identity.*

10. Ongoing documentation should provide information about FHR, including baseline rate in beats per minute (bpm), presence of variability, response to uterine contractions (accelerations or decelerations), procedures performed, changes in position, and the like, as well as any therapy initiated.

    **RATIONALE:**    *A full description of fetal monitoring analysis is beyond the scope of this manual. Refer to your textbook for further information.*

# Assessment of Fetal Well-Being

Fetal assessment techniques are available to evaluate the well-being and maturity of a developing fetus as well as the pregnant woman's well-being. These prenatal tests can alert the woman and her healthcare providers to problems that might be related to the fetus so that appropriate intervention can be initiated if needed. Nurse practitioners, certified nurse-midwives, and physicians all perform these tests. Nurses assist the healthcare providers and support the woman during these tests.

## SKILL 2–7  Assessment of Fetal Well-Being: Non-Stress Test (NST)

### PREPARATION

1. Identify the woman, comparing the name and medical record number appearing in the electronic medical record against identification arm band information.

2. Verify the correct procedure as ordered by the healthcare provider for the correct woman.

3. Explain the procedure, purpose, and implications of the procedure to the woman and her support person. The purpose of the non-stress test is to assess fetal well-being by monitoring fetal activity and concurrent fetal heart rate (FHR) response to fetal activity.

4. Allow time for and encourage any questions the woman and her support person may have. Reinforce any teaching as necessary.

### EQUIPMENT AND SUPPLIES

- External fetal heart rate and contraction monitors (ultrasound transducer and tocodynamometer)
- Ultrasonic gel

### PROCEDURE

1. Have the woman empty her bladder before the procedure begins.

2. Have the woman in a left-tilted semi-Fowler sitting position or in the left lateral position, comfortably, with pillows for support if needed.

    **RATIONALE:**    *These positions displace the uterus to prevent compression of the vena cava and/or aorta. These positions also have more fetal movement and are more likely to have a reactive tracing.*

3. Apply fetal heart rate and contraction monitors as instructed in Skill 2–6: External Electronic Fetal Monitoring.

4. Monitor the fetal heart rate and any contraction activity for at least 20 minutes. Note any fetal movement.

    **RATIONALE:**    *Accelerations in fetal heart rate should occur in response to fetal movement and spontaneously.*

5. If there are no accelerations in 20 minutes, continue monitoring for 20 more minutes.

    **RATIONALE:**    *The fetus may be in a sleep cycle in which there are usually no heart rate accelerations.*

6. If there are no accelerations or fetal movement during the testing period, stimulation of the fetus may be necessary (acoustic stimulation [Figure 2–9], maternal intake of cold liquids).

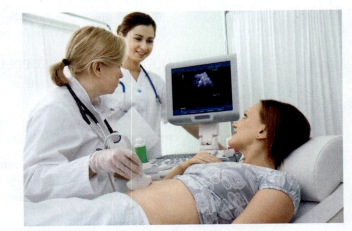

**Figure 2–9**  *Fetal acoustic stimulation testing.*

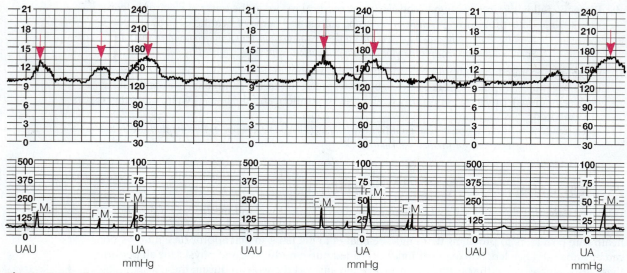

**Figure 2–10** *Example of a reactive non-stress test (NST).*

## TEST INTERPRETATION

**Reactive NST (normal):** Shows at least two accelerations of FHR with fetal movements of 15 beats per minute, lasting 15 seconds or more, over 20 minutes. See Figure 2–10.

**Nonreactive NST:** Accelerations are not present or do not meet the reactive criteria. For example, the accelerations do not meet the requirements of 15 beats per minute or do not last 15 minutes. If the test is considered nonreactive (nonreassuring), further testing may be needed.

## DOCUMENTATION

Document the procedure, results, any intervention(s) needed, and any need for further testing in the woman's medical record, and notify the ordering healthcare provider of the results of the NST per agency policy.

## SKILL 2–8  Assessment of Fetal Well-Being: Contraction Stress Test (CST)

### PREPARATION

1. Identify the woman, comparing the name and medical record number appearing in the electronic medical record against identification arm band information.

2. Verify the correct procedure as ordered by the healthcare provider for the correct woman.

3. Explain the procedure, purpose, and implications of the procedure to the woman and support person. The purpose of the CST is to determine fetal heart rate response to contractions.

4. Ensure privacy.

5. Allow time for and encourage any questions the woman and her support person may have. Reinforce any teaching as necessary.

### EQUIPMENT AND SUPPLIES

- External fetal heart rate and contraction monitors (ultrasound transducer and tocodynamometer)
- Ultrasonic gel

### PROCEDURE

1. Position the woman in a semi-Fowler or side-lying position.
   RATIONALE: *The uterus should be displaced and not compressing the vena cava and/or aorta.*

2. Apply electronic fetal monitor (EFM) transducers and obtain, at minimum, a 20-minute tracing.

3. Assess maternal vital signs.

4. Contact the physician before beginning the CST if any of the following are noted:

   a. Three or more palpable contractions that last 40 seconds or more (a spontaneous CST)

   b. A reactive non-stress test (a CST may not be needed)

   c. Late decelerations

5. Induction of uterine contractions either via breast stimulation (either by nipple self-stimulation or application of an electric breast pump) or infusion of oxytocin (Pitocin) intravenously.

   *Nipple stimulation:* Instruct the woman to massage, roll, or lightly brush her fingertips across the nipple of one breast over her clothing for 2 minutes. Rest for 2 to 5 minutes. Repeat on the opposite breast. The complete cycle is repeated up to 4 times. Nipple stimulation should be stopped during a contraction, then started again after the contraction ends to avoid hypersystole of the uterus. Record each nipple stimulation in the electronic medical record.
   If no contractions occur, begin stimulation of both nipples for 2 minutes. Rest for 2 minutes. Repeat. Bilateral stimulation may be used for 10 minutes. Notify the healthcare provider if inadequate contractions are achieved after nipple stimulation cycles are completed.
   When three palpable contractions lasting 40 to 60 seconds occur in a 10-minute period, stop nipple stimulation and interpret the FHR pattern. The CST is complete.

   *Pitocin infusion (oxytocin challenge test):* Initiate intravenous Pitocin infusion per agency policy for Pitocin induction of labor. Stop Pitocin infusion when three palpable contractions have occurred in 10 minutes, lasting 40 to 60 seconds.

## TEST INTERPRETATION

**Negative (reassuring):** Has three contractions of good quality lasting 40 or more seconds in 10 minutes without evidence of late decelerations.
**Positive (nonreassuring):** Repetitive late deceleration with more than 50% of the uterine contractions.
**Suspicious (equivocal):** Where less than 50% of the contractions on the strip are late decelerations. Variability is usually good.
**Hyperstimulation:** Uterine contraction frequency of every 2 minutes or contraction lasting greater than 90 seconds with a late deceleration occurring.

## DOCUMENTATION

Document the procedure, results, and any intervention(s) needed in the woman's medical record and notify the ordering healthcare provider of the results of the CST per agency policy.

## SKILL 2–9  Assessment of Fetal Well-Being: Biophysical Profile (BPP)

### PREPARATION

1. Identify the woman, comparing the name and medical record number appearing in the electronic medical record against identification arm band information.

2. Verify the correct procedure as ordered by the healthcare provider for the correct woman.

3. Explain the procedure, purpose, and implications of the procedure to the woman and her support person.

4. Allow time for and encourage any questions the woman and her support person may have. Reinforce any teaching as necessary.

### EQUIPMENT AND SUPPLIES

- Ultrasound equipment
- Ultrasonic gel

### PROCEDURE

This is performed by an ultrasonographer or registered nurse who has had extensive education in ultrasonography for the purpose of obstetric ultrasound surveillance. Some healthcare providers may perform the procedure at the bedside.

1. Perform ultrasound scanning to assess for the following:

   a. Fetal breathing movement

   b. Fetal movement of body or limbs

   c. Fetal tone (extension and flexion) of extremities

   d. Amniotic fluid volume (visualized as pockets of fluid around fetus)

   e. Reactive non-stress test (Reactive FHR with activity)

| TABLE 2–1 | Criteria for Biophysical Profile Scoring | |
|---|---|---|
| **Component** | **Normal (score = 2)** | **Abnormal (score = 0)** |
| Fetal breathing movements | ≥1 episode of rhythmic breathing lasting ≥30 sec within 30 min | ≤30 sec of breathing in 30 min |
| Gross body movements | ≥3 discrete body or limb movements in 30 min (episodes of active continuous movement considered as single movement) | ≤2 movements in 30 min |
| Fetal tone | ≥1 episode of extension of a fetal extremity with return to flexion, or opening or closing of hand | No movements or extension/flexion |
| Amniotic fluid volume | Single vertical pocket >2 cm | Largest single vertical pocket ≤2 cm |
| | Amniotic fluid index (AFI) >5 cm | AFI <5 cm |
| Non-stress test | ≥2 accelerations of ≥15 beats/min for ≥15 sec in 20–40 min | 0 or 1 acceleration in 20–40 min |

2. Perform a non-stress test using either an external fetal monitor or ultrasound equipment.

3. A score of 2 is given to each normal finding and a score of 0 is given to each abnormal finding, for a maximum total score of 10. Scores of 8 to 10 are considered normal (see Table 2–1).

### DOCUMENTATION

Document the procedure, results, and any intervention(s) needed in the woman's electronic medical record and notify the ordering healthcare provider of the results of the BPP per agency policy.

# Chapter 3
# Intrapartum

## ∨ Skills

### Intrapartal Vaginal Examination

**3–1** Performing an Intrapartal Vaginal Examination, page 21

### Amniotomy

**3–2** Assisting With Amniotomy (AROM: Artificial Rupture of Membranes), page 24

### Leopold Maneuvers

**3–3** Performing Leopold Maneuvers, page 25

### Fetal Heart Rate

**3–4** Auscultating Fetal Heart Rate, page 27

### Electronic Fetal Monitoring

**3–5** Internal Electronic Fetal Monitoring: Applying a Fetal Scalp Electrode, page 28

### Induction of Labor

**3–6** Assisting With and Monitoring the Woman Undergoing Labor Induction With Pitocin (Oxytocin) and Cervical Ripening Agents, page 30

### Epidural During Labor

**3–7** Assisting With and Caring for the Woman With an Epidural During Labor, page 31

### Prolapsed Cord

**3–8** Care of the Woman With Prolapsed Cord, page 33

# Intrapartal Vaginal Examination

An intrapartal vaginal examination provides valuable information about cervical dilatation and effacement, membrane status, characteristics of amniotic fluid, fetal position, and station. Most labor nurses become highly skilled at using this important intrapartum assessment tool.

Intrapartal vaginal examination should not be performed in the presence of unexplained vaginal bleeding because of the risk of causing a major hemorrhage if the woman has placenta previa. Consult your textbook for an explanation of this potentially serious complication of pregnancy.

## SKILL 3–1 Performing an Intrapartal Vaginal Examination

### PREPARATION

1. Explain the procedure, the indications for the examination, what the examination may feel like, and that it may cause discomfort.

2. Assess for latex allergies.

3. Position the woman with her thighs flexed and abducted. Instruct her to put the heels of her feet together. Drape the woman with a sheet, leaving a flap to access the perineum.
   **RATIONALE:** *This position provides access to the woman's perineum. The drape ensures privacy.*

4. Encourage the woman to relax her muscles and legs.
   **RATIONALE:** *Relaxation decreases muscle tension and increases comfort.*

5. Inform the woman before touching her. Be gentle.

**CLINICAL TIP**

Use nonlatex gloves if the woman has a latex allergy.

## EQUIPMENT AND SUPPLIES

- Clean, disposable gloves if membranes are not ruptured
- Sterile gloves if membranes are ruptured
- Lubricant
- Nitrazine test tape
- Slide
- Sterile cotton-tipped swab (Q-tip)

## BEFORE THE PROCEDURE

### Test for Fluid Leakage

If fluid leakage has been reported or noted, use Nitrazine test tape and a Q-tip with a slide for the fern test before performing the examination.

- The fern test is done by inserting the swab in the pool of fluid in the posterior vagina and then applying the fluid to a slide.

  RATIONALE: *As long as lubricant has not been used, Nitrazine tape registers a change in pH if amniotic fluid is present.*

## PROCEDURE

1. Pull glove on dominant hand.

   RATIONALE: *A single glove is worn when membranes are intact. If a sterile examination is needed, both hands will be gloved with sterile gloves.*

2. Using your gloved hand, position the hand with the wrist straight and the elbow tilted downward. Insert your well-lubricated second and index fingers of the gloved hand gently into the vagina until they touch the cervix. Use care when positioning your hand.

   RATIONALE: *This position allows the fingertips to point toward the umbilicus and find the cervix.*

3. If the woman expresses discomfort, acknowledge it and apologize. Pause for a moment and allow her to relax before progressing.

   RATIONALE: *This validates the woman's discomfort and helps her feel more in control.*

4. To determine the status of labor progress, perform the vaginal examination during and between contractions.

   RATIONALE: *Cervical effacement, dilatation, and fetal station are affected by the presence of a contraction.*

**CLINICAL TIP**

Women with a history of sexual abuse or sexual assault often have significant anxiety with pelvic examinations. Encourage the woman to take slow breaths, and explain each step of the examination process to decrease stress and anxiety.

5. Palpate for the opening, or a depression, in the cervix. Estimate the diameter of the depression to identify the amount of dilatation (see Figure 3–1).

   RATIONALE: *This allows determination of effacement and dilatation.*

6. Determine the status of the fetal membranes by observing for leakage of amniotic fluid. If fluid is expressed, test for amniotic fluid.

7. Palpate the presenting part (see Figure 3–2).

   RATIONALE: *Determining the presenting part is necessary to assess the position of the fetus and to evaluate fetal descent.*

8. Assess fetal descent (see Figure 3–3) and station by identifying the position of the fetal presenting part in relation to the ischial spines. Station progresses from −5 to +4.

9. Record findings on the woman's chart and on the fetal monitor strip if a fetal monitor is being used.

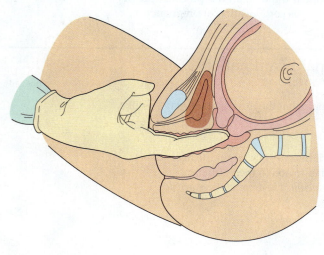

**Figure 3–1** *To gauge cervical dilatation, place the index and middle fingers against the cervix and determine the size of the opening. Before labor begins, the cervix is long (approximately 2.5 cm), the sides feel thick, and the cervical canal is closed, so an examining finger cannot be inserted. During labor, the cervix begins to dilate, and the size of the opening progresses from 1 to 10 cm in diameter.*

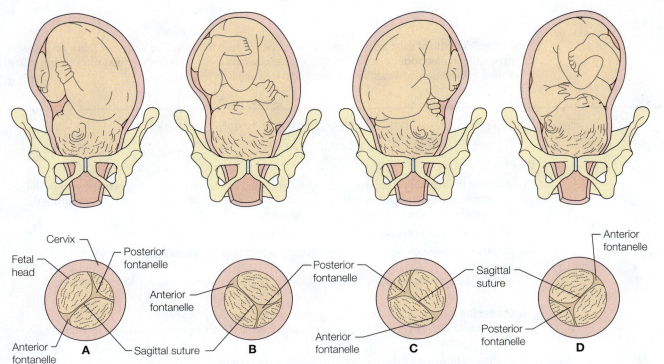

Figure 3–2 *Palpating the presenting part (portion of the fetus that enters the pelvis first). A, Left occiput anterior (LOA). The occiput (area over the occipital bone on the posterior part of the fetal head) is in the left anterior quadrant of the woman's pelvis. When the fetus is LOA, the posterior fontanelle (located just above the occipital bone and triangular in shape) is in the upper-left quadrant of the maternal pelvis. B, Left occiput posterior (LOP). The posterior fontanelle is in the lower-left quadrant of the maternal pelvis. C, Right occiput anterior (ROA). The posterior fontanelle is in the upper-right quadrant of the maternal pelvis. D, Right occiput posterior (ROP). The posterior fontanelle is in the lower-right quadrant of the maternal pelvis.*

Note: The anterior fontanelle is diamond shaped. Because of the roundness of the fetal head, only a portion of the anterior fontanelle can be seen in each of the views, so it appears to be triangular in shape.

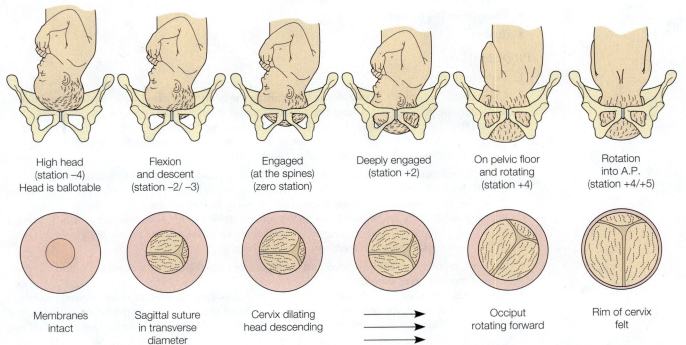

Figure 3–3 *Top: The fetal head progressing through the pelvis. Bottom: The changes that will be detected on palpation of the occiput through the cervix while doing a vaginal examination.*

Source: From Myles, M. F. (1975). *Textbook for midwives* (p. 246). Edinburgh, Scotland: Churchill-Livingstone.

# Amniotomy

Amniotomy (artificial rupture of membranes) is performed to induce or augment labor or to insert an internal fetal electrode or an intrauterine pressure catheter for electronic fetal monitoring. Most labor nurses become highly skilled at using this intrapartum technique.

## SKILL 3–2 Assisting With Amniotomy (AROM: Artificial Rupture of Membranes)

### PREPARATION

1. Identify the woman, comparing the name and medical record number appearing within the electronic medical record against identification on arm band. Some facilities may require that the nurse scan the arm band to confirm identity.

2. Verify the correct procedure for the correct woman.

3. Explain the procedure, its purpose, and implications of the procedure to the woman and support person.
   RATIONALE: *Anticipatory guidance will decrease the woman's anxiety and facilitate cooperation during the procedure.*

4. Assist the woman to the lithotomy position, maintaining privacy.
   RATIONALE: *Proper positioning provides easier access to the cervix and enhances the woman's ability to relax.*

5. Assess FHR prior to, during, and following amniotomy.
   RATIONALE: *Rupturing the amniotic membranes changes the pressure inside the uterus and also causes risk of a prolapsed cord.*

6. Encourage and answer any questions the woman or her support person(s) may have at this time. Reassure the woman that amniotic fluid is constantly produced, as she may worry about a "dry birth."

### EQUIPMENT AND SUPPLIES

- Sterile vaginal examination glove (for healthcare provider)
- Sterile gloves (for nurse)
- Sterile amniotomy hook
- Sterile water-soluble lubricant
- Doppler or monitor (external or internal)
- Waterproof linen/barrier
- Towels

### PROCEDURE

1. Don sterile gloves.

2. Using sterile technique, apply sterile lubricant to the healthcare provider's sterile gloved hand, and open the package containing the amnio hook for the healthcare provider to grasp.
   RATIONALE: *Lubricant decreases friction between the gloved hand and vaginal wall during the procedure. Sterile technique is essential during amniotomy to prevent potential contamination and decrease the risks of maternal and fetal infections.*

3. In some facilities, the nurse may be trained to perform amniotomies. In this case, the sterile gloves should be preopened and the lubricant and amnio hook should be placed on the sterile field. The sheet should be adjusted to obtain access to the perineum.
   RATIONALE: *A sterile field should be set up to maintain sterility of the gloves and amnio hook to prevent infection. The sheet covering the woman should be adjusted so the nurse's gloves are not contaminated while accessing the perineal area.*

4. Once the membranes are ruptured and fluid is seen, note the color, amount, odor, and the presence of meconium or blood.
   RATIONALE: *Amniotic fluid should be clear or slightly cloudy and without any odor. Meconium-stained or bloody amniotic fluid indicates or places the fetus at risk for complications. Foul-smelling fluid may indicate infection. Absent, decreased, or increased amounts of amniotic fluid may indicate fetal stress.*

5. Assess fetal heart rate immediately before and after the rupture of membranes.
   RATIONALE: *Fetal well-being must be confirmed prior to and after amniotomy to assess fetal tolerance to the procedure.*

6. Maternal temperature should be assessed every 2 hours or more frequently if febrile and/or healthcare provider ordered.
   RATIONALE: *A rise in maternal temperature might indicate an intrauterine infection (chorioamnionitis).*

7. While wearing disposable gloves, cleanse the perineum with a warm washcloth and dry the perineal area, and change the waterproof linen pads as needed.
   RATIONALE: *A dry underpad enhances maternal comfort.*

8. Keep vaginal examinations to a minimum.
   RATIONALE: *To prevent introducing ascending infections*

9. Assist the woman to a comfortable position.

### DOCUMENTATION

Document date, time of ruptured membranes, color, amount and odor (if applicable), who performed the procedure, cervical examination results, fetal heart rate, and how the client tolerated the procedure.

> **CLINICAL TIP**
>
> If the fetal heart rate is irregular after the amniotomy, continuous electronic fetal heart rate monitoring is warranted.

# Leopold Maneuvers

Leopold maneuvers are a systematic way to evaluate the woman's abdomen to determine fetal position and presentation. Frequent practice increases the examiner's skill. Leopold maneuvers may be difficult to perform on a woman with a multiple pregnancy, obese woman, or a woman who has excessive amniotic fluid.

## SKILL 3–3  Performing Leopold Maneuvers

### PREPARATION

1. Have the woman empty her bladder.
   RATIONALE: *Palpating the abdomen may be uncomfortable if the woman's bladder is full. A full bladder may also make it difficult to complete the third and fourth maneuvers. See later discussion.*

2. Ask the woman to lie on her back with her feet on the bed and her knees bent.
   RATIONALE: *This position provides good access to the woman's abdomen. Flexing the knees helps relax the abdominal muscles.*

3. Complete the procedure between contractions.
   RATIONALE: *It is difficult to identify fetal parts when the abdominal muscles are contracted.*

### EQUIPMENT AND SUPPLIES

- Gloves

### PROCEDURE

1. Don gloves.

2. *First maneuver:* Done to determine whether the fetal head or breech (fetal buttocks) occupies the uterine fundus.

   Facing the woman, palpate the upper abdomen with both hands. Note the shape, consistency, and mobility of the palpated part. See Figure 3–4.
   RATIONALE: *The fetal head is firm, hard, and round and moves independently of the trunk. The breech (fetal buttocks) feels softer and symmetric and has small bony prominences; it moves with the trunk.*

3. *Second maneuver:* Done to determine the location of the fetal back.

   After determining whether the head or breech (fetal buttocks) occupies the fundus, try to determine the location of the fetal back. Still facing the woman, palpate the abdomen with gentle but deep pressure, using the palms. Hold the right hand steady while the left hand explores the right side of the uterus. Then repeat the maneuver, holding the left hand steady while exploring the left side of the woman's abdomen with your right hand. See Figure 3–5.
   RATIONALE: *The fetal back, on one side of the abdomen, feels firm and smooth and should connect what was found in the fundus with a mass in the outlet. The fetal extremities, which feel small and knobby, should be found on the other side.*

4. *Third maneuver:* Done to determine what fetal part is lying just above the pelvic outlet.

   To do this, gently grasp the abdomen with the thumb and fingers just above the symphysis pubis. Note whether the presenting part feels like the fetal head or buttocks and whether it is engaged. See Figure 3–6.

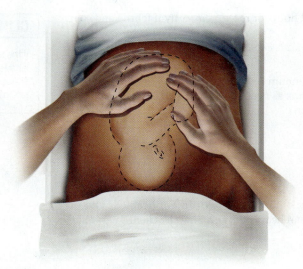

**Figure 3–4** *First maneuver.*

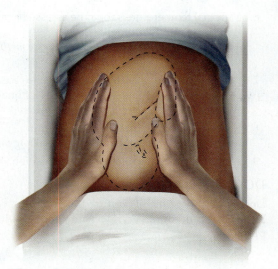

**Figure 3–5** *Second maneuver.*

RATIONALE: *This maneuver yields the opposite information from that gained with the first maneuver and validates the presenting part. If the head is presenting and is not engaged, it may be gently pushed back and forth.*

5. *Fourth maneuver:* Done to determine the location of the cephalic prominence.

Facing the woman's feet, place both hands on the lower abdomen and move the hands gently down the sides of the uterus toward the pubis. Attempt to locate the cephalic prominence, or brow. See Figure 3–7.

RATIONALE: *The brow is located on the side where there is the greatest resistance to the descent of the fingers toward the pubis. It is located on the side opposite the fetal back if the head is well flexed. However, when the fetal head is extended, the occiput is the first cephalic prominence felt, and it is located on the same side as the fetal back. Thus, when completing the fourth maneuver, if the first cephalic prominence palpated is on the same side as the back, the head is not flexed. If the cephalic prominence is found opposite the back, the head is well flexed.*

**CLINICAL TIP**

Many nurses do the fourth maneuver first in order to identify the part of the fetus in the pelvic inlet.

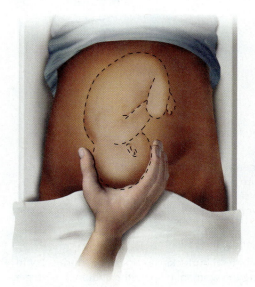

**Figure 3–6** *Third maneuver.*

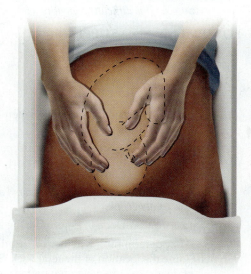

**Figure 3–7** *Fourth maneuver.*

# Fetal Heart Rate

The fetal heart rate (FHR) provides vital information about the status of the fetus and is typically assessed using a handheld Doppler device, which provides a clearly audible heartbeat.

## SKILL 3–4  Auscultating Fetal Heart Rate

### PREPARATION

1. Explain the procedure, the indications for it, and the information that will be obtained.
2. Uncover the woman's abdomen.

### EQUIPMENT AND SUPPLIES

- Doppler device
- Ultrasonic gel

### PROCEDURE

1. To use the Doppler:
   - Place ultrasonic gel on the diaphragm of the Doppler. Gel is used to maintain contact with the maternal abdomen and enhances the conduction of sound.
   - Place the Doppler diaphragm on the woman's abdomen halfway between the umbilicus and symphysis and in the midline. You are most likely to hear the FHR in this area. Listen carefully for the sound of the fetal heartbeat.
2. Check the woman's pulse against the fetal sounds you hear. If the rates are the same, reposition the Doppler and try again.
   RATIONALE: *If the rates are the same, you are probably hearing the maternal pulse and not the FHR.*
3. If the rates are not similar, count the FHR for 1 full minute. Note that the FHR has a double rhythm and only one sound is counted.
4. If you do not locate the FHR, move the Doppler laterally (see Figure 3–8).
5. Auscultate the FHR between, during, and for 30 seconds following uterine contractions.
6. Frequency recommendations are as follows:
   - Low-risk women: Every 30 minutes in the first stage and every 15 minutes in the second stage.
   - High-risk women: Every 15 minutes in the first stage and every 5 minutes in the second stage.
     RATIONALE: *This evaluation provides the opportunity to assess fetal status and the response to labor.*
7. Document FHR data (rate and rhythm), characteristics of uterine activity, and any actions taken as a result of the FHR.

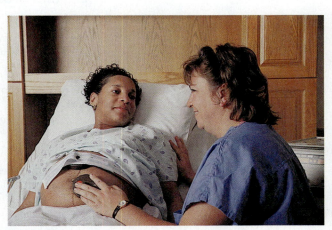

> **CLINICAL TIP**
>
> The FHR is heard most clearly through the fetal back. Locate the fetal back using Leopold maneuvers. (See Skill 3–3.)

**Figure 3–8**  *When the fetal heartbeat is picked up by the electronic monitor, the sound can be heard by everyone in the room.*

# Electronic Fetal Monitoring

Electronic fetal monitoring provides a continuous tracing of uterine contractions (UCs) and of the fetal heart rate (FHR), which allows visualization of many characteristics of the FHR. Electronic monitoring of UCs provides continuous data. In many birth settings, electronic monitoring is routine for high-risk women and for women who are having oxytocin-induced labor; other facilities monitor all laboring women. Specific high-risk factors that would warrant fetal monitoring include the presence of one or more of the following:

- Previous history of a stillborn (fetus dies in the uterus) at 38 or more weeks' gestation
- Presence of a complication of pregnancy (e.g., preeclampsia-eclampsia, placenta previa, abruptio placentae, multiple gestation, prolonged or premature rupture of membranes)
- Induction of labor (labor that is begun as a result of some type of intervention such as an intravenous infusion of oxytocin)

**CLINICAL TIP**

Evaluating the FHR tracing provides information about fetal status and response to the stress of labor. The presence of reassuring characteristics is associated with good fetal outcomes. Rapid identification of nonreassuring characteristics allows prompt interventions and the opportunity to determine the fetal response to the interventions.

- Preterm labor (gestation less than 37 completed weeks)
- Decreased fetal movement
- Fetal stress or nonreassuring fetal status
- Meconium staining of amniotic fluid (meconium has been released into the amniotic fluid by the fetus, which may indicate a problem)

In addition to FHR information, external monitoring provides a continuous recording of the frequency and duration of uterine contractions and is noninvasive.

External fetal monitoring does not accurately record the intensity of the uterine contraction, and it is difficult to obtain an accurate FHR in some women, such as those who are very obese, those who have hydramnios (an abnormally large amount of amniotic fluid), or those with a very active fetus. In addition, the woman may be bothered by the belt if it requires frequent readjustment when she changes position. See Skill 2–6 for a description of external electronic fetal monitoring.

Internal monitoring using an electrode attached directly to the fetal scalp provides more accurate information. The internal scalp electrode is applied by a healthcare provider.

## SKILL 3–5 Internal Electronic Fetal Monitoring: Applying a Fetal Scalp Electrode

### PREPARATION

1. Identify the woman, comparing name and medical record number appearing in the chart against identification arm band information.

2. Verify correct procedure for correct client.

3. Explain the procedure, purpose, and implications of using a fetal scalp electrode to the client and support person.
   RATIONALE: *This method of monitoring provides more accurate continuous data than external monitoring because the signal is clearer and movement of the fetus or woman does not interrupt it.*

4. Assist the woman into lithotomy position, providing privacy.

5. The woman's membranes must have already ruptured spontaneously or have been ruptured by the healthcare provider.
   RATIONALE: *The fetal scalp electrode cannot be applied to the scalp if the membranes are covering the scalp, and registered nurses (RNs) are not allowed to rupture membranes.*

### EQUIPMENT AND SUPPLIES

- Sterile examination glove
- Sterile water-soluble lubricant
- Spiral fetal scalp electrode apparatus
- Fetal monitor
- Scalp electrode cable
- Grounding pad (usually found in electrode packaging)

### PROCEDURE

1. Using sterile technique, open the lubricant package, don a sterile glove on the dominant hand, and apply lubricant to the glove with the nondominant hand.
   RATIONALE: *Sterile technique is essential to decrease the risk of intrauterine infection.*

2. Perform the vaginal examination to determine dilatation and presentation of the fetus. Ensure presenting part is vertex.
   RATIONALE: *The fetal scalp electrode is placed on the fetal occiput. To do so, the membranes must be ruptured, the cervix must be dilated at least 2 cm, the presenting part must be known, and the presenting part must be down against the cervix.*

3. Apply the fetal scalp electrode according to the package directions on a firm area of the fetal vertex, avoiding, for example, fontanelles, face, or genitals. This usually involves inserting the electrode within the firm plastic guide. Place the end of the guide/electrode against a firm area of the scalp, and rotate the electrode end clockwise until resistance is met. Release the guide according to the package directions and discard.

    RATIONALE: *Care must be taken to avoid attaching the monitor to soft tissue, which could result in fetal trauma.*

4. Connect the spiral electrode wire to a leg plate taped to mother's inner thigh with a grounding pad per package instructions. This in turn is attached to the electronic fetal monitor. See Figure 3–9.

5. Verify that the fetal heart rate is tracing before discontinuing the intermittent or continuous external monitor.

6. To remove the fetal scalp electrode, disconnect the electrode wire from the cable and rotate the lead counterclockwise. Once removed, visually examine the electrode to ensure it is intact. If unable to remove the electrode before going for a cesarean birth, tape the electrode wire to the mother's thigh and notify the surgeon.

7. Document the date and time of application and removal, including the condition of the electrode (intact).

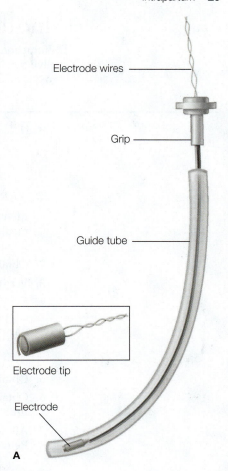

Electrode wires

Grip

Guide tube

Electrode tip

Electrode

**A**

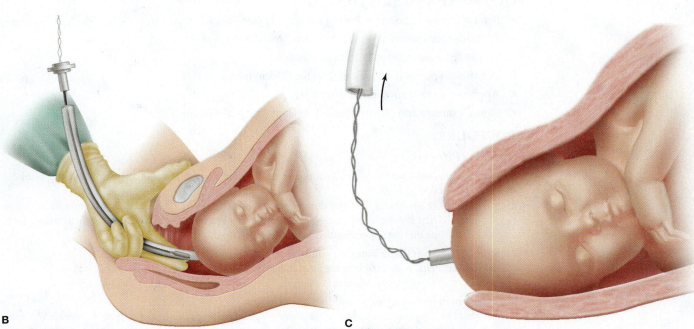

**B**

**C**

**Figure 3–9** *Technique for internal, direct fetal monitoring. A, Spiral electrode. B, Attaching the spiral electrode to the scalp. C, Attached spiral electrode with the guide tube removed.*

# Induction of Labor

Induction of labor is used to stimulate the onset of uterine contractions, which will facilitate progressive cervical effacement and dilatation and descent of the fetus. The decision to initiate labor using oxytocin should be made only after risk factors, cervical readiness, and fetal maturity are evaluated.

## SKILL 3–6 Assisting With and Monitoring the Woman Undergoing Labor Induction With Pitocin (Oxytocin) and Cervical Ripening Agents

### PREPARATION

1. Identify the woman, comparing name and medical record number appearing in the electronic medical record (EMR) against identification arm band information. Scan in identification band if required by facility.

2. Obtain an order for the procedure, and have a written order in the chart.

3. Verify correct procedure as ordered by healthcare provider for the correct woman.

4. Explain the procedure, purpose, and implications of the procedure to the woman and her support person.
   RATIONALE: *The mother and her family need to be aware that induction of labor may take longer than spontaneous labor. They also need to know that there may be limitations on food intake and activity, continuous fetal monitoring, and frequent assessments due to the method of induction.*

5. Obtain informed consent per agency policy.

6. Obtain Pitocin premixed bag from pharmacy or mix 10 units Pitocin per 1000 mL secondary fluid. Obtain cervical ripening agent.

7. Allow time for and encourage any questions the woman and her support person may have. Reinforce any teaching as necessary.

### EQUIPMENT AND SUPPLIES

- Fetal and contraction monitoring equipment (for Pitocin infusion)
- IV fluids (per agency policy, healthcare provider orders)
- IV administration sets (for Pitocin infusion)
- IV infusion pump (two if available) for Pitocin infusion
- Appropriate induction medications
- Sterile examination gloves, sterile lubricant (cervical ripening)

### PROCEDURE

#### Oxytocin (Pitocin)

1. Apply fetal and contraction monitors per unit policy. Assess for reactive or reassuring fetal heart rate tracing.
   RATIONALE: *A baseline of fetal well-being and uterine activity should be established before induction so that the nurse will recognize complications associated with oxytocin administration, such as uterine hyperstimulation and fetal distress.*

2. Start IV infusion using aqueous solution at 125 mL/hr.
   RATIONALE: *This is done to keep the woman hydrated and to have an intravenous line available when the oxytocin infusion is stopped.*

3. Assess maternal vital signs and hydration status.
   RATIONALE: *Ongoing assessment of the woman's fluid balance (intake and output) is necessary because oxytocin has an antidiuretic effect.*

4. Attach secondary line to an infusion pump.
   RATIONALE: *An intravenous infusion pump must be used during oxytocin induction to ensure that an accurate volume and dosage of oxytocin are administered to the woman.*

5. Start Pitocin infusion per agency policy and increase accordingly. One suggested method is to begin at 1 to 2 mU/min and increase by 1 to 2 mU/min every 15 to 40 minutes.

6. Evaluate fetal heart rate pattern, contraction pattern, and maternal vital signs before each increase in Pitocin.

RATIONALE: *Accurate monitoring of uterine contraction frequency, duration, and intensity and uterine resting tone is essential to evaluate the effect of each oxytocin dosage level and determine the need to increase the infusion rate.*

7. Increase the Pitocin rate until adequate labor is established and then maintain at the current rate. Decrease the Pitocin rate if hypersystole occurs, per agency policy.

   RATIONALE: *Because the half-life of oxytocin is very short (1 to 6 minutes), stopping an oxytocin infusion may quickly reverse the effects of excessive uterine activity and improve fetal oxygenation.*

## Misoprostol (Cytotec)

1. Don sterile glove.

2. Monitor fetal heart rate and contractions per agency policy.

3. Have IV infusion or IV access established per agency policy.

4. Have the woman empty her bladder prior to insertion of cervical ripening agent.

5. Perform sterile vaginal examination, establishing that the cervix is "unfavorable" for induction using Pitocin only (1 cm or less, little to no effacement).

6. Remove glove, wash hands, don sterile glove, apply minimal lubricant, and insert two fingers (second and third digits) into the vagina with 25 micrograms (1/4 tablet) misoprostol at end of fingers. It is placed in the posterior vaginal fornix.

7. The woman should remain in bed for 30 minutes following insertion and then may be up to void.

8. This process may be repeated every 3 to 6 hours for up to 24 hours. The healthcare provider should be notified if hyperstimulation occurs or if there is no onset of labor.

9. Pitocin should not be administered less than 4 hours after the last Cytotec dose.

10. The fetal heart rate/contraction pattern should be evaluated for 3 hours following the insertion of misoprostol.

11. Monitor closely for uterine hyperstimulation.

## Dinoprostone (PGE$_2$) (Cervidil or Prepidil)

Same procedures as for misoprostol except as follows:

1. Cervidil (10 mg): Administer as vaginal insert, × 1 dose. Monitor for 2 hours after insertion.

2. Prepidil (0.5 mg): Administer intracervically. Monitor for 1 to 2 hours. May repeat after 6 hours. No more than 3 doses in 24 hours. If hypersystole occurs, remove medication by gently pulling attached string out of vagina.

## DOCUMENTATION

Document the procedures, results, vital signs, fetal heart rate/contraction patterns, and labor progress in the woman's medical record, including date and times of administration of medication and any complications.

# Epidural During Labor

Regional epidural pain blocks are used during labor and birth to offer local pain control. An epidural block can be given as soon as active labor begins and allows the laboring woman to be alert and be part of the birth process.

---

## SKILL 3–7  Assisting With and Caring for the Woman With an Epidural During Labor

### PREPARATION

1. Identify the woman, using the name and medical record number and comparing the medical record with the identification arm band. Verify the correct procedure with the correct woman. Document informed consent by the woman. Ensure that the anesthesia personnel and/or the obstetrician explain possible side effects and complications.

2. Explain the procedure and interventions that may be required because of the epidural: continuous intravenous infusion, continuous fetal monitoring, complete bed rest, indwelling or intermittent urinary catheterization, frequent blood pressure assessments, and other interventions according to hospital policy.

> RATIONALE: *The woman may be focused on pain relief and not aware of further interventions that will be required due to epidural infusion.*

3. Obtain the healthcare provider order for epidural.

4. After obtaining results of blood work, notify anesthesia personnel per hospital policy.

5. Throughout the procedure and following, allow time to answer any questions the woman or her support person may have. Follow up with further teaching regarding any matter that may have been unforeseen or out of the ordinary.

### EQUIPMENT AND SUPPLIES

- Fetal heart rate and contraction monitoring equipment as ordered
- Intravenous fluid and apparatus as ordered and per hospital policy
- Epidural administration set
- Anesthetic medications per anesthesia department protocol, if certified registered nurse anesthetist (CRNA) or anesthesiologist does not provide it
- High-pressure volumetric pump if epidural will be a continuous infusion
- Ephedrine syringe; dosage according to hospital protocol

### PROCEDURE

1. Obtain maternal baseline vital signs, fetal heart rate, and variability. The fetal heart rate tracing should show a reassuring tracing before starting the epidural process.

2. Administer an IV fluid bolus per hospital protocol before the epidural is begun (usually 500 to 1000 mL lactated Ringer).
   > RATIONALE: *This is to avoid maternal hypotension associated with vasodilation common with epidurals.*

3. Assist and support the woman in position per anesthesia personnel request (usually sitting up on side of bed with back flexed or side-lying with knees flexed is occasionally used).
   > RATIONALE: *This will assist the anesthesia personnel in locating the correct vertebrae between which to administer the epidural.*

4. Assess BP, heart rate, and fetal heart rate before and after test doses and frequently thereafter according to hospital policy, often every 5 minutes throughout the procedure and immediately following, then regularly according to hospital policy.

5. Have ephedrine at bedside in case of hypotensive or fetal bradycardia episode. Administer according to unit protocol and physician orders.

6. Assess the bladder for distention every 30 minutes. Catheterize with intermittent catheter if birth is imminent or indwelling if not.
   > RATIONALE: *A full bladder can slow the descent of the fetus, as well as risk damage to the bladder.*

7. Assess maternal position (from side to side) and body alignment frequently, changing position at least every hour.
   > RATIONALE: *Maximize uteroplacental blood flow, increase circulation, promote comfort, and avoid a one-sided block.*

8. Periodically assess the level of anesthesia and pain control. Notify anesthesia personnel as needed for changes in epidural infusion.

9. Change syringes as needed per hospital policy.

10. After birth, per hospital policy, a qualified RN may remove the epidural catheter.

### DOCUMENTATION

Document the procedure throughout administration of the epidural and removal of the catheter. Document time of removal, condition of epidural puncture site, catheter condition (intact), any dressing applied (if applicable), and how the woman tolerated the procedure.

# Prolapsed Cord

Prolapsed umbilical cord results when the umbilical cord precedes the fetal presenting part. When this occurs, pressure is placed on the umbilical cord as it is trapped between the presenting part and the maternal pelvis. Consequently, the cord vessels carrying blood to and from the fetus are compromised. Prolapse of the cord can occur with rupture of the membranes if the presenting part is not well engaged in the pelvis. The labor nurse must recognize this situation and intervene quickly in this obstetric emergency.

## SKILL 3–8 Care of the Woman With Prolapsed Cord

### PREPARATION

A prolapsed cord is an unexpected event and an emergency. Preparation can only consist of calmly teaching the woman and her support person the rationale for interventions, what to expect, and the plan of care. Although difficult at times with this particular situation, privacy is to be maintained. Allow time for questions from the laboring woman, her support person, and any other family members who may be present. Another RN may need to answer questions if the woman's RN is busy with the woman's care.

### EQUIPMENT AND SUPPLIES

- Sterile examination glove
- Sterile lubricant
- Sterile gauze pad moistened with saline solution, if cord is outside of vagina
- Oxygen and mask
- Fetal monitor/Doppler

### PROCEDURE

1. Don sterile glove.

2. If the cord is visualized extending through the vagina, a sterile gauze moistened with sterile saline must be placed on the cord immediately to prevent the cord from drying. Do not handle the cord.
   RATIONALE: *Handling the cord may cause it to spasm.*

3. Notify the healthcare provider immediately.

4. Place the woman in the knee-chest position (Figure 3–10).
   RATIONALE: *This position uses gravity to relieve umbilical cord pressure.*

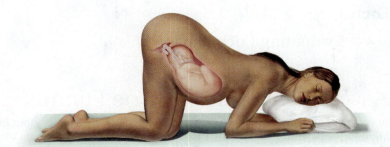

**Figure 3–10** *The knee-chest position is used to relieve cord compression during a cord prolapse emergency.*

5. If the cord is palpated during vaginal examination (using sterile glove and lubricant), place two fingers on either side of the cord or both fingers on one side of the cord to avoid compressing it. Exert upward pressure against the presenting part to relieve pressure on the cord.

6. Continue assessing fetal heart rate to determine if interventions and the position of the fingers are successful in keeping fetal heart rate between 110 and 160 bpm.
   RATIONALE: *A fetal heart rate in this range indicates that fetal well-being has not been compromised by cord compression.*

7. Start oxygen via face mask at 10 L/min.

8. **The examiner's fingers must be kept on the presenting part while exerting pressure on the part to prevent uterine contractions from compressing the cord until the baby is born, usually via cesarean.** This may require the examiner to travel to the operating room (OR) on the bed with the mother to maintain the position of the fingers and the presenting part. **The woman's position must be maintained until birth or arrival to the OR and placement on the OR table.** Although difficult, privacy should be maintained during transport to surgery. This may require extra personnel and sheets to cover the woman.

### DOCUMENTATION

Document the course of events, interventions, and maternal and fetal response to interventions in the medical record per agency policy. If there is a poor fetal outcome, further quality assurance documentation may be necessary.

# Chapter 4
# Postpartum

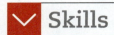 **Skills**

## Assessment of the Uterine Fundus

## Perineal Assessment

## Assessment of the Uterine Fundus

Assessment of the uterine fundus provides valuable information about the woman's condition during the postpartum period. This assessment is especially important during the first 1 to 4 hours when the woman is at greatest risk for hemorrhage.

---

### SKILL 4–1  Assessing the Uterine Fundus Following Vaginal or Cesarean Birth

#### PREPARATION

1. Consider offering to premedicate 30 to 45 minutes before assessing the fundus, especially if the woman has had a cesarean section.
   RATIONALE: *The postoperative area will be very tender, and she may be very fearful of the potential pain.*

2. Explain the procedure, the information it provides, and what it might feel like.

3. Ask the woman when she last voided. Ask her to void if it has been longer than 1 hour.
   RATIONALE: *A full bladder can cause uterine atony.*

4. Have the woman lie flat in bed with her head on a pillow. If the procedure is uncomfortable, she may find that it helps to flex her legs. Flexing the legs and providing support under them with folded pillows is especially helpful with women who have had a cesarean.
   RATIONALE: *The supine position prevents falsely high assessment of fundal height. Flexing the legs relaxes the abdominal muscles.*

#### EQUIPMENT AND SUPPLIES

- A clean perineal pad (see Skill 4–2)
- Clean gloves

#### PROCEDURE

1. Gently place one hand on the lower segment of the uterus for support. Using the side of the other hand, palpate the abdomen until you locate the top of the fundus.
   RATIONALE: *One hand stabilizes the uterus while the other hand locates the top of the fundus. (Support of the uterus prevents stretching of the ligaments that support the uterus.)*

2. Determine whether the fundus is firm. If it is, it will feel hard and round like a firm grapefruit in the abdomen. If it is not firm, massage the abdomen lightly until it becomes firm, then check for bleeding.
   RATIONALE: *A firm fundus indicates that the uterine muscles are contracted and bleeding will not occur.*

> **CLINICAL TIP**
>
> Gloves may be put on before assessing the abdomen and fundus or when you are ready to assess the perineum and lochia.

3. Measure the top of the fundus in fingerbreadths above, below, or at the fundus. See Figure 4–1.
   RATIONALE: *Fundal height gives information about the progress of involution.*

4. Determine the position of the fundus in relation to the midline of the body. If it is not in the midline, locate it and then evaluate the bladder for distention.
   RATIONALE: *The fundus may deviate from the midline when the bladder is full because the enlarged bladder pushes the uterus aside.*

5. If the bladder is distended, use nursing measures to help the woman void. If she is not able to void after a specified period of time, catheterization may be necessary.

6. Measure urine output for the next few hours until normal elimination is established.
   RATIONALE: *During the postpartum period as diuresis occurs, the bladder may fill far more rapidly than normal, putting the woman at risk for uterine atony and hemorrhage. (A diminished tone of the uterus may cause loss of the urge to void.)*

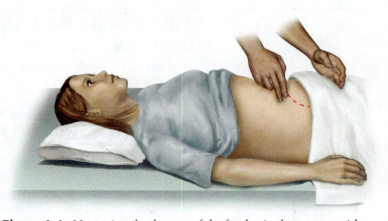

**Figure 4–1** *Measuring the descent of the fundus in the woman with a vaginal birth. In this case, the fundus is located two fingerbreadths below the umbilicus.*

7. Assess the lochia (see Skill 4–2).

8. During the first few hours postpartum, if the fundus becomes boggy frequently or is located high above the umbilicus and the woman's bladder is empty, the uterine cavity may be filled with clots of blood. In this case, do the following:

   ▪ Release the front of the perineal pad and lay it back so that you can see the perineum and the pad lying between the woman's legs.

   ▪ Massage the uterine fundus until it is firm.

   ▪ Keep one hand in position, stabilizing the lower portion of the uterus. With the hand you used to massage the fundus, put steady pressure on the top of the now-firm fundus and see if you are able to express any clots. (Watch the pad between her legs for clots to pass from the vagina.)
   RATIONALE: *If the woman's uterus is filled with blood, it acts as an irritant and the uterus will not remain contracted. When the muscle fibers relax, bleeding results, further aggravating the problem. Pushing on a uterus that is not firm is dangerous because it is possible to cause the uterus to invert, a true emergency.*

9. If measurement of the blood is needed, the perineal pad and absorbent pad can be weighed.

10. Provide the woman with a clean perineal pad.

11. Record findings. Fundal height is recorded in fingerbreadths (e.g., "2 FB ↓ U" or "1 cm ↑ U"). If fundal massage was necessary, note that fact: "Uterus boggy → firm with light massage."

12. Communicate bogginess or heavy flow to primary healthcare provider.

13. If the woman is post–cesarean section, inspect the abdominal incision for signs of healing, such as approximation or bleeding, and for any signs of infection, including drainage, edema, foul odor, or redness. Observe whether internal sutures, Steri-Strips, or staples are intact. If dressing is in place over the incision, observe for the dressing to be clean, dry, and intact.
   RATIONALE: *If drainage is present on the dressing, mark the outline of the drainage and reevaluate 30 minutes later for further bleeding or drainage.*

14. Document the findings according to hospital or unit policy.

15. Communicate active bleeding, increasing drainage, redness, foul odor, or incision edges not approximated to primary provider.

# Lochia

The uterus rids itself of the debris remaining after birth through a discharge called *lochia*, which is classified according to its appearance and contents. Lochia rubra, which is dark red, occurs for the first 2 to 3 days. Lochia serosa is a pinkish color and follows from about day 3 until the 10th day. Lochia alba, a creamy or yellowish discharge, lasts for an additional 1 to 2 weeks.

The type, amount, and consistency of lochia determine the stage of healing of the placental site. A progressive change from bright red at birth to dark red to pink to creamy white or clear discharge should occur. Persistent discharge of lochia rubra or a return to lochia rubra indicates subinvolution or late postpartum hemorrhage. See your textbook for discussion of these complications.

## SKILL 4–2 Evaluating Lochia

### PREPARATION

1. Explain why lochia occurs, why it is assessed, how it is assessed, and how it changes during the postpartum.

2. Ask the woman to void.
   RATIONALE: *A full bladder can cause uterine atony and increase the amount of lochia.*

3. Complete the assessment of uterine fundal height and firmness.
   RATIONALE: *In almost all cases, fundal height and firmness are evaluated with an assessment of lochia. This practice provides a more thorough assessment.*

4. If she has not already done so for the fundal assessment, ask the woman to flex her legs. Then ask her to spread her legs apart. Use the bed sheet as a drape to preserve her modesty.
   RATIONALE: *This position allows you to see the perineum and the perineal pad more effectively.*

### EQUIPMENT AND SUPPLIES

- Clean perineal pad
- Clean gloves
  NOTE: *Gloves are put on before assessing the perineum and lochia.*

### PROCEDURE

1. Don gloves.

2. Lower the perineal pad and observe the amount of lochia on the pad. Because women's pad-changing practices vary, ask her about the length of time the current pad has been in use, whether the amount of lochia is changed, and whether any clots were passed before this examination, such as during voiding.
   RATIONALE: *During the first 1 to 3 days the woman's lochia should be rubra, which is dark red. A few small clots are normal and occur as a result of blood pooling in the vagina when the woman is lying down. The passage of large clots is abnormal, and the cause should be investigated immediately.*

3. If the woman reports heavy bleeding or clots, ask her to put on a clean perineal pad and then reassess the pad in 1 hour. Also, ask her to call you before flushing any clots she passes into the toilet during voiding.

4. When the uterine fundus is firm and stabilized with the nondominant hand, press down on it with the dominant hand while watching to see if any clots are expelled. (See Skill 4–1, step 8.)

5. Determine the amount of lochia, using the following guide (see Figure 4–2):
   - Heavy amount—Perineal pad has a stain larger than 6 inches in length within 1 hour; 30- to 80-mL lochia.
   - Moderate amount—Perineal pad has a stain less than 6 inches in length within 1 hour; 25- to 50-mL lochia.
   - Small amount—Perineal pad has a stain less than 4 inches in length after 1 hour; 10- to 25-mL lochia.
   - Scant amount—Perineal pad has a stain less than 1 inch in length after 1 hour or lochia is only on tissue when the woman wipes.
     RATIONALE: *Lochia should never exceed a moderate amount such as four to eight partially saturated perineal pads daily. Using a consistent standard for measuring lochia improves the accuracy of the information charted and conveyed to others.*

6. In most cases, a woman is discharged while her lochia is still rubra. Provide her with information about lochia serosa and lochia alba.
   RATIONALE: *Accurate discharge information enables the woman to assess herself more accurately and enables her to judge better when to contact her healthcare provider.*

7. Document the findings specifically according to hospital/unit policy. For example, "Uterus firm, 1 FB ↓ U. Lochia moderate rubra, no clots passed."

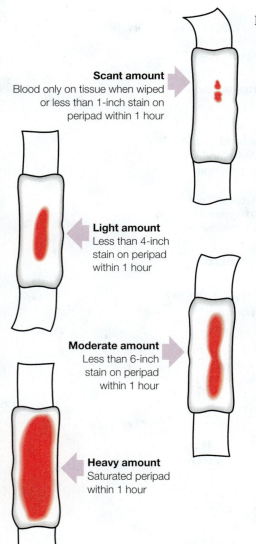

**Scant amount**
Blood only on tissue when wiped or less than 1-inch stain on peripad within 1 hour

**Light amount**
Less than 4-inch stain on peripad within 1 hour

**Moderate amount**
Less than 6-inch stain on peripad within 1 hour

**Heavy amount**
Saturated peripad within 1 hour

**Figure 4–2** *Suggested guidelines for assessing lochia volume.*
Source: From Jacobson, H. (1985, May). A standard for assessing lochia volume. *Maternal–Child Nursing,* May–June.

# Perineal Assessment

During the early postpartum period the soft tissue in and around the perineum may appear edematous with some bruising. If an episiotomy is present, the edges should be drawn together (well approximated).

Perineal assessment is an important part of normal postpartum assessment and provides important information about the woman's recovery following childbirth.

---

## SKILL 4–3  Postpartum Perineal Assessment

### PREPARATION

1. Explain the purpose and the procedure for assessing the perineum during the postpartum period.

2. Complete the assessment of fundal height and lochia as described in Skills 4–1 and 4–2.

   **RATIONALE:** *Typically, perineal assessment is the final step of the postpartum assessment.*

3. At this point in a postpartum assessment, the woman is lying on her back with her knees flexed. Her perineal pad has already been lifted away from her perineum to permit inspection of the lochia. If an episiotomy was performed or if the birth was difficult, the woman may be using an ice pack on her perineum to reduce swelling. The ice pack would also have been removed for inspection of the lochia.

4. Ask her to turn onto her side with her upper knee drawn forward and resting on the bed (Sims position).

   **RATIONALE:** *When the woman is supine, even with her knees flexed, it is very difficult to expose the posterior portion of the perineum. Thus, Sims position makes it easiest to inspect the perineum and anal area.*

### EQUIPMENT AND SUPPLIES

- Clean perineal pad, clean ice pack if desired/needed
- Small light source such as a penlight may be necessary
- Clean gloves

### PROCEDURE

1. Use a systematic approach to assessment.

   **RATIONALE:** *A systematic approach helps ensure that you do not overlook a significant finding.*

2. In evaluating the perineum, begin by asking the woman's perceptions. How does she describe her discomfort? Does it seem excessive to her? Has it become worse since the birth? Does it seem more severe than you would expect?

   **NOTE:**    *Pain that seems disproportionately severe may indicate that the woman is developing a vulvar hematoma.*

   **RATIONALE:** *Information from the woman herself often helps identify developing problems.*

3. After talking with the woman, assess the condition of the tissue. To allow for full visualization, it may be helpful to ask the woman to lift the knee of her upper leg to expose her perineum more fully. In some cases, it may help to use the nondominant hand to lift the buttocks and tissue. Note any swelling (edema) and bruising (ecchymosis). (Use the REEDA scale to recall what to assess.)

   **RATIONALE:** *The tissue is often traumatized by the birth, and mild bruising is not unusual. However, excessive bruising may indicate that a hematoma is developing.*

---

**CLINICAL TIP**

In evaluating the perineum, use the REEDA scale as a quick reminder of what to assess. Specifically:

   R = redness

   E = edema or swelling

   E = ecchymosis or bruising

   D = drainage

   A = approximation (how well the edges of an incision—the episiotomy—or a repaired laceration seem to be holding together)

Be prepared to respond appropriately to findings.

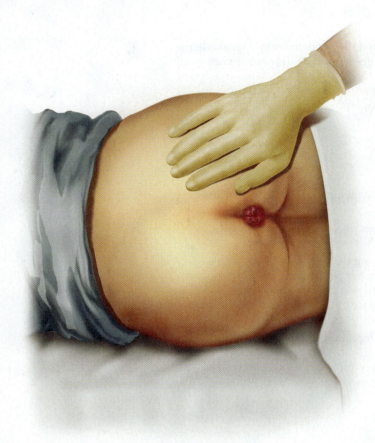

**Figure 4–3** *Intact perineum with hemorrhoids. Note how the nurse's hand raises the upper buttocks to expose the anal area fully.*

4. Evaluate the episiotomy, if there is one, or any repaired laceration for its state of healing. Is it reddened? Note the edges of the incision. Are they well approximated? Tell the woman that you are going to palpate the incision gently, and then do so. Note any areas of hardness. Note whether the incision is warmer to the touch than the surrounding tissue.

   RATIONALE: *Gentle palpation should elicit minimal tenderness and there should be no redness, warmth, or areas of hardness, which suggest infection. Both bruising and infection interfere with normal healing. Typically, within 24 hours the edges of the incision should be well approximated and "glued" together.*

5. During the assessment be alert for odors. Typically, the lochia has an earthy, but not unpleasant, smell that is easily identifiable.

   RATIONALE: *A foul odor associated with drainage often indicates infection.*

6. Finally, assess for hemorrhoids. To visualize the anal area, lift the upper buttocks (see Figure 4–3). If hemorrhoids are present, note the size, number, and pain or tenderness.

   RATIONALE: *Hemorrhoids often develop during pregnancy or labor and can cause considerable discomfort. If hemorrhoids are present, the woman may benefit from available comfort measures.*

7. During the assessment, talk to the woman about the effectiveness of comfort measures being used. Provide teaching about care of the episiotomy, hemorrhoids, and the like.

   RATIONALE: *Health teaching is an important part of nursing care. Many women have concerns about the episiotomy and may not know, for example, that the suture used is dissolvable. This is an excellent time to provide information about good healthcare practices in both the short and long term.*

8. Provide the woman with a clean perineal pad. Replenish the ice pack if necessary.

9. Document findings according to hospital/unit policy. For example: "Midline episiotomy; no edema, ecchymosis, or tenderness. Skin edges well approximated. Woman reports pain-relief measures are controlling discomfort," or "Perineal repair is approximated, minimal edema, no ecchymosis or tenderness; ice pack to perineum relieves pain."

## SKILL 4–4  Assisting With Breastfeeding After Childbirth

Breastfeeding provides newborns and infants with immunologic, nutritional, and psychosocial advantages. It also promotes involution in women who have just given birth. Newborns who are put to breast soon after their birth benefit from the physical warmth of the mother's body, from the stimulation of sucking and swallowing, from replenishment of nutrients, and from the opportunity to interact intimately with their mothers. As long as the mother is tolerating the birth well and her newborn is adjusting to extrauterine life without complication, breastfeeding can be promoted in the first hour of life when the newborn is usually alert and ready to nurse.

### PREPARATION

1. Wash hands.

### EQUIPMENT AND SUPPLIES

- None required

### PROCEDURE

1. Assist the mother to a comfortable position. Support her head, shoulders, and arms as necessary for comfort.

   RATIONALE: *A position of comfort allows the new mother to focus on breastfeeding.*

**A  Modified cradle position**

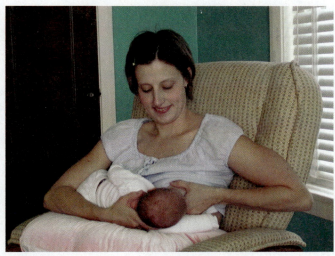

- Have the mother sit comfortably in an upright position using good body alignment. Use pillows for support (may use Boppy, body pillow, or standard bed pillows). Lap pillow should help bring the baby up to breast level so the mother does not lean over baby.
- Place the baby on the mother's lap and turn the baby's entire body toward the mother (the baby is in side-lying position). Position the baby's body so that the baby's nose lines up to the nipple. Maintain the baby's body in a horizontal alignment.
- To feed at left breast, the mother supports the baby's head with her right hand at nape of the baby's neck (allow head to slightly lag back); the mother's right thumb by the baby's left ear, and right forefinger near the baby's right ear.
- With the mother's free left hand, she can offer her left breast.

**Figure 4–4**  *Four common breastfeeding positions.* **A,** *Modified cradle.* **B,** *Cradle.* **C,** *Football (or clutch) hold.* **D,** *Side-lying position.*
Source: Courtesy of Brigette Hall, MSN, IBLCL.

2. Help the mother to wash her hands using a washcloth with soap and water, then rinse well and dry.
   RATIONALE: *Hands carry a variety of organisms, including* Staphylococcus aureus, Escherichia coli, Streptococcus *species, and* Haemophilus influenzae, *which are all common causes of mastitis, an infection of the breast.*

3. Provide warmed bath blankets to wrap around the mother and newborn together.

4. Help the mother to place the baby skin-to-skin against her body. Encourage a position that is comfortable for the mother (see Figure 4–4).
   RATIONALE: *The mother should hold the newborn in a way that feels natural and provides her with a free hand.*

5. Instruct the mother to use the thumb and first two fingers of her dominant hand to make a C-shape around her breast with the nipple in the center of the C-shape and to steadily support her breast (see Figure 4–5).
   RATIONALE: *This C-hold hand position enables the mother to position the breast correctly in the newborn's mouth.*

6. Help the mother to hold her newborn so that the mouth is in alignment with her breast at the level of the nipple. She then lightly tickles the baby's mouth with the nipple until the baby's mouth opens. She then brings the baby closely in to her breast. It is important that the baby takes the whole nipple into the mouth so that the gums are on the areola. Provide firm steady support as the newborn begins to suckle. If sucking does not begin, stroke the baby's cheek gently to elicit the suck–search response and then offer the breast again. Instruct the mother to be sure that the breast tissue does not occlude the newborn's nares.
   RATIONALE: *The newborn's gums need to be positioned over the areola because this allows the baby's jaws to compress the milk ducts located directly beneath the areola as the newborn suckles.*

7. If the newborn is sufficiently responsive, have the newborn suckle at both breasts. Initially, some newborns suck well; others may simply lick or nuzzle the nipple. Reassure the mother that this is a positive interaction.
   RATIONALE: *Even simple breast stimulation promotes the release of oxytocin, which aids uterine involution and lactation.*

8. Document in the medical record the time and duration of the breastfeeding, the quality of the latch, and interactions between the mother and newborn. Note any difficulties such as flat or inverted nipples, and initiate referral to a lactation consultant.

---

**CLINICAL TIP**

Be patient and allow the newborn and mother to experience breastfeeding in a relaxed way. Your calmness and support can help the mother feel confident and in control.

**B  Cradle position**

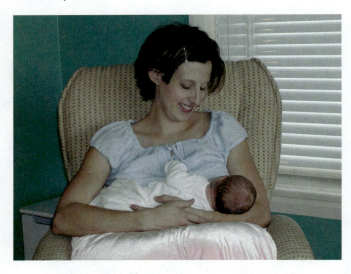

- Have the mother sit comfortably in an upright position using good body alignment. Use pillows for support (may use Boppy, body pillow, or standard bed pillows). Lap pillow should help bring the baby up to breast level so the mother does not lean over the baby.
- Place the baby on the mother's lap and turn the baby's entire body toward the mother (the baby is in side-lying position). Position the baby's body so that the baby's nose lines up to the nipple. Maintain the baby's body in a horizontal alignment.
- If feeding from the left breast, have the mother cradle the baby's head near the crook of her left arm while supporting her baby's body with her left forearm.
- With the mother's free right hand, she can offer her left breast.

**C  Football hold position**

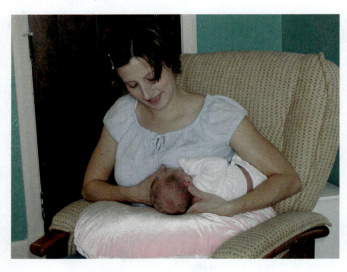

- Have the mother sit comfortably and use pillows to raise the baby's body to breast level. If using a Boppy and the Boppy is in "normal" position on the mother's lap, turn it counterclockwise slightly (if feeding at left breast) to provide extended support for the baby's body resting along the mother's left side and near the back of the mother's chair.
- If feeding at the left breast, place the baby on the left side of the mother's body, heading the baby into position feet first. The baby's bottom should rest on the pillow near the mother's left elbow.
- Turn the baby slightly on her side so that she faces the breast.
- The mother's left arm clutches the baby's body close to the mother's body. The baby's body should feel securely tucked in under the mother's left arm.
- Have the mother support the baby's head with her left hand. With the mother's free right hand, she can offer her breast. (Good position for the mother with a C-section.)

**D  Side-lying position**

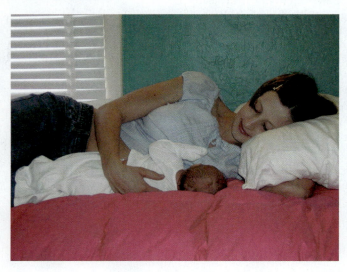

- Have the mother rest comfortably lying on her side (left side for this demonstration). Use pillows to support the mother's head and back, and provide support for the mother's hips by placing a pillow between her bent knees.
- Place the baby in side-lying position next to the mother's body. The baby's body should face the mother's body. The baby's nose should line up to the mother's nipple. Place a roll behind the baby's back, if desired.
- With the mother's free right hand, she can offer her left breast. After the baby is securely attached, mom can rest her right hand anywhere that is comfortable for her.

**C-hold hand position**

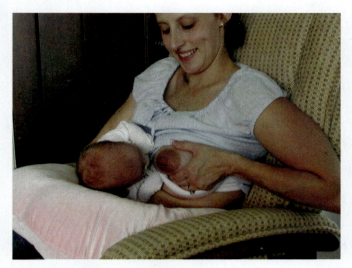

**Figure 4–5** *C-hold hand position.*
Source: Courtesy of Brigette Hall, MSN, IBLCL.

To be ready to draw the baby's mouth onto the mother's breast, as soon as the baby opens her mouth widely enough, the mother needs to have her hand supporting her breast in the ready position. She can use various hand holds, but she needs to keep her fingers well behind the areola. One such hand position is called the "C-hold." In this hold, the thumb is placed on top of the breast near the 12:00 position and the other four fingers are placed on the underside of the breast near the 6:00 position (depends on mother's hand size and length of fingers). The key point is to keep the fingers at least 1½ inches back from the base of the nipple as the fingers support the breast. Mothers are not often aware of where they place their fingers especially on the underside of the breast. If the fingers are too far forward (too close to the nipple), then the infant cannot grasp a large amount of areola in her mouth and this results in a "shallow" latch. A shallow latch is associated with nipple pain and ineffective drainage of the breast.

An alternate handhold not shown is a "U-hold" hand position. The thumb and forefinger are near the 3 and 9 position on the breast again with fingers at least 1½ inches back from the base of the nipple; the body of the hand rests on the lower portion of the breast. Using this handhold, the mother's arm position is down at her side rather than sticking outward as it is when supporting the breast using the C-hold position.

# Chapter 5
# Newborn

## Skills

## Nasal Pharyngeal Suctioning

Immediately following birth, look for mucus in the newborn's nose and mouth and remove it with a bulb syringe as needed. If there is excessive mucus or respiratory distress, suction the newborn with a mucus trap, as described in this procedure.

### SKILL 5–1 Performing Nasal Pharyngeal Suctioning

**PREPARATION**

1. Suction equipment is always available in the birthing area to clear secretions from the newborn's nose or oropharynx if respirations are depressed or if amniotic fluid was meconium stained.

2. Tighten the lid on the DeLee mucus trap or other suction device collection bottle.

   RATIONALE: *This avoids spillage of secretions and prevents air from leaking out of the lid.*

3. Connect one end of the DeLee tubing to low suction.

**EQUIPMENT AND SUPPLIES**

- DeLee mucus trap or other suction device
- Clean gloves

**PROCEDURE**

1. Don gloves.

2. Without applying suction, insert the free end of the DeLee tubing 3 to 5 inches into the newborn's nose or mouth (Figure 5–1).

   RATIONALE: *Applying suction while passing the tube would interfere with smooth passage of the tube.*

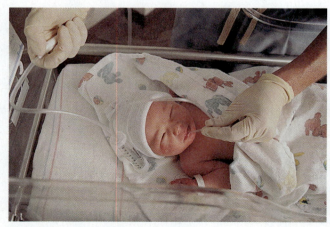

**Figure 5–1** *DeLee mucus trap.*
Source: Courtesy of Wilson Garcia.

3. Place your thumb over the suction control and begin to apply suction. Continue to suction as you slowly remove the tube, rotating it slightly.

    RATIONALE: *Suctioning during withdrawal removes fluid and avoids redepositing secretions in the newborn's nasopharynx.*

4. Continue to reinsert the tube and provide suction for as long as fluid is aspirated.

    RATIONALE: *Excessive suctioning can cause vagal stimulation, which decreases the heart rate.*

5. If it is necessary to pass the tube into the newborn's stomach to remove meconium secretions that the newborn swallowed before birth, insert the tube through the newborn's mouth into the stomach. Apply suction and continue to suction as you withdraw the tube.

    RATIONALE: *Because the newborn's nares are small and delicate, it is easier and faster to pass the suction tube through the mouth.*

6. Document the completion of the procedure and the amount and type of secretions.

    RATIONALE: *This documentation provides a record of the intervention and the status of the baby at birth.*

# Newborn Apgar

The Apgar score is used to evaluate the physical condition of the newborn at birth. The score summarizes the newborn's progress toward independent function specifically in relation to heart rate, respiratory effort, muscle tone, cry, and irritability. A score of 7 to 10 indicates that the newborn is in good condition and requires only nasopharyngeal suctioning. If the Apgar score is between 4 and 7, this indicates the need for stimulation. A score under 4 indicates the need for resuscitation.

---

## SKILL 5–2  Assigning Newborn Apgar Scores

### PREPARATION

1. Identify the person responsible to assign the Apgar score.

2. Preheat the radiant warmer to 36.5°C.

3. Prewarm blankets under the warmer.

### EQUIPMENT AND SUPPLIES

- Apgar timer or digital timer that counts seconds or a timepiece with a second hand
- Infant warmer with infant servo control (ISC) and probe preheated
- Clean gloves
- Stethoscope
- Sterile baby blanket

### PROCEDURE

1. Don gloves.

    RATIONALE: *A newborn is wet with amniotic fluid, vernix, and secretions. Consequently, universal precautions are indicated when handling the newborn until the initial bath is completed.*

2. Using the following five criteria, determine a score in each and assign an Apgar score within 1 minute and then at 5 minutes.

    - *Heart rate*—Palpate the pulse at the base of the umbilical cord for 6 seconds and multiply by 10, or use the stethoscope to auscultate the heart rate. Score as follows:

        0—no heart rate detected

        1—heart rate below 100 beats/min

        2—heart rate greater than 100 beats/min

    - *Respiratory effort*—Observe respirations and cry. Score as follows:

        0—no respiratory effort or cry

        1—slow to breathe, irregular, weak cry

        2—robust cry, good respiratory effort

    - *Muscle tone*—Assess flexion of extremities and quality of muscle tone. Score as follows:

        0—flaccid

        1—some flexion of extremities

        2—active motion

> **CLINICAL TIP**
>
> Heart rate and respirations are the two most significant categories to evaluate.

- *Reflex irritability*—Assess response to noxious stimuli such as vitamin K injection. Score as follows:

  0—no response

  1—grimace, noticeable facial movement

  2—cry, coughs, sneezes, pulls away when touched

- *Color*—Assess skin color and score as follows:

  0—generally poor color, pale or cyanotic

  1—body is pink with some pallor or cyanosis over extremities, around mouth or eyes

  2—pink body and extremities

  RATIONALE: *Assessing these five parameters provides a quick indication of the newborn's adaptation to extrauterine life. With practice, healthcare providers become skilled at assigning an accurate score within minutes. Repeat the score at 5 minutes and again at 10 minutes, as indicated.*

3. Document appropriately in the electronic medical record.

# Thermoregulation of the Newborn

A neutral thermal environment is essential to minimize the newborn's need for increased oxygen consumption and the use of calories to maintain body heat. If the newborn becomes hypothermic, the body's response can lead to metabolic acidosis, hypoxia, and shock.

---

## SKILL 5–3 Thermoregulation of the Newborn

### PREPARATION

1. Prewarm the incubator or radiant warmer. Make sure warm towels and/or lightweight blankets are available.

2. Maintain the temperature of the birthing room at 22°C (71°F), with a relative humidity of 60% to 65%.

   RATIONALE: *The change from a warm, moist intrauterine environment to a cool, dry, drafty environment stresses the newborn's immature thermoregulation system.*

### EQUIPMENT AND SUPPLIES

- Prewarmed towels or blankets
- Stocking cap for baby
- Servo control probe
- T-shirt and diaper
- Open crib
- Clean gloves

### PROCEDURE

1. Don gloves.

   RATIONALE: *Gloves are worn whenever there is the possibility of contact with body fluids—in this case, a newborn wet with amniotic fluid, vernix, and maternal blood.*

2. Place the newborn under the radiant warmer. Wipe the newborn free of blood, fluid, and excess vernix, especially from the head, using prewarmed towels.

   RATIONALE: *The radiant warmer creates a heat-gaining environment. Drying is important to prevent the loss of body heat through evaporation.*

3. If the newborn is stable, wrap the newborn in a prewarmed blanket, apply a stocking cap, and carry the baby to the mother. Alternatively, carry the newborn wrapped to the mother, loosen the blanket, and place the baby skin-to-skin on the mother's chest under a warmed blanket. The mother and her support person can hold and enjoy the newborn together.

   RATIONALE: *Use of a prewarmed blanket reduces convection heat loss and facilitates maternal–newborn contact without compromising the newborn's thermoregulation. Skin-to-skin contact with the mother or father helps maintain the newborn's temperature.*

4. After the newborn has spent time with the parents, return the baby to the radiant warmer. Leave the newborn uncovered (except for the cap and diaper) under the radiant warmer.

   RATIONALE: *Radiant heat warms the outer skin surface, so the skin needs to be exposed.*

5. Tape a servo control probe on the newborn's anterior abdominal wall, with the metal side next to the skin. Do not place it over the ribs. Secure the probe with porous tape or a foil-covered aluminum heat deflector patch. Figure 5–2 shows a newborn with a skin probe. Note that in this picture the newborn is no longer wearing a stocking cap.

6. Turn the heater to servo control mode so that the abdominal skin is maintained at 36.0°C to 36.5°C (96.8°F to 97.7°F).

7. Monitor the newborn's axillary and skin probe temperatures per agency protocol.

   RATIONALE: *The temperature indicator on the radiant warmer continually displays the newborn's probe temperature. The axillary temperature is checked to ensure that the machine is accurately recording the newborn's temperature.*

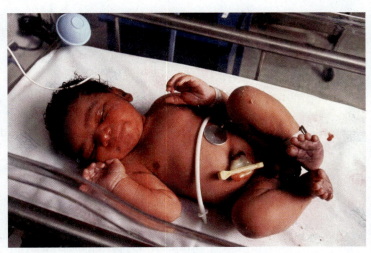

**Figure 5–2** *Temperature monitoring for the newborn. A skin thermal sensor is placed on the newborn's abdomen, upper thigh, or arm and secured with porous tape or a foil-covered foam pad.*
Source: © Tom McCarthy/Photoedit.

8. When the newborn's temperature reaches 37°C (98.6°F), add a T-shirt, double-wrap the baby (two blankets), and place the baby in an open crib.

9. Recheck the newborn's temperature in 1 hour and regularly thereafter according to agency policy.

   RATIONALE: *It is important to monitor the newborn's ability to maintain own thermoregulation.*

10. If the newborn's temperature drops below 36.1°C (97.0°F), rewarm the baby gradually. Place the baby (unclothed except for a diaper) under the radiant warmer with a servo control probe on the anterior abdominal wall.

    RATIONALE: *Rapid heating can lead to hyperthermia, which is associated with apnea, insensible water loss, and increased metabolic rate.*

11. Recheck the newborn's temperature in 30 minutes, then hourly.

12. When the temperature reaches 37.0°C (98.6°F), dress the newborn, remove from the radiant warmer, double-wrap, and place in an open crib. Check the temperature hourly until stable, then regularly according to agency policy.

    NOTE: *A newborn who repeatedly requires rewarming should be observed for other signs and symptoms of illness, and a healthcare provider should be notified because it may warrant screening for infection.*

---

### CLINICAL TIP

Take action to help the newborn maintain a stable temperature:

- Keep the newborn's clothing and bedding dry.
- Double-wrap the newborn and put on a stocking cap.
- Use the radiant warmer during procedures.
- Reduce the newborn's exposure to drafts.
- Warm objects that will be in contact with the newborn (e.g., stethoscopes).
- Encourage the mother to snuggle with the newborn under blankets or to breastfeed the newborn with hat and light cover on.

---

# Umbilical Cord Care

Secure clamping of the umbilical cord is necessary for the transition to extrauterine circulatory patterns and to prevent hemorrhage. Routine care of the umbilical cord helps to promote drying and sloughing of the cord and thus helps to prevent infection.

## SKILL 5–4  Umbilical Cord Clamp: Application, Care, and Removal

**PREPARATION**

1. Obtain necessary supplies.

**EQUIPMENT AND SUPPLIES**

- Cord clamp
- Prescribed preparations; Triple dye, bacitracin ointment, isopropyl alcohol or air drying for initial cord care
- Cord clamp remover or scissors
- Gloves

**PROCEDURE**

### Cord Clamp Application

The goal of applying the cord clamp is to prevent bleeding and promote adaptation to the extrauterine circulation pattern.

1. Place a disposable clamp at the base of the cord about 1 inch distal to the skin demarcation line.
2. Secure the clamp by pressing until it clicks and locks.
3. Cut away excess cord distal to the disposable clamp.
4. Examine the cord and count the vessels.
5. Wash the umbilical area with tap water to remove debris, and dry to remove excess moisture. Apply agency-specified antimicrobial agent if required.
   RATIONALE: *Antimicrobial ointments may be used for initial cord care in an attempt to minimize microorganisms and promote drying but have not shown to be more effective in preventing infection than just keeping the cord clean and dry (Association of Women's Health, Obstetrics and Neonatal Nurses [AWHONN], 2013).*
6. Document status of the clamp and cord in the electronic medical record.

### Routine Cord Care

The goal of routine cord care is to promote drying and sloughing of the cord and to prevent infection.

1. Apply diapers so that they are folded below the umbilical cord and do not dampen the cord with urine.
2. Change the diaper frequently to prevent urine from soaking the diaper and cord.
3. Keep the site clean and dry per agency protocol (Figure 5–3).
   RATIONALE: *Wetness and moistness promote growth of microorganisms.*
4. Assess the cord for signs and symptoms of infection (foul smell, redness, and greenish yellow drainage, localized heat and tenderness) or bleeding.
5. Document the condition of the cord in the electronic medical record as part of routine assessment.

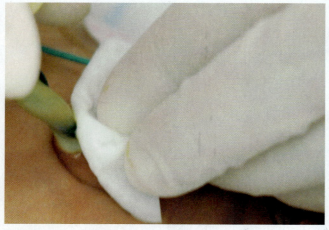

**Figure 5–3** *The umbilical cord base is carefully cleaned.*

### Cord Clamp Removal

Cord clamps are removed once the site is dry and before discharge. The cord should look dark and dried up before falling off.

1. Verify that the stump is thoroughly dry.
2. Apply the cord clamp removal device or insert scissors into the loop at the base of the clamp.
3. Cut through the loop, directing the tool away from the cord and baby.
4. Observe for any oozing or bleeding.
5. Instruct parents regarding care of the site. Advise them to contact their primary healthcare provider if bleeding, oozing, or odor is noticed, or if the area remains unhealed 2 to 3 days after the cord has sloughed off.
6. Document the condition of the cord and teaching in the electronic medical record.

# Circumcision Care

Circumcision is performed on male newborns whose parents elect to have the procedure performed. It is performed once the baby has demonstrated the ability to maintain his own temperature and in most cases prior to discharge.

---

## SKILL 5–5  Assisting With Circumcision and Providing Circumcision Care

### PREPARATION

1. Obtain or verify parental consent.
2. Medicate the baby for pain.
3. Plan for distraction.
4. Plan for safe positioning.
5. Plan to prevent unnecessary heat loss.
6. Obtain necessary supplies.
7. Coordinate timing to avoid performing the procedure within 3 to 4 hours after feeding.

### EQUIPMENT AND SUPPLIES

- Infant warmer
- Circ board
- Iodine skin prep
- Circ tray
- Analgesia medications
- Pacifier
- Sucrose solution
- Petroleum (Vaseline) gauze or ointment
- Clean diaper
- Gloves

### PROCEDURE

#### Assisting With Circumcision

The goal of assisting with circumcision is to provide for the safety of the newborn and to relieve discomfort during the procedure.

1. Check the identity of the newborn, comparing the ID number on the security bands with the number in the electronic medical record with the circumcision order.
2. Confirm that consent has been obtained and documented properly.
3. Confirm that the newborn has been NPO as ordered.
4. Have equipment and medications available for medicating the newborn for pain as ordered.
5. Prepare the baby by removing diaper and secure the baby to a padded circ board using Velcro straps or other restraint devices; restrain only the legs. Apply warm blankets to the upper body.
6. Prepare site with skin disinfectant.
7. Assess the newborn's response to dorsal penile nerve block (DPNB) or ring block.
8. Before and during procedure, provide sucrose as ordered for comfort. Offer a pacifier for non-nutritive sucking. Lightly stroke the baby's head.

#### Care Following Circumcision

The goal of care following circumcision is to reduce trauma to the surgical site and to observe for signs of complications.

1. Following procedure, completely remove any disinfectant with sterile water or saline. Pay special attention to leg creases, the lower back, and the buttocks, where pools form during the procedures.

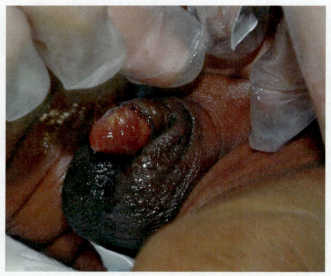

**Figure 5–4** *Following circumcision, petroleum ointment may be applied to the site for the next few diaper changes.*

2. Apply petroleum gauze or ointment to the head of the penis (Figure 5–4).
   RATIONALE: *Prevent the diaper from adhering to the surgical site and avoid trauma.*

3. Apply a clean diaper. Fasten diaper over penis snugly enough so that it does not move and rub the tender glans.

4. Assess the ability to void. Document urination following the procedure in the electronic medical record.
   RATIONALE: *Swelling or damage may obstruct the urethral opening.*

5. Return the newborn to his parents. Explain the procedure.

6. Teach parents to apply petroleum ointment to the site and to prevent adherence of the diaper to the surgical site (unless a Plastibell is in place).
   RATIONALE: *Dressings and petroleum are usually not indicated when a Plastibell is used because they could cause the plastic shield to move out of place.*

7. Monitor temperature.

8. Check the site hourly till discharge. Note any bleeding, discharge, temperature, or inability to void in the electronic medical record.

9. The glans is sensitive; avoid placing the newborn on his stomach for the first day after the procedure.

# Newborn Bath

At birth the newborn is wet and slippery. The nurse dries the baby under the radiant warmer, wiping away amniotic fluid and blood using prewarmed towels. This may help to minimize the risk of infection (AWHONN, 2013). The initial bath is generally delayed until the newborn's temperature and other vital signs are stable. Until after the first bath, use standard precautions. Depending upon agency policy and the mother's condition and degree of fatigue, the initial bath may be done by the parents in the birthing room with the nurse's assistance or by the nurse in the nursery.

## SKILL 5–6  Initial Newborn Bath

### PREPARATION

1. The baby should be resting in a radiant warmer, an incubator, or at room temperature (26°C to 27°C [79°F to 81°F]).

2. Prewarm all baby blankets to be used.

3. Gather equipment and supplies.

### EQUIPMENT AND SUPPLIES

- Clean gloves
- Warm water
- Washcloths
- Blankets or towels for drying

### PROCEDURE

1. Assess newborn temperature. Once the newborn has demonstrated the ability to maintain a stable temperature greater than 36.6°F, a first bath can be given. It is ideal to wait at least 2 hours when possible (AWHONN, 2013).
   RATIONALE: *Temperature instability introduces a threat to newborn adaptation that can lead to serious complications, including respiratory distress, hypoglycemia, and acidosis. Preventing cold stress is an important goal for newborn care.*

2. Bathe the baby under the radiant warmer. If feasible, position the warmer close to a sink for a source of warm water. Alternatively, fill a basin with warm (38°C to less than 40°C [100°F to less than 104°F]) water.
   RATIONALE: *Human newborns cannot maintain their temperature independently but require protection against heat loss in the form of warm, dry blankets and hats, or an external heat source such as the warmth of the mother's body or a warmer.*

3. Using a clean, warm, wet washcloth, clean the eyes, washing from the inner to outer canthus of each eye, moving to a clean portion of the washcloth for each eye.

4. Wash the remainder of the face, cleaning the washcloth after each use.

5. A minimal amount of mild (pH-neutral or slightly acidic) soap may be used for the remainder of the bath. Gently wash the folds of skin in the neck and axilla. Wash chest, back, arms, and between the fingers. Dry and cover upper body.

6. Wash the belly, extremities, and back. Wash the groin and diaper area. Dry the baby after each area is washed.

7. For initial bath, leave as much vernix as possible on the skin. Do not vigorously scrub to remove all vernix. Keep bath to a minimum of 5 to 10 minutes.

8. Complete cord care according to agency policy.

9. The hair and scalp can be washed using a mild shampoo, typically at a sink. To do so, wrap the baby in a warm blanket with arms tucked inside the blanket out of the way. Hold the baby in a football hold with head extended over the sink. Use the free, cupped hand to bring water from the faucet to the baby's head. Wet the scalp, apply a small quantity of shampoo, lather, and rinse, again using a cupped hand to bring water to the newborn's head. Dry the head thoroughly and apply a cap. (*Note:* The head may also be shampooed over a basin.)
   RATIONALE: *The newborn is wrapped for the shampooing to prevent excessive heat loss. Because significant heat loss can occur through the scalp, it is important to work quickly and to dry the head thoroughly. The cap helps retain heat.*

10. Repeat assessment of temperature. If the temperature is normal and stable, dress the newborn in a shirt, diaper, and cap. Wrap the baby and return to parents in an open crib. If the baby's axillary temperature is below 36.8°C (98.6°F), return the baby to the radiant warmer.

11. Document the bath, any significant findings, and temperature in the electronic medical record.

> **CLINICAL TIP**
>
> Use only a small amount of mild soap. Excessive soap and lather can be difficult to rinse off.

> **CLINICAL TIP**
>
> Some nurses prefer to begin the bath with the shampoo.

# Jaundice/Bilirubin

The most common abnormal physical finding in newborns is jaundice. Jaundice is a yellowish discoloration of the skin and sclerae of the eyes that develops from the deposit of the yellow pigment bilirubin in fat tissue. Unchecked, hyperbilirubinemia can have toxic effects on the newborn's central nervous system.

## Phototherapy

Phototherapy is the exposure of the newborn to high-intensity light. It may be used alone or in conjunction with an exchange transfusion to reduce serum bilirubin levels.

## SKILL 5–7 The Newborn Receiving Phototherapy

### PREPARATION

1. Explain the purpose of phototherapy, the procedure (including the need to use eye patches), and possible side effects such as dehydration.

2. Note evidence of jaundice in the skin, sclerae, and mucous membranes (in newborns with darkly pigmented skin). Be sure that recent serum bilirubin levels are available.
   RATIONALE: *The decision to use phototherapy is based on a careful assessment of the newborn's condition over a period of time. The most recent results prior to starting therapy serve as a baseline to evaluate the effectiveness of therapy.*

### EQUIPMENT AND SUPPLIES

- Bank of phototherapy lights
- Eye patches
- Small scale to weigh diapers

### PROCEDURE

1. Obtain vital signs, including the axillary temperature.
   RATIONALE: *This provides baseline data.*

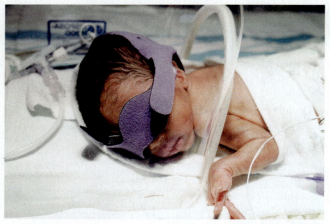

**Figure 5–5** *Newborn receiving phototherapy. The phototherapy light is positioned over the incubator or crib. Bilateral eye patches are always used during photo light therapy to protect the baby's eyes.*
Source: Courtesy of Lisa Smith-Pedersen, RNC, MSN, NNP-BC.

**CLINICAL TIP**

If the area of jaundice about the eyes begins to disappear, it is probable that the eye patches are allowing light to enter and better eye protection is needed.

2. Remove all of the baby's clothing except the diaper.
   RATIONALE: *Exposure of the newborn to high-intensity light (a bank of fluorescent lightbulbs or bulbs in the blue-white spectrum) decreases serum bilirubin levels in the skin by aiding biliary excretion of unconjugated bilirubin. Because the tissue absorbs the light, the best results are obtained when there is maximum skin surface exposure.*

3. Apply eye coverings (eye patches or a Bili-mask) to the baby according to agency policy.
   RATIONALE: *Eye coverings are used because it is not known if phototherapy injures delicate eye structures, particularly the retina.*

4. Place the newborn in an open crib or isolette (more commonly used in preterm babies and babies who are sicker) about 12 to 16 in. below the bank of phototherapy lights. (See Figure 5–5.) Reposition every 2 hours (Glomella, 2013).
   RATIONALE: *The isolette helps the newborn maintain body temperature while undressed. Repositioning exposes different areas of skin to the lights, prevents the development of pressure areas on the skin, and varies the stimulation the baby receives.*

5. Monitor vital signs every 4 hours with axillary temperatures.
   RATIONALE: *Temperature assessment is indicated to detect hypothermia or hyperthermia. Deviation in pulse and respirations may indicate developing complications.*

6. Check the lights using a bilimeter to ensure safe, effective treatment.

7. Cluster care activities.
   RATIONALE: *Care activities are clustered to help ensure that the newborn has maximum time under the lights.*

8. Discontinue phototherapy and remove eye patches at least every 2 to 3 hours when feeding the baby and when the parents visit.
   RATIONALE: *Eye patches are removed to assess for signs of complications such as excessive pressure, discharge, or conjunctivitis. Patches are also removed to provide some social stimulation and to promote parental attachment.*

9. Maintain adequate fluid intake. Evaluate the need for IV fluids.

10. Monitor intake and output carefully. Weigh diapers before discarding. Record quantity and characteristics of each stool.
    RATIONALE: *Newborns undergoing phototherapy treatment have increased water loss and loose stools as a result of bilirubin excretion. This increases their risk of dehydration.*

11. Assess specific gravity with each voiding. Weigh the newborn daily.
    RATIONALE: *Specific gravity provides one measure of urine concentration. Highly concentrated urine is associated with a dehydrated state. Weight loss is also a sign of developing dehydration in the newborn.*

12. Observe the baby for signs of perianal excoriation, and institute therapy if it develops.
    RATIONALE: *Perianal excoriation may develop because of the irritating effect of diarrhea stools.*

13. Ensure that serum bilirubin levels are drawn regularly according to orders or agency policy. Turn the phototherapy lights off while the blood is drawn.
    RATIONALE: *Serum bilirubin levels provide the most accurate indication of the effectiveness of phototherapy. They are generally drawn every 12 hours, but at least once daily. The phototherapy lights are turned off to ensure accurate serum bilirubin levels.*

14. Examine the newborn's skin regularly for signs of developing pressure areas, bronzing, maculopapular rash, and changes in degree of jaundice.
    RATIONALE: *Pressure areas may develop if the baby lies in one position for an extended period. A benign, transient bronze discoloration of the skin may occur with phototherapy when the newborn has elevated direct serum bilirubin levels or liver disease. A maculopapular rash is another transient side effect of phototherapy that develops occasionally.*

15. Avoid using lotion or ointment on the exposed skin.
    RATIONALE: *Lotion and ointments on a newborn receiving phototherapy may cause skin burns.*

16. Provide parents with opportunities to hold the newborn and assist in the baby's care. Answer their questions accurately and keep them informed of developments or changes.

**RATIONALE:** *A sick newborn is a source of great anxiety for parents. Information helps them deal with their anxiety. Moreover, they have a right to be kept well informed of their baby's status so that they are able to make informed decisions as needed.*

17. Alternatively, provide phototherapy using lightweight fiberoptic blankets ("biliblankets"). The baby is wrapped in the blanket, which is plugged into an outlet (Figure 5–6).

    **NOTE:**    *With fiberoptic blankets, the newborn is readily accessible for care, feedings, and diaper changes. The baby does not get overheated, and fluid and weight loss are not complications of this system. The baby is accessible to the parents, and the procedure seems less alarming to parents than standard phototherapy. A combination of a fiberoptic light source in the mattress under the baby and a standard phototherapy light source above is also used by some agencies. In addition, many agencies and pediatricians use fiberoptic blankets for home care.*

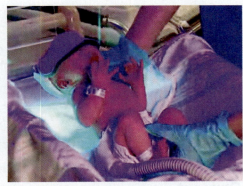

**Figure 5–6** *Newborn on fiberoptic "bili" mattress and under phototherapy lights. A combination of fiberoptic source mattress and standard phototherapy light source may also be used.*
Note: The color is distorted because of the reflection of the bililight mattress.

# Chapter 6
# Informed Consent

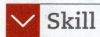 **Skill**

## General Guidelines for Obtaining Informed Consent

**6–1** Pediatric Considerations for
Obtaining Informed Consent,
page 53

## General Guidelines for Obtaining Informed Consent

Informed consent involves explaining a specific procedure to the parent (or legal guardian), and when appropriate to the child as well, and then obtaining written permission from the parent/guardian to perform that procedure.

Before a procedure, the parent or legal guardian and child (to the level of the child's ability) must be given enough information to clearly understand the condition, a detailed description of the procedure or treatment to be performed, the possible benefits and significant risks associated with the procedure or treatment involved, and alternative methods available to achieve the same end. The parent or guardian is also informed of the right to refuse treatment on behalf of the child. In some cases, the judicial system may intervene to mandate life-saving treatment for a child if the parents refuse treatment for the child. See your textbook for information about obtaining consent for research projects with children.

It is both legally and ethically necessary to obtain informed consent. Without signed permission for medical management, the healthcare provider could be found guilty of assault and battery. Most often physicians obtain consent, especially for invasive procedures and surgery. Occasionally another healthcare provider, such as a dentist or advanced practice nurse, may obtain consent. Know your agency policy about who is designated to obtain consent for procedures.

Guidelines have been established to ensure that informed consent is obtained for medical care:

- Information must be presented to the individual responsible for making an informed decision to allow this person to weigh the benefits of the proposed treatment or procedure against the potential for complications. This information should be presented in simple, easy-to-understand terms. All questions and concerns should be answered honestly and completely.

- The person making a healthcare decision must be over the age of majority (i.e., the age at which full civil rights are accorded—18 years in most states) and must be competent (i.e., must be able to make a decision based on the information received). The person needs to understand the proposed medical management and any risks. Know the parameters of the state law where you practice nursing.

- The decision reached must be voluntary. The person making the decision must not be coerced, forced, under medication that can influence judgment, or placed under duress while considering the options.

Although general written consent for care is obtained within the hospital setting during the admission process, specific consent must be obtained for procedures or treatments that include the following:

- Major surgery
- Minor surgery such as a cutdown, incision and drainage, closed reduction of a fracture, or fracture pinning
- Invasive diagnostic tests such as lumbar puncture, bone marrow aspiration, biopsy, cardiac catheterization, or endoscopy

- Treatments that may involve high risk, such as radiation therapy, chemotherapy, or dialysis
- Any procedure or treatment that falls under the auspices of research
- Photographing clients, even when done for educational purposes

## SKILL 6–1 Pediatric Considerations for Obtaining Informed Consent

### PREPARATION

1. Assess the parent's knowledge about the procedure so that during the discussion with the healthcare provider, correct information can be reinforced and misconceptions can be clarified.

2. Assess the child's ability to understand information and participate in the decision-making process.

   - If the child is a *minor* (has not reached the age of majority—under the age of 18 years in most states) the parent or legal guardian must give consent for all procedures or treatments. Children should become more actively involved in decision making about treatment procedures as their reasoning skills develop. Children too young to give informed consent can be given age-appropriate information about their condition and asked about their care preferences. Their parents, however, make ultimate decisions regarding their care. *Mature minors* (14- and 15-year-old adolescents who are able to understand treatment risks) can give consent for treatment or refuse treatment in some states, particularly for birth control and substance abuse treatment; this often does not include the ability to consent for major medical procedures (Coleman & Rosoff, 2013).

     RATIONALE: *By 7 or 8 years of age, a child is able to understand concrete explanations about informed consent for research participation. By age 11 years, a child's abstract reasoning and logic are advanced. By age 14 years, an adolescent can weigh options and make decisions regarding consent similar to an adult.*

   - Some states provide for the rights of nonemancipated teens to make certain healthcare decisions. The child may give permission for those conditions identified in state law, and at the ages specified by that particular state. The developmental level and understanding of the adolescent, best interests of the adolescent, and family context are all considered in decision making for health care (Padon & Baren, 2011; Unguru, 2011; Wooley, 2011). Some examples of the treatments that many states permit adolescents to sign for include birth control, treatment of sexually transmitted infections, contraceptive and abortion counseling and services, prenatal care, parenting issues, substance use and other mental health conditions, and participation in research. Check the law in your state for specific guidelines.

   - If the child is an *emancipated minor* (under the age of 18 years but legally independent from the parents), the child may give informed consent for medical care. Common examples of emancipated minors include teenagers who are married, in the military, living apart from their parents and financially independent, or pregnant or parents themselves. Emancipation is a title given by courts of law, and the adolescent will have a legal document verifying the emancipation.

3. If a parent or guardian is not available, determine that an authorized adult can give informed consent.

   - When a parent or guardian is unavailable to provide consent for treatment, the person in charge of the child (e.g., relative, babysitter, teacher, or camp counselor) may give consent for emergency treatment if the person has signed written permission from the parent/guardian to authorize care in the parent's/guardian's absence. When the parent or guardian can be contacted by telephone, verbal consent can be obtained with two witnesses listening simultaneously. The consent should be recorded for later signature. Under the federal

Emergency Medical Treatment and Labor Act (EMTALA), a minor can be examined, treated, stabilized, and even transferred to another hospital for emergency care when the parent or legal guardian is not available to provide consent (for more information, consult https://www.cms.gov/Regulations-and-Guidance/Legislation/EMTALA/index.html?redirect=/EMTALA/).

## EQUIPMENT AND SUPPLIES

- Private area to comply with HIPAA regulations (see Chapter 1)
- Appropriate forms and educational materials
- Pen

## PROCEDURE

1. Notify the physician or other healthcare provider that the family is available to discuss the procedure.

2. Obtain necessary forms and written explanations of the procedure.

3. Find a quiet and private place where the physician or other designated healthcare provider and nurse can confidentially explain the forms and procedure to the child and/or family.

4. Accompany the physician to serve as a witness and to assist with answering the family's questions.

   RATIONALE: *The nurse's role is to serve as a witness for the physician or other designated healthcare provider that the family members were fully informed about the procedure and their right to consent to or refuse treatment. The nurse also assists by ensuring that the information provided is understood by the family and put into a context that has meaning to the family.*

5. Ask the family members several questions to evaluate their understanding. Provide additional information when any points need to be clarified.

6. When the family members appear to have no more questions, ask if they are prepared to give consent for the procedure or need more time to consider their options.

7. When the family members are prepared to give consent, the physician or other designated healthcare provider and the nurse obtain their signatures and serve as witnesses to the consent.

# Chapter 7
# Physical Assessment

## ⌄ Skills

# Growth Measurements

The accurate assessment of growth is important throughout childhood to ensure the child's health or to identify the impact of disease on the child. Growth charts for infants and children of both genders are provided in Appendix A.

---

### SKILL 7–1  Length

Until 2 years of age, length is measured with the infant and child in the supine position, even if the child is able to stand independently. The length measurement is the standard for accurate assessment of growth in children under 2 years of age. A difference in length and height measurements for children does exist. If height were plotted on a length-based growth chart, a true assessment of the young child's growth over time would be inaccurate.

#### PREPARATION

1. Have the parent remove any hat or shoes the infant is wearing.

#### EQUIPMENT AND SUPPLIES

- Measuring board or other length-measuring device

#### PROCEDURE

1. When using a measuring board, ask the parent or an assistant to place and hold the top of the infant's head against the top of the board.
2. After positioning the infant's head, gently push down on the infant's knees until the legs are straight.
   RATIONALE: *Because of the normally flexed posture of the infant, the body must be extended to obtain an accurate measurement.*
3. Position the heels of the feet on the footboard, and record the length to the nearest 0.5 cm or 0.25 inch (Figure 7–1).
4. Repeat the measurement for accuracy. If a difference between the two readings is found, take the average reading for documentation.
5. Plot the measurement for the child's age on the standardized growth curve. See Appendix A.

If such a measuring device is not available, place the infant on a paper sheet, stabilizing the infant in the same manner as when using the board. Carefully holding the pen so that it touches the child's head and feet at a right angle to the surface, make one mark at the vertex of the head and another at the heel. Then measure the distance between the two marks. Record the length in centimeters or inches.

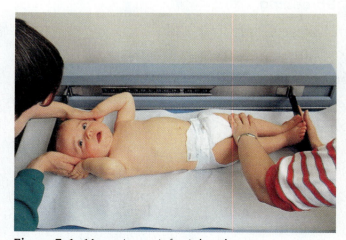

**Figure 7–1**  *Measuring an infant's length.*

## SKILL 7–2  Height

After 2 years of age, height is measured with the child standing upright against a wall with a stadiometer (Figure 7–2).

### PREPARATION

1. Have the child remove shoes and hat.

### EQUIPMENT AND SUPPLIES

- Stadiometer or platform scale with stature-measuring device

### PROCEDURE

1. Have the child stand straight with the back to the wall and the head held erect in the midline position.
2. The shoulders, buttocks, and heels should touch the wall. The outer canthus of the eyes should be on the same horizontal plane as the top of the external ear.
   RATIONALE: *Positioning the head properly helps ensure consistency in placement of the headpiece on the crown of the head.*
3. Move the headpiece down to touch the crown.
4. Make the height reading to the nearest 0.5 cm or 0.25 inch.
5. Plot the measurement for the child's age on the standardized growth curve. See Appendix A.

In the older child and adolescent, height is often measured using a platform scale with an attached stature-measuring device. Have the child stand erect, facing forward. Move the stature-measuring device to the top of the head. Have the child step off the scale, and read the height in centimeters or inches.

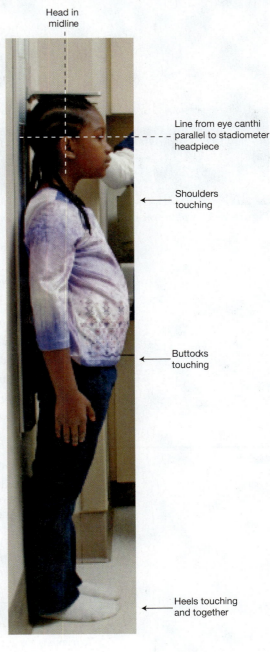

Head in midline

Line from eye canthi parallel to stadiometer headpiece

Shoulders touching

Buttocks touching

Heels touching and together

**Figure 7–2** *Measuring a child's height. Position the head in an erect and midline position while the shoulders, buttocks, and heels touch the wall. Move the headpiece down to touch the crown.*

## SKILL 7–3  Weight

Infants and children are weighed on a scale that measures only in kilograms (kg) to reduce errors in calculating medication dosages (American Academy of Pediatrics Committee on Drugs, 2015). Infants are placed on a platform scale (Figure 7–3), in either a supine or sitting position, depending on their age. Take care to ensure the infant's safety. Keep the room warm for comfort.

### PREPARATION

1. Check the balance of the scale before using it.
2. Have the parent or assistant remove all of the infant's clothing and diaper. Weigh toddlers in their underclothes. Weigh older children in their street clothes after heavy clothing and shoes are removed. Toddlers with acute diarrheal disease or chronic health problems may need to be weighed nude for accuracy.
   RATIONALE: *It is important to minimize the amount of clothing worn by children when being weighed to improve comparisons with previous weights taken.*
3. Clean the infant scale tray between uses. Place a paper cover over the scale tray.

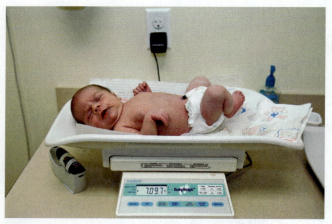

**Figure 7–3** *A platform scale is used to weigh an infant.*

## EQUIPMENT AND SUPPLIES

- Infant scale for infants
- Paper
- Standing scale for older children

## PROCEDURE

### *Infants*

1. Place the infant on the scale and keep a hand close.
   RATIONALE: *Infants move quickly and it is essential to protect them from falling.*
2. Distract the infant to reduce movement, and take the reading when the infant stops moving.
   RATIONALE: *It takes a few seconds of inactivity for the scale to settle on the infant's actual weight.*
3. Record the weight in the nearest 10 grams.
4. Plot the weight measurement for the infant's age in months on the standardized growth curve. See Appendix A.
5. Convert the weight to pounds and inform the parent.

### *Older Children*

The older child can be weighed on a standing scale.

1. Provide privacy for the older child and adolescent.
2. Have the child stand still on the scale.
3. View the digital reading or move the weights until the scale is balanced for the child's weight.
4. Record the weight to the nearest 0.1 kg.
5. Convert the weight to pounds and inform the parent.

## SKILL 7–4  Body Mass Index

The body mass index (BMI) uses a formula of kilograms per meter squared ($kg/m^2$) to assess nutritional status and total body weight relative to height. Beginning at age 2 years, the child's BMI can be easily determined after plotting the length and weight, or height and weight, on the standardized growth curves. See Appendix A. An online BMI calculator for weight in kilograms or pounds and is available at http://www.cdc.gov/healthyweight.
   RATIONALE: *Tracking the change in BMI can often provide clues to nutritional problems, including obesity, health promotion issues, or illness.*

---

### CLINICAL TIP

To manually calculate body mass index (BMI), follow these steps:

1. Be sure that weight is in kilograms.
2. Change height measurement to meters. Because 1 meter = 39.37 inches (or 0.0254 meter = 1 inch), you need to multiply the child's height in inches by 0.0254 to obtain height in meters.
3. Now square the number of meters.
4. You are ready to calculate BMI. Divide kilograms of weight by height in meters squared. For example, the child's weight is 12 kg. The child's height is 34.5 in. or 0.8763 m. Then $m^2$ = 0.7679. Divide 12 by 0.7679, resulting in the BMI = 15.63.

---

## SKILL 7–5  Head Circumference

Head circumference is usually measured at regular intervals until the child's second birthday.

## PREPARATION

1. Remove any hat, hair binders, or barrettes the infant is wearing.

## EQUIPMENT AND SUPPLIES

- Disposable, nonstretching measuring tape with centimeter and millimeter markings

## PROCEDURE

1. Wrap the tape around the head at the supraorbital prominence above the eyebrows, above the ears, and around the occipital prominence (Figure 7–4). This is usually the point of largest circumference of the head. Take care to prevent the tape from slipping or causing a paper cut.

2. Record the circumference to the nearest 0.5 cm or 0.2 in. Repeat the measurement to confirm the reading.

3. Plot the measurement for the child's exact age in months on the standardized growth curve. See Appendix A.

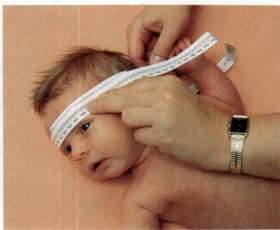

**Figure 7–4** *Measuring head circumference.*

## SKILL 7–6  Abdominal Girth

Abdominal girth may occasionally be measured in children to monitor abdominal size, which can vary with conditions such as ascites or edema from cardiac or renal disease.

### PREPARATION

1. Remove all clothing from the abdomen.

### EQUIPMENT AND SUPPLIES

- Disposable, nonstretching measuring tape with centimeter and millimeter markings

### PROCEDURE

1. Wrap the tape around the abdomen at the level of the umbilicus, taking care to prevent a paper cut.

2. If the measurement is taken at another location on the abdomen, place ink marks at the location of the measurement.
   RATIONALE: *This action will enable you or another nurse to take a future measurement at the same location.*

3. Record the measurement to the nearest 0.5 cm or 0.2 in. Compare the reading to those taken previously to determine a change in size.

# Vital Signs

## SKILL 7–7  Heart Rate

The procedure for assessing the heart rate is similar to that for adults. However, an apical heart rate is assessed in infants and young children.

### PREPARATION

1. Move clothing away from the anterior chest.

2. Give the infant a pacifier or use other distraction to get a resting pulse rate.

### EQUIPMENT AND SUPPLIES

- Stethoscope

### PROCEDURE

*Infants*

1. Place the cleaned stethoscope on the anterior chest at the fifth intercostal space in a midclavicular position (Figure 7–5).
   RATIONALE: *The apical heart rate is preferred in infants and young children, and it is also used for older children when the condition warrants it. In infants and young children, palpating the pulse in an extremity consistently enough to count the rate may be difficult.*

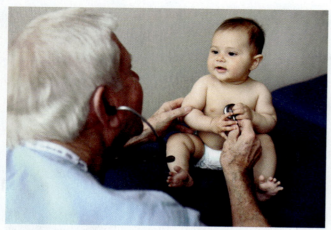

**Figure 7–5** *Assessing the apical heart rate.*

2. Count the beats (each "lub-dub" sound) for 1 full minute in young children. In older children, count for 30 seconds and multiply by 2.
3. While auscultating the heart rate, note if the rhythm is regular or irregular.

### Children

Pulse rates may be palpated in children over 3 years of age, even though an apical heart rate may be used in older children. Palpation sites commonly used include the brachial, radial, femoral, and dorsalis pedis. In addition, the pulse rhythm, strength, and amplitude may be checked.

- Note if the rhythm is regular or irregular.
- Compare the distal and proximal pulses in an extremity for strength.
- Document the rate, rhythm, and character of the pulsation (normal, bounding, or thready).

The range of normal heart rates by age is listed in Table 7–1.

| TABLE 7–1 | Normal Heart Rates for Children at Different Ages | |
|---|---|---|
| **Age** | **Heart Rate Range (beats/min)** | **Average Heart Rate (beats/min)** |
| Newborns | 100–170 | 120 |
| Infants to 2 years | 80–130 | 110 |
| 2–6 years | 70–120 | 100 |
| 6–10 years | 70–110 | 90 |
| 10–16 years | 60–100 | 85 |

## SKILL 7–8 Respiratory Rate

The procedure for measuring a child's respiratory rate is the same as for an adult. However, keep in mind these points:

- Observe the abdomen, rather than the chest, rise and fall in an infant or young child.
  **RATIONALE:** *Because the respirations of an infant or young child are diaphragmatic, the abdomen moves more than the chest with breathing.*
- Abdominal movement in a child will be irregular.
- Count breaths for 1 full minute in young children due to rate variability. In older children count for 30 seconds and multiply by 2.

The range of normal respiratory rates based on age is listed in Table 7–2.

| TABLE 7–2 | Normal Respiratory Rates for Different Age Groups |
|---|---|
| **Age** | **Respiratory Rate per Minute** |
| Newborn | 30–80 |
| 1 year | 20–40 |
| 3 years | 20–30 |
| 6 years | 16–22 |
| 10 years | 16–20 |
| 17 years | 12–20 |

# SKILL 7–9 Blood Pressure

The procedure to measure the blood pressure for the child is the same as that for an adult. Whether manual or electronic equipment is being used, the correctly sized blood pressure cuff must be selected to obtain an accurate reading (Figure 7–6). The child should sit quietly for 3 to 5 minutes before taking the blood pressure (Flynn, Pierce, Miller, et al., 2012).

## PREPARATION

1. To select the proper cuff size, compare the cuff to the size of the child's upper arm or thigh.
2. The bladder of the cuff should encircle the extremity used and have a width that covers two thirds of the length of the extremity used (Daniels, 2012).
   RATIONALE: *If the bladder of the cuff is too small, the blood pressure reading will be falsely high.*
3. Inform the child that the cuff will hug and squeeze the arm and then release.

## EQUIPMENT AND SUPPLIES

- Various sizes of blood pressure cuffs with air squeezed out of the bladder
- Electronic blood pressure monitor
- Sphygmomanometer and stethoscope
- A chart with blood pressure values by age, gender, and height percentiles (Appendix B)

## PROCEDURE

### With Oscillometry

Electronic equipment is often used to obtain the systolic blood pressure for infants and young children. With this equipment, a transducer measures oscillations or the force of blood movement in the arterial wall from the heart contraction to identify the mean arterial pressure and then uses an algorithm to estimate the systolic and diastolic blood pressure (Schrauf, 2012) (Figure 7–7A).

1. Wrap the cuff around the right arm or upper leg directly against the skin with the center of the bladder over the artery of the extremity. The lower edge of the cuff should be 2 to 3 cm above the antecubital or popliteal fossa.
   RATIONALE: *The right arm is preferred, as this extremity was used for standardizing the blood pressure tables. While the upper leg is not a preferred site to obtain the blood pressure, it may be used when comparing arm and leg blood pressures to detect coarctation of the aorta.*
2. Place the arm with the antecubital fossa at heart level with muscles relaxed. Stabilize the arm, as movement interferes with the reading.
3. Ensure that the tubing is free of kinks, and activate the equipment according to the manufacturer's recommendations.
4. Pressure is recorded as the number over "D."
5. Document the blood pressure reading and compare to values for age, gender, and height percentile (Appendix B). When a blood pressure reading over the 90th percentile for age, gender, and height percentiles is measured, repeat the measurement in 5 to 10 minutes. Confirm an elevated blood pressure measurement with a manual sphygomomanometer.

> ### CLINICAL TIP
>
> To choose the appropriate cuff size for a newborn, measure the newborn's limb circumference with a measuring tape around the midpoint of the limb used. If the blood pressure cuff has marks to determine fit, use these lines to ensure that the cuff is not too small. The cuff should fit between the joints of the extremity used. Place the artery mark on the cuff over the brachial artery.

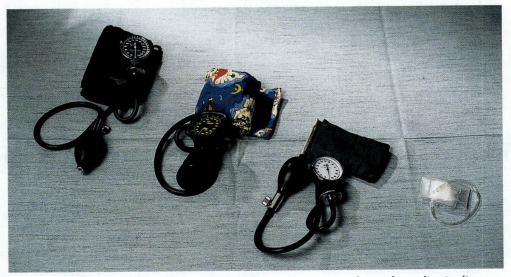

**Figure 7–6** *Blood pressure cuffs are available in various types and sizes for pediatric clients.*

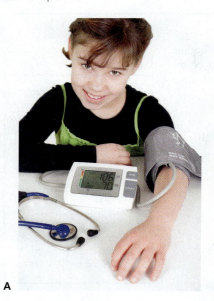

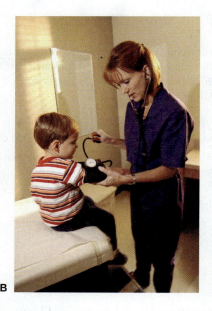

**Figure 7–7** *A, Measuring blood pressure using the oscillometric technique. B, Measuring blood pressure with a manual cuff. Note that the arm is at the same level as the heart.*
Source: A, courtesy of the photographer: Elena Dorfman.

### *With a Manual Sphygmomanometer*

1. Wrap the cuff snugly around the desired extremity directly against the skin with the bladder centered over the extremity's artery.

2. Hold the arm with the antecubital fossa at heart level (Figure 7–7B). If taking the blood pressure in the thigh, the child should be lying down flat.

3. Palpate for the pulse and inflate the cuff until the pulse is occluded and no longer felt. Note the reading. Release the cuff pressure. This is the palpated systolic blood pressure, and it can be recorded as blood pressure over "P."

4. Wait a minute and place the stethoscope over the pulse area. Avoid using too much pressure against the pulse area to improve the quality of sounds heard.

5. Close the air escape valve. Pump the cuff with the bulb until the gauge rises 30 mmHg above the level of the palpated systolic blood pressure. Slowly release the air through the valve at 2 to 3 mm/sec while watching the falling gauge.
   RATIONALE: *The palpated reading helps improve accuracy in the recognition of the first Korotkoff sound.*

6. Note the number at which the first Korotkoff sound is heard; this is the systolic pressure.

7. Continue slowly releasing the air. The fifth Korotkoff sound (the disappearance of all sound) is the diastolic pressure. It may be 0 in children under age 12 years. For these children, the fourth Korotkoff sound is considered the diastolic pressure.

8. Document the systolic and diastolic blood pressure readings and compare to values for age, gender, and height percentiles (see Appendix B).

## Body Temperature

Body temperature can be measured in two scales: Celsius or Fahrenheit. Follow the manufacturer's guidelines for the use of electronic thermometers.

The five routes for measuring body temperature are oral, rectal, axillary, tympanic, and temporal.

---

### HOME AND COMMUNITY CARE CONSIDERATIONS

Ask parents what type of thermometer they use at home, and provide instructions on its correct use. They may not know how long to insert the thermometer or how to clean and store it after use. Nurses in schools and childcare centers should assess the knowledge of healthcare providers in these settings and provide teaching as needed.

If the parents still have a mercury thermometer, instruct them to replace it with another type. Encourage parents to safely dispose of the mercury thermometer at an approved collection site.

## SKILL 7–10  Oral Route

The oral route for temperature measurement may be used for the child over 3 years of age who is able to cooperate by holding the thermometer with the mouth closed. The expected temperature is 37°C (98.6°F).

### PREPARATION

1. Assess the cooperation of the child to hold the thermometer in the mouth, under the tongue with the mouth closed.

### EQUIPMENT AND SUPPLIES

- An electronic nonbreakable probe is preferred.

### PROCEDURE

1. Cover the oral probe with the protective sheath.
2. Place the oral probe or an electronic thermometer under the tongue, and have the child close the mouth (Figure 7–8).
3. Turn on the scanner. It will sound a tone or beep when finished. Remove the probe.
4. Read and record the temperature.

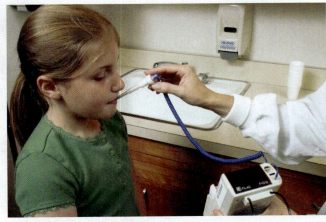

**Figure 7–8** *Measuring the oral temperature.*

## SKILL 7–11  Rectal Route

The rectal route should be used only when no other route is possible due to the risk of rectal perforation and because most children view this as an intrusive procedure. The rectal temperature is often estimated to be one degree higher than the axillary temperature. The rectal temperature may be recommended to obtain the best temperature reading when assessing for fever in infants and children less than 3 years of age (Stine, Flook, & Vincze, 2012).

### PREPARATION

1. Place the infant or child prone on a bed or the parent's lap; turn the older child on the side.

### EQUIPMENT AND SUPPLIES

- Electronic thermometer with sheath
- Water-soluble lubricant
- Clean gloves

### PROCEDURE

1. Don gloves and cover the tip of the electronic thermometer protective sheath with a water-soluble lubricant.
2. For the infant, place the tip 1 cm (0.5 in.) into the rectum. For the child, place the tip 2.5 cm (1 in.) into the rectum.
   RATIONALE: *This reduces the risk of rectal perforation.*
3. Turn on the scanner and follow the manufacturer's recommendations. It will tone or beep when finished. Remove the probe.
4. Read and record the temperature.

## SKILL 7–12  Axillary Route

The axillary route is often used for newborns and for children who are seizure-prone, unconscious, or immunosuppressed, or who have a structural abnormality that precludes an alternative route. The axillary temperature reading is generally 0.6°C (1.0°F) lower than the oral or rectal temperature. The axillary route may miss a low-grade fever because of its usual lower reading (Stine et al., 2012).

### PROCEDURE

1. Cover the thermometer probe with a protective sheath. Place the thermometer tip in the highest area of the axilla and hold it with the arm pressed close to the body (Figure 7–9).
2. Turn on the scanner. It will sound a tone or beep when finished. Remove the probe.
3. Read and record the temperature.

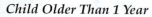

**Figure 7–9** *Measuring the axillary temperature.*

## SKILL 7–13 Tympanic Route

The tympanic route is a convenient and fast method for taking temperatures in infants and children. Infrared technology provides a rapid reading of the temperature of the blood flowing through the carotid artery, a reflection of core body temperature (Gasim, Musa, Abdien, et al., 2013). The tympanic thermometer is easy to use, provides a rapid reading, and is less invasive.

### PREPARATION

1. Place the infant in a supine position on a flat surface. Stabilize the infant's head, and turn the infant's head 90 degrees for easy access.
2. Position the child on the parent's or assistant's lap with the head secured.

### EQUIPMENT AND SUPPLIES

- Tympanic thermometer with clean, disposable probe fitted without wrinkles

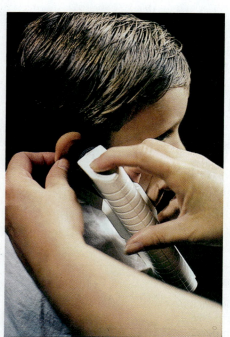

**Figure 7–10** *Position for inserting a thermometer when the tympanic route is used. The pinna is pulled up and back to straighten the ear canal in this young child.*

### PROCEDURE

#### Child Younger Than 1 Year

1. If using the child's right ear, hold the thermometer in your right hand. For the child's left ear, hold the thermometer in your left hand.
2. Pull the pinna of the ear straight back and downward. Approach the ear from behind to direct the thermometer tip anteriorly, aimed toward the tympanic membrane (Figure 7–10).
   RATIONALE: *An inaccurate reading may occur if the thermometer is not directed at the tympanic membrane.*
3. Place the probe in the ear as far as possible to seal the canal. Turn on the scanner.
4. Leave the probe in the ear according to the manufacturer's recommendations. It will sound a tone or beep when finished.
5. Remove the probe, and read and record the temperature.

#### Child Older Than 1 Year

1. Pull the pinna up and back in children beginning at about age 3 years, but pull the pinna downward and back in children under age 3 years.
   RATIONALE: *This helps to straighten the auditory canal so the tympanic membrane is in alignment with the thermometer scanner.*
2. Place the probe and continue as described previously for the child younger than 1 year.
3. Read and record the temperature.

## SKILL 7–14 Temporal Route

The temporal artery thermometer contains an infrared scanner that collects skin temperature readings over the forehead and temporal artery and calculates the temporal artery reading. A potential inaccuracy in readings may occur in newborns and preterm infants (Smith, Alcock, & Usher, 2013). The reading is quickly obtained and is noninvasive.

### PREPARATION

1. Position the child on the parent's or assistant's lap with the head secured.

### EQUIPMENT AND SUPPLIES

- Temporal artery thermometer with a sensor that was cleaned with an alcohol swab

### PROCEDURE

1. Move the thermometer sensor across the forehead over the temporal artery (Figure 7–11).
2. Read and record the temperature.

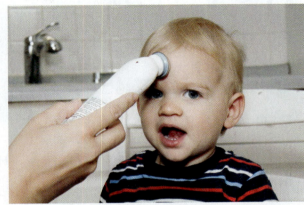

**Figure 7–11** *Measuring the temperature with a temporal artery thermometer.*
Source: Wilson Photo/Custom Medical Stock.

# Visual Acuity Screening

Vision acuity screening should begin at about 3 years of age, when the child can cooperate with the procedure. Several procedures may be used to screen visual acuity in children.

> ### HOME AND COMMUNITY CARE CONSIDERATIONS
>
> Most states have laws regulating the ages or school grades at which children must have vision screening performed, and what passing standards are accepted. Check your state laws or codes for guidelines.

## SKILL 7–15 Snellen Letter Chart

The Snellen letter (alphabet) chart (Figure 7–12*A*) is the most commonly used assessment tool for visual acuity in school-aged children. It consists of lines of letters in decreasing size.

- Most charts are designed for reading from a distance of 20 feet. When the child reads the line designated "20 feet" while standing 20 feet away, vision is 20/20. If, however, the child can only read the line labeled "40 feet" while standing 20 feet away, vision is 20/40.
- Charts are also available that can be used at a distance of 10 feet. A child who stands 10 feet from this chart and reads the 10-foot line (10/10) has vision equivalent to that of 20/20 when using the 20-foot chart.

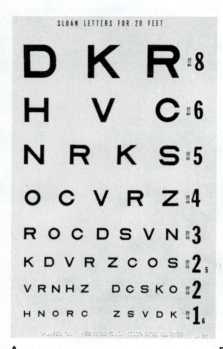

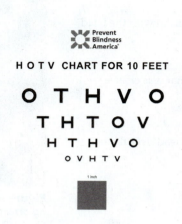

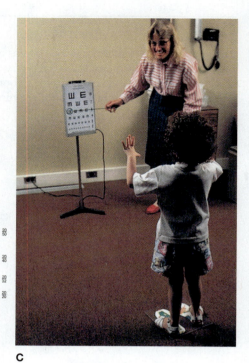

**A**  **B**  **C**

**Figure 7–12** *Visual acuity charts. A, Snellen letter chart. B, HOTV chart. C, Snellen E chart.*
Source: A and B courtesy of the National Society to Prevent Blindness.

## SKILL 7–16  HOTV, Snellen E, or Picture Chart

For toddlers and children who have not yet mastered the alphabet, the HOTV, Snellen E (Figure 7–12*B* and *C*), or picture chart may be used. Position the child either 10 or 20 feet away, matching the guidelines on the chart. Young children may have improved testing when the 10-foot eye chart is used (Hered, 2011).

- The HOTV test uses a chart with the letters H, O, T, and V placed in random order on lines in decreasing size. The child either names the letters or points to them on a card held close by the examiner as the assistant points to the letters on the chart. The procedure followed is the same as with the Snellen test, but because children can point to the letters on the chart in front of them, they do not need to know the alphabet. After a practice session, the HOTV test can also be used with children who do not speak English.

- In the Snellen E chart, the capital letter E is shown facing in different directions. The child is asked to point in the direction of the "legs" of the E. Another option is to give the child a paper with an E on it and have the child turn it in the direction the E is pointing on the chart.

- The Lea Symbols are commonly identified simple pictures (e.g., heart, square, circle, house). The child is asked to identify the pictures or point to the picture on a card held close by the examiner as the assistant points to the picture on the chart.

### PREPARATION

1. The procedure is explained to the child and parent. With a young child, make a game of identifying the letter, the direction of the E's legs, or the picture. Practice with the child before starting, providing positive feedback for correct responses.
   RATIONALE: *This ensures that the child understands the directions for the test to improve the chances of an accurate screening test result.*

2. Place the chart at the child's eye level and ensure that it is well lit.

### EQUIPMENT AND SUPPLIES

- Screening chart
- Card or other item to cover one eye
- Card with HOTV letters, E, or Lea Symbols

## PROCEDURE

1. Place the heels of the child at the 20-foot mark (or 10-foot mark if using that chart).

2. Assess each eye separately and then both together. If the child wears glasses, check the vision both with and without glasses. If the child is wearing contacts, leave them in and note that the results were with contacts.

   RATIONALE: *It is important to detect significant differences in visual acuity between the eyes of children under 5 years. When one eye has poorer vision than the other, the brain may decide to stop using the eye with poor vision, leading to further vision deterioration. Corrective lenses are required to enable the child to use both eyes and to preserve vision.*

3. While one eye is being tested, use the child's hand, a patch, or a piece of cardboard to cover the other eye. Tell the child to keep the covered eye open during the testing. Use a different eye cover for each child to minimize the spread of infection among children.

4. Observe for squinting, moving the head forward (to be closer to the chart), excessive blinking, or tearing during the examination.

   RATIONALE: *These may be signs that the child has a vision problem.*

5. Document the last line the child can read correctly (i.e., the smallest line on which the child correctly reads at least three of five symbols). Refer the child to the pediatrician or other healthcare provider (e.g., ophthalmologist or optometrist) if the following findings are noted (American Association for Pediatric Ophthalmology and Strabismus, 2014):

   - Age 3 to 4 years—20/50 or less in either eye
   - Age 4 to 5 years—20/40 or less in either eye
   - After age 5 years—20/32 or less in each eye
   - A difference in vision between the eyes of two lines or more on the eye chart, for example, 20/20 in one eye and 20/40 in the other eye, even when one eye is within the expected range

## SKILL 7–17 Autorefractor Vision Screening

The refraction, or direct visual acuity measurement, can be performed automatically with a tabletop or handheld photoscreening device. Autorefraction uses automated wavefront technology to evaluate the refractive error of each eye. A photoscreening device uses optical images of the eye's red reflex to detect estimates of myopia, hyperopia, opacity, eye alignment, and astigmatism (American Academy of Pediatrics Section on Ophthalmology, 2012). Minimal cooperation from the child is needed because of the short time needed for assessment, usually less than a minute.

### PREPARATION

1. Follow the guidelines in the device user manual to obtain accurate results.

2. The procedure is explained to the child and parent. Explain that a camera will take pictures of the child's eyes and the child needs to look at the lights on the camera. If necessary, have an assistant to help hold the child's head still.

### EQUIPMENT AND SUPPLIES

- Handheld or tabletop autorefraction or photoscreening device

### PROCEDURE

1. For a handheld screening device, place the child on a chair of adult height, and sit on a child-sized chair at a distance from the child guided by the instrument manual (e.g., 1 foot or 1 meter).

   RATIONALE: *The lower position puts the nurse at a better level to target the handheld device at the pupils of the child's eyes.*

2. Hold the device in a position to have both eyes visible on the screen. A series of beeps and lights helps keep the child's focus on the device. Another beep sounds when the eye assessment has been completed. The second eye is then evaluated without the child or nurse needing to change position.

3. For the tabletop screening device, position the seated child to look directly into the eye pieces of the device (Figure 7–13).

4. Print out the results of the refraction screening or record in the child's electronic medical record.

5. Use the referral guidelines in Skill 7–16 to identify children who need additional evaluation.

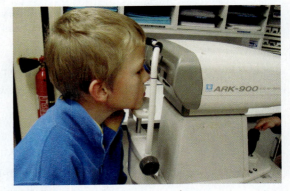

**Figure 7–13** *Use of an autorefractor vision screening device.*

# Hearing Acuity Screening

It is important to perform hearing acuity screening to ensure that infants and children are able to hear for speech and language development to occur. Newborn hearing screening is performed prior to discharge from the hospital. Several procedures may be used to screen hearing acuity in children. Various conditions during childhood, such as frequent ear infections, could result in a hearing loss.

---

### HOME AND COMMUNITY CARE CONSIDERATIONS

Each state has an early hearing and intervention program with a goal of having all infants screened for hearing loss as early as possible. Each state also has specific laws mandating when children attending school should be screened for hearing acuity and the hertz and decibel levels to be included. Consult your state school code for guidance about local requirements.

---

## SKILL 7–18 Otoacoustic Emission Screening

An otoacoustic emission (OAE) test is used to screen for hearing loss in newborns by evaluating cochlear and hair cell function rather than cranial nerve VIII function. The miniature microphone probe detects and records a faint echo from the cochlea in response to a short clicking stimulus.

### PREPARATION

1. Select a time when the newborn is calm and not hungry to perform the test.
2. Swaddle the newborn and consider using a pacifier to promote comfort.
3. Use a room with minimal environmental noise.

### EQUIPMENT AND SUPPLIES

- An otoacoustic emission screening ear probe with a soft flexible tip attached to computer cable, which is attached to the computer

### PROCEDURE

1. Turn the newborn's head to the side. Gently pull back on the ear canal and inspect it to make sure it is free of debris.
   RATIONALE: *OAE is especially affected by vernix in the ear canal and middle ear effusion.*
2. Select a probe that fits snugly in the ear canal to seal it and block out background noises.
3. Insert the probe in the direction of the ear canal and obtain a seal.
4. Position the cable connected to the computer where it has less chance of being disconnected.
5. When the newborn is quiet, remove your hand from the probe and turn on the sound stimulus.
   RATIONALE: *Holding the probe may add background noise that interferes with the test results. The tip should stay in place if inserted correctly.*
6. Remove the probe, clean off any debris, and then complete the process with the same probe in the other ear.
7. Document the results with the computer printout and write either "pass" or "refer" in the newborn's record.

---

## SKILL 7–19 Automated Auditory Brainstem Screening

Automated auditory brainstem response (AABR) records brain activity in response to sounds. It detects cranial nerve VIII, cochlear, and auditory brainstem activity.

### PREPARATION

1. Select a time to perform the test when the newborn is calm and not hungry.
2. Swaddle the newborn and consider using a pacifier to promote comfort.
   RATIONALE: *Movement by the newborn may interfere with the test results.*
3. Use a location with minimal environmental noise for the test.

### EQUIPMENT AND SUPPLIES

- Occlusive headphones for sound transmission with cables attached to the computer
- Three sensors with wires that are attached to the module with a cable connected to the computer
- Skin cleaner for electrode sites

## PROCEDURE

1. Clean the skin where electrodes will be attached with approved cleanser.

2. Attach the three sensors to the baby's head according to manufacturer's directions, one behind each ear and one at midline on the top of the head.

3. Connect the sensor wires to the module.

4. Cover the baby's ears with the occlusive headphones (Figure 7–14).

5. Turn on the sound stimulus (series of clicking sounds) for the amount of time designated by the manufacturer.

   RATIONALE: *The computer registers samples of electrical activity over a fixed period of time (Chung & Morgan, 2013).*

6. When the test is complete, remove the headphones and sensors and dispose of them.

7. Document the results with the computer printout and state either "pass" or "refer" in the newborn's record.

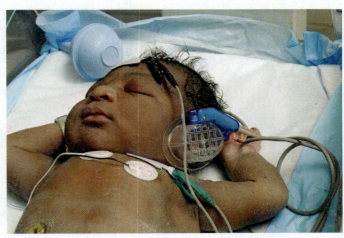

**Figure 7–14** *Newborn being evaluated for hearing loss with the automated auditory brainstem response screening process.*

## SKILL 7–20  Pure Tone Audiometry

This procedure screens for hearing using air conduction in cooperative children over the age of 3 years. It can detect sensorineural hearing loss, but it does not detect fluid in the middle ear.

### PREPARATION

1. When screening a large group of children, such as in a school, the machine may be taken to the classroom for demonstration and practice.

2. Check the transmission of sound to be sure both earphones work properly.

3. Explain the procedure in terms the child can understand. Show the earphones. Turn the sound loud enough for the child to hear and practice raising a hand or putting a block in a basket in response to the sound, which will improve test accuracy.

4. If a soundproof room is not available, the audiometer should be set up in a quiet environment.

   RATIONALE: *It is important to reduce exposure to other sources of sound that could interfere with the child's response to the audiometer's sounds.*

5. Clean the earphones with alcohol swabs between children for infection control.

### EQUIPMENT AND SUPPLIES

- Calibrated audiometer
- Scoring sheet
- Alcohol swabs

### PROCEDURE

1. Position the child so that the back is toward the machine and faced away from the tester.

   RATIONALE: *In this position, the child cannot receive cues from the examiner's face or see the examiner press the lever to present the sound.*

2. Place the headset on the child's head and adjust for a proper fit. Note the right and left indicators on the earphones.

3. Follow the manufacturer's directions for using the audiometer. Deliver sounds and watch for the child to raise a hand or put a block in a basket when heard. Use a random order to give the sound cues when testing the ears.

   RATIONALE: *A random order does not allow the child to anticipate the sound and potentially cause an inaccurate interpretation of the screening test.*

4. Test each ear at the following pitches—500, 1000, 2000, and 4000 Hz—at increasing levels of loudness (decibels).

5. If the young child does not seem to understand what to do once screening begins, remove the headphones and practice more. Have blocks ready and instruct the child to place a block in a basket when hearing the sound. Turn up the decibel level slightly and practice until the child understands. Then turn the decibel level back to the appropriate screening level.

> **CLINICAL TIP**
>
> The sounds of the audiometer are delivered at hertz levels, or the frequency of sound in cycles per second. Lower numbers indicate lower sounds, such as speech tones. Higher numbers indicate higher sounds, such as heard in music. The decibel level, or loudness of the sounds, can also be controlled by the audiometer.

| TABLE 7–3 | Passing Standards for Hearing Acuity With Pure Tone Audiometer |
|---|---|
| Hertz | Decibels |
| 500 | 20–25 |
| 1000 | 20–25 |
| 2000 | 20–25 |
| 4000 | 25 |

6. If the child does not pass the screening with both ears, retest the child in 2 weeks. If the child still does not pass, refer for further evaluation (Table 7–3).
   RATIONALE: *The child with an upper respiratory infection may not hear well and needs time for the infection to improve. Continued failure of the screening may indicate a hearing problem.*

7. Document the results of the hearing test.

## SKILL 7–21 Tympanometry

Tympanometry provides an estimate of middle ear pressure and an indirect measure of tympanic membrane compliance (movement). Older infants and children can be tested. Abnormal findings often indicate fluid accumulation in the middle ear that prevents the efficient transmission of sound to the inner ear. This can result in hearing loss over time.

### PREPARATION

1. Explain the procedure to the child and parents and the need for the child to hold still.

### EQUIPMENT AND SUPPLIES

- Calibrated tympanometer
- Disposable earpiece
- Graph paper

### PROCEDURE

1. Encourage the child to hold still during the test. The infant and young child may need assistance in holding still.
   RATIONALE: *This reduces the chance of pain or injury from the earpiece in the auditory canal.*

2. Gently insert the earpiece with the tympanometer probe into the auditory canal until the canal is sealed and airtight.
   RATIONALE: *The canal must be sealed tight to get an accurate measurement of the pressure it takes to move the tympanic membrane.*

3. Turn on the tympanometer according to manufacturer instructions and emit the tone. The pressure is measured by the probe and then plotted on a graph (Figure 7–15A and B).

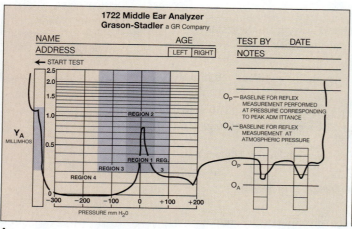
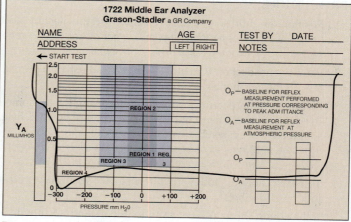

**A**  **B**

**Figure 7–15** *A, This tympanogram demonstrates normal hearing as evidenced by the curve showing the tympanic membrane's movement when a sound wave is emitted into the ear canal. Mobility is between 0.2 and 1.0 mL, the normal range. B, In contrast, note the flat pattern in the second tympanogram, which shows very restricted mobility of the tympanic membrane in response to sound.*

4. Repeat the procedure in the other ear.

5. Insert the printout into the child's medical record and document the results of the test.

# Fluid and Electrolyte Balance: Intake and Output

Intake and output (I and O) is a measurement of fluid and electrolyte balance in the body. Input is measured as for adults, recording the fluids delivered to the child through parenteral or oral routes in milliliters (mL).

Output is a measurement of what is expelled, drained, secreted, or suctioned from the body. Output sources include urine, stool, vomitus, sweat, drainage from wounds, and nasogastric suction. Output for infants can be measured by weighing the diaper. Output for older children can be measured as for adults with a graduated cylinder, and recorded in cubic centimeters (cc) or milliliters (mL).

Accurate measurement of I and O is documented for many children, such as those receiving IV fluids or certain medications, after major surgery, and those with serious infections, renal disease or kidney damage, congestive heart failure, diabetes mellitus, dehydration or hypovolemia, or severe thermal burns.

---

## SKILL 7–22 Urine Output Measurement

### PREPARATION

1. Weigh the diapers to be worn by the infant, and mark the weight in grams on the diapers, or zero the scale to the weight of a clean diaper.

### EQUIPMENT AND SUPPLIES

- Scale with gram measurement
- Urine toilet collection device, urinal
- Graduated cylinder
- Clean gloves

### PROCEDURE

#### Infants

1. When a precise measurement of output for infants is needed, don gloves and weigh the diaper after the infant has voided or had a stool. Disadvantages to this procedure include the inability to differentiate between urine and stool weights because the two substances may mix in the diaper, and due to the evaporation of urine that takes place after about 30 minutes.
   RATIONALE: *For each 1-g increase in weight of the diaper, 1 mL of liquid has been excreted by the infant.*

2. Count the number of wet diapers. The amount of micturition is fairly standard during infancy and early toddlerhood. Four to eight wet diapers per day is usually normal.
   RATIONALE: *This general guideline is used when a precise measurement is not needed.*

3. A urine bag may be used to obtain a fairly accurate measurement. Watch for any leakage. See Chapter 11: Specimen Collection for application of a urine bag.

4. Document the output in the medical record.

#### Toddlers and Older Children

Once the child is toilet trained, urine is collected in a toilet collection device or urinal. The output is measured as for adults with a graduated cylinder.

See Chapter 11: Specimen Collection for output measurement when a urinary catheter is in place.

# Chapter 8
# Pain Assessment and Management

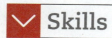 **Skills**

## Pain Assessment

## Special Pain Management Techniques

## Pain Assessment

Pain is considered a vital sign, and every child has the right to be assessed for pain and receive pain management. The goal of pain assessment is to provide accurate information about the location and intensity of pain and its effects on the child's functioning. Various pain scales have been developed to assess pain in children. Some pain assessment scales rely on the nurse's observation of the child's behavior if the child is nonverbal. Other scales depend on the child's report of pain intensity. For more information, refer to your textbook.

---

### SKILL 8–1 Selected Pediatric Pain Scales

***Neonatal Infant Pain Scale (NIPS)***

- Use in preterm and term infants up to 6 weeks after birth.
- Observe the infant's facial expression, cry quality, breathing pattern, arm and leg position, and state of arousal (Table 8–1).

| TABLE 8–1 | Neonatal Infant Pain Scale (NIPS) |

| Characteristic | Scoring Criteria |
|---|---|
| **Facial Expression** | |
| 0 = Relaxed muscles | ■ Restful face with neutral expression |
| 1 = Grimace | ■ Tight facial muscles; furrowed brow, chin, and jaw (Note: At low gestational ages, infants may have no facial expression.) |
| **Cry** | |
| 0 = No cry | ■ Quiet, not crying |
| 1 = Whimper | ■ Mild moaning, intermittent cry |
| 2 = Vigorous cry | ■ Loud screaming, rising, shrill, and continuous (Note: Silent cry may be scored if infant is intubated, as indicated by obvious facial movements.) |
| **Breathing Patterns** | |
| 0 = Relaxed | ■ Relaxed, usual breathing pattern maintained |
| 1 = Change in breathing | ■ Change in breathing, irregular, faster than usual, gagging, or holding breath |
| **Arm Movements** | |
| 0 = Relaxed/restrained | ■ Relaxed, no muscle rigidity, occasional random (with soft restraints) movements of arms |
| 1 = Flexed/extended | ■ Tense, straight arms; rigid; or rapid extension and flexion |
| **Leg Movements** | |
| 0 = Relaxed/restrained | ■ Relaxed, no muscle rigidity, occasional random (with soft restraints) movements of legs |
| 1 = Flexed/extended | ■ Tense, straight legs; rigid; or rapid extension and flexion |
| **State of Arousal** | |
| 0 = Sleeping/awake | ■ Quiet, peaceful, sleeping; or alert and settled |
| 1 = Fussy | ■ Alert and restless or thrashing; fussy |

Source: From Lawrence, J., Alcock, D., McGrath, P., et al. (1993). The development of a tool to assess neonatal pain. *Neonatal Network, 12*(6), 61; and Taddio, A., Hogan, M. E., Moyer, P., Girgis, A., Gerges, S., Wang, L., & Ipp, M. (2011). Evaluation of the reliability, validity and practicality of 3 measures of acute pain in infants undergoing immunization injections. *Vaccine, 29,* 1390–1394.

## FLACC Pain Scale

- This scale is designed to measure acute pain in infants and young children following surgery or while sleeping. It may also be used for older children who are nonverbal or developmentally challenged.
- FLACC is an acronym for the five categories that are assessed: **f**ace, **l**egs, **a**ctivity, **c**ry, and **con**solability (Table 8–2).
- Use until the child is able to self-report pain with another pain scale.

| TABLE 8–2 | FLACC Behavioral Pain Assessment Scale | | |
|---|---|---|---|

| | Scoring | | |
|---|---|---|---|
| **Categories** | **0** | **1** | **2** |
| Face | No particular expression or smile | Occasional grimace or frown; withdrawn, disinterested | Frequent to constant frown, clenched jaw, quivering chin |
| Legs | Normal position or relaxed | Uneasy, restless, tense | Kicking or legs drawn up |
| Activity | Lying quietly, normal position, moves easily | Squirming, shifting back and forth, tense | Arched, rigid, or jerking |
| Cry | No cry (awake or asleep) | Moans or whimpers, occasional complaint | Crying steadily, screams or sobs; frequent complaints |
| Consolability | Content, relaxed | Reassured by occasional touching, hugging, or being talked to; distractible | Difficult to console or comfort |

### How to Use the FLACC

**In infants or children who are awake:** Observe for 1 to 5 minutes or longer. Observe legs and body uncovered. Reposition client or observe activity. Assess body for tenseness and tone. Initiate consoling interventions if needed.

**In infants or children who are asleep:** Observe for 5 minutes or longer. Observe body and legs uncovered. If possible, reposition the client. Touch the body and assess for tenseness and tone.

### Face

Score 0 if the client has a relaxed face, makes eye contact, shows interest in surroundings.
Score 1 if the client has a worried facial expression, with eyebrows lowered, eyes partially closed, cheeks raised, mouth pursed.
Score 2 if the client has deep furrows in the forehead, closed eyes, an open mouth, deep lines around nose and lips.

### Legs

Score 0 if the muscle tone and motion in the limbs are normal.
Score 1 if client has increased tone, rigidity, or tension; if there is intermittent flexion or extension of the limbs.
Score 2 if client has hypertonicity, the legs are pulled tight, there is exaggerated flexion or extension of the limbs, tremors.

### Activity

Score 0 if the client moves easily and freely, normal activity or restrictions.
Score 1 if the client shifts positions, appears hesitant to move, demonstrates guarding, a tense torso, pressure on a body part.
Score 2 if the client is in a fixed position, rocking; demonstrates side-to-side head movement or rubbing of a body part.

### Cry

Score 0 if the client has no cry or moan, awake or asleep.
Score 1 if the client has occasional moans, cries, whimpers, sighs.
Score 2 if the client has frequent or continuous moans, cries, grunts.

### Consolability

Score 0 if the client is calm and does not require consoling.
Score 1 if the client responds to comfort by touching or talking in 30 seconds to 1 minute.
Score 2 if the client requires constant comforting or is inconsolable.

Whenever feasible, behavioral measurement of pain should be used in conjunction with self-report. When self-report is not possible, interpretation of pain behaviors and decisions regarding treatment of pain require careful consideration of the context in which the pain behaviors are observed.

### Interpreting the Behavioral Score

Each category is scored on the 0–2 scale, which results in a total score of 0–10.

| | |
|---|---|
| 0 = Relaxed and comfortable | 4–6 = Moderate pain |
| 1–3 = Mild discomfort | 7–10 = Severe discomfort or pain or both |

Source: From Merkel, S. I., Voepel-Lewis, T., Shayevitz, J. R., & Malviya, S. (1997). The FLACC: A behavioral scale for scoring postoperative pain in young children. *Pediatric Nursing, 23*(3), 293–297; and Gomez, R. J., Barrowman, N., Elia, S., Manias, E., Royle, J., & Harrison, D. (2013). Establishing intra- and inter-relater agreement of the Faces, Legs, Activity, Cry, Consolability scale for evaluating pain in toddlers during immunization. *Pain Research & Management, 18*(6), e124–e128. The FLACC scale was developed by Sandra Merkel, MS, RN, Terri Voepel-Lewis, MS, RN, and Shobha Malviya, MD, at C. S. Mott Children's Hospital, University of Michigan Health System, Ann Arbor, MI.

### Oucher Scale

- Use in children between 3 and 12 years of age. Select the scale that matches the child's ethnic background—White, African American, Hispanic, or Asian (Figure 8–1).
- The child selects the face that matches the level of pain. The older child can select a number between 0 and 10.

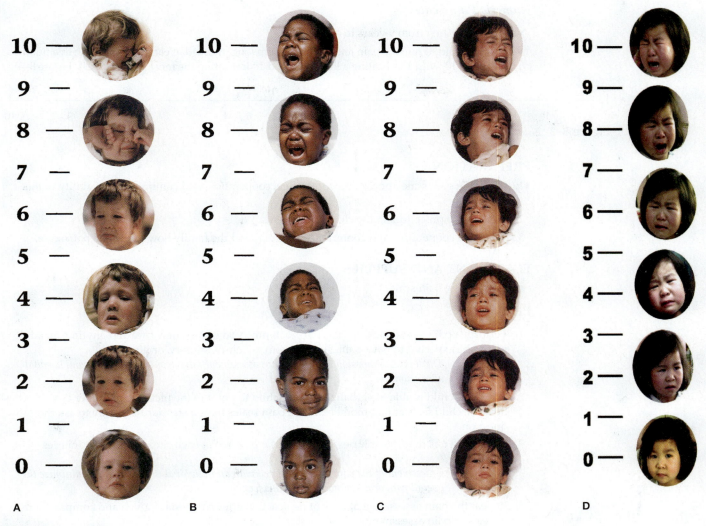

**Figure 8–1** *Oucher Scale 3–12 years.*
Note: In the form presented in this book, the Oucher Scale is for educational purposes only and cannot be used for client care. *A,* The White version of the Oucher Scale, developed and copyrighted by Judith E. Beyer, RN, Ph.D., 1983. *B,* The African American version of the Oucher Scale, developed and copyrighted by Mary J. Denyes, RN, Ph.D., and Antonio M. Villarruel, RN, Ph.D., 1990. Cornelia P. Porter, RN, Ph.D., and Charlotta Marshall, RN, MSN, contributed to the development of the scale. *C,* The Hispanic version of the Oucher Scale, developed and copyrighted by Antonio M. Villarruel, RN, Ph.D., and Mary J. Denyes, RN, Ph.D., 1990. *D,* The Asian version of the Oucher Scale, developed and copyrighted by C. H. Yeh, RN, Ph.D., and C. H. Wang, BSN, 2003. http://www.oucher.org.

### Faces Pain Rating Scale

- Use in children from 3 years through adolescence.
- The child selects the face that is the closest match to the amount of pain felt (Figure 8–2).

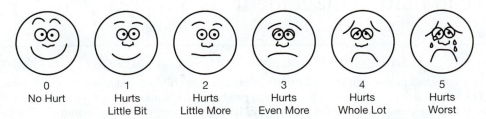

**Figure 8–2** *Faces Pain Rating Scale. After determining that the child has an understanding of number concepts, teach the child how to use the scale. Point to each face and use the words under the picture to describe the amount of pain the child feels. Then ask the child to select the face that comes closest to the amount of pain felt.*
Source: Used with permission from Wong, D. L., & Baker, C. M. (1988). Pain in children: Comparison of assessment scales. *Pediatric Nursing, 14,* 9–16.

*Numeric Pain Scale*

- Use in children from 9 years to adult.
- Ask the child to rate the pain felt on a line 10 cm long, marked at each centimeter with a number from 0 to 10, with 1 indicating a little pain and 10 indicating the most pain ever felt (Figure 8–3).

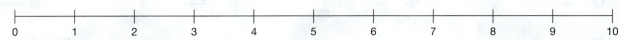

**Figure 8–3** *Numeric pain scale.*

### PREPARATION

1. Select the pain scale appropriate for the age, cooperation, and communication ability of the child.
2. Explain the procedure to the child and parents.
3. Teach the cooperative and communicative child and the family how to use the pain scale.

### EQUIPMENT AND SUPPLIES

- Copy of the pain scale

### PROCEDURE

1. Perform a pain assessment with a child each time you initiate new care and anytime an adult would be expected to have pain, such as from an injury, surgery, or illness.
   RATIONALE: *The Joint Commission requires a pain assessment during outpatient visits and hospital admissions.*

2. When the child is able to verbalize, ask the child to point to the picture or number that matches how the child feels at that moment. Some pain scales have a standardized way to ask the question.

3. If the child has multiple injuries, ask about the pain felt at each site, and then all injuries together.
   RATIONALE: *Assessment of the pain only associated with an individual injury site may minimize the overall pain or discomfort the child is feeling.*

4. Repeat the pain assessment at time of peak action after analgesia is given and compare with the earlier pain assessment.
   RATIONALE: *This action determines the effectiveness of the analgesia provided and facilitates individualized pain management.*

5. Document the pain assessment method, score, and time performed.

---

**GROWTH AND DEVELOPMENT**

Even newborns and infants feel and remember pain. Children may not complain about pain because they fear the method to relieve pain is worse than the pain, or they may believe you already know about the pain they have.

---

## Special Pain Management Techniques

### SKILL 8–2 Administering Patient-Controlled Analgesia (PCA) Pumps

Specially designed pumps can be used to deliver analgesia to children and adolescents for pain control. The pumps use an intravenous line and a syringe or syringe and bag with ordered medication locked inside the pump. After initial pain control has been achieved with a continuous IV infusion of morphine (basal dose), the child presses a button to receive a smaller analgesic dose (bolus dose) for episodic pain relief (Figure 8–4). The pump is set by the nurse for doses and timing to prevent the child from receiving an overdose of medication. In addition, the pump can be set to administer a specific amount of medication at designated time intervals without the child pushing the button. This allows for pain control even during sleep or for young children.

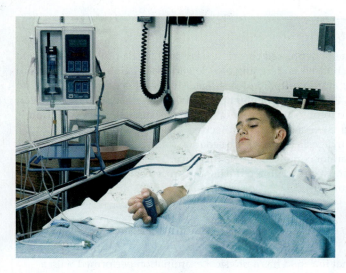

**Figure 8–4** *This boy was instructed preoperatively in use of the PCA pump. Being able to administer his own analgesia when it is needed offers him a sense of control and contributes to successful pain management.*

## PREPARATION

1. Identify the child (often 5 years and older) who may be selected to use patient-controlled analgesia (PCA). The child should be able to self-report pain with a pain scale and understand that pushing the button will give medication to relieve pain. Educate the child and parent about the use of PCA before the surgery.

    RATIONALE: *This will enhance the child's understanding because the child is not in pain or less alert during immediate postoperative period.*

2. Once the PCA is ordered, check the medication order and compute the maximum 24-hour dose to verify safety.

3. Prepare the tubing and pump according to manufacturer's directions. Prime the tubing with IV fluid and medication and attach with a Y connector to the client's IV line.

    RATIONALE: *Priming the IV tubing enables the child to receive pain medication as soon as the pump is turned on or the button is pushed.*

## EQUIPMENT AND SUPPLIES

- Pump
- Tubing
- IV fluid
- Medication
- Alcohol swabs
- Clean gloves

## PROCEDURE

1. Complete a thorough pain and physical assessment.

    RATIONALE: *Baseline data are used to evaluate pain control effectiveness and any side effects from the medication.*

2. Bring the prepared tubing, pump, and medication to the child.

3. Don gloves.

4. Attach the tubing as directed to the child's IV line.

5. Unlock the pump door and follow protocol for programming the pump delivery.

6. Deliver a loading dose if ordered.

    RATIONALE: *Loading doses begin the medication process and allow pain control to be effective.*

7. Verify that the pump is locked. When the pump is locked with a key, remove it from the room.

    RATIONALE: *Inadvertent entry of unauthorized persons into the pump mechanism must be avoided.*

8. Continue to reassess the child's pain to ensure adequate pain control, and make the needed adjustment to the care plan.

## SKILL 8–3 Sedation Monitoring

Sedation is a medically controlled state of depressed consciousness used for painful diagnostic and therapeutic procedures. It is used in children undergoing a wide variety of painful diagnostic and treatment procedures in the hospital and in outpatient settings. **Moderate sedation** occurs with lower doses of sedatives and enables the child to maintain protective reflexes and a patent airway, and to make an appropriate response to physical stimuli or verbal commands. **Deep sedation** is a controlled state of depressed consciousness in which protective airway reflexes are lost, but the child can respond to painful stimuli. Analgesia is given with sedation for invasive procedures, as the sedated child can still feel pain but cannot communicate its presence. The child receiving sedation must be properly prepared; the child must be monitored during the procedure and while recovering consciousness after the procedure is completed.

### PREPARATION

1. Inform the child (if old enough to understand) and parents. Ensure that informed consent is obtained.

2. Obtain a health history. Ensure that the child has a physical examination performed with a focused airway assessment by an anesthetist or anesthesiologist.

3. Evaluate recent food and fluid intake.
   **RATIONALE:** *The desired time for the child to be NPO prior to a procedure varies for type of food or fluid: a light meal and/or milk is 6 hours, for breastmilk 4 hours, and for clear liquids 2 hours (Allison & George, 2014).*

4. Insert an IV line for medication administration.

5. Verify sedation orders.

### EQUIPMENT AND SUPPLIES

- Have drugs to be used prepared and available. Prepare emergency drugs. Have opioid and benzodiazepine reversal agents (naloxone, flumazenil, nalmefene) available if these medications are used for sedation.
  **RATIONALE:** *The practitioner using sedation must be trained in use of the medication and in airway management. An additional support person must be present to monitor the child. All personnel present should be trained in advanced life support in emergency situations.*

- A pediatric code cart, resuscitation drugs, oxygen, and suction must be available, in addition to a pulse oximeter and cardiopulmonary monitor.

- Make sure syringes and IV lines and fluids are available.

- Clean gloves, sterile gloves

### PROCEDURE

#### During Procedure

1. Record all drugs administered, doses, and times.

2. Don gloves. Monitor oxygen saturation and heart rate continuously throughout the procedure, and visually confirm respiratory effort, color, and vital signs.

3. Assess level of sedation throughout the procedure.
   **RATIONALE:** *It is important to recognize when a child progresses from moderate to deep sedation so that the needed respiratory support can be provided.*

4. Record all assessments on flow sheet according to facility policy.

5. Check procedural immobilizer and head position throughout the procedure.

#### After Procedure

1. Perform assessments and monitoring while keeping suction and emergency equipment available.

2. Take vital signs and complete other monitoring according to agency guidelines, such as every 5 minutes until the client is awake and then every 15 minutes until stable and discharged.

---

**CLINICAL TIP**

Common medications used for sedation include the following:

- Benzodiazepines: diazepam (Valium), midazolam (Versed), and lorazepam (Ativan); antagonist agent is flumazenil

- Hypnotics or barbiturates: thiopental, pentobarbital, methohexital

- Ketamine

- Propofol (Diprivan) or etomidate

- Dexmedetomidine

- Analgesics: Fentanyl, Alfentanil; antagonist medications are naloxone and nalmefene

---

**CLINICAL TIP**

Discharge criteria from unit after sedation:

- Satisfactory and stable cardiovascular function and airway patency.

- Easily arousable, with protective reflexes intact.

- Adequately hydrated.

- Able to stand and walk without assistance, or the infant holds the head up and sits up unassisted if old enough to do so.

- Discharge status is the same as admission status.

# SKILL 8–4 Regional and Local Pain Management

Regional and local pain management are increasingly being used during surgery or other procedures to offer local pain control. Commonly, microtubing is inserted into a site such as the lumbar or caudal space for regional pain management or into the popliteal or interscalene (muscle of the cervical vertebrae) area for local pain blocks. The tubing is wrapped securely and attached to an infusion pump with pain medication (Figure 8–5). Regional and local pain blocks allow the child to be alert and interactive while achieving excellent pain control.

## PREPARATION

1. Have an infusion pump ready when the child may return from surgery with a regional or local block.

2. Review the child's operative and recovery records, and the medication noted on the infusion bag.

## EQUIPMENT AND SUPPLIES

- Medication and pain assessment records
- Infusion pump
- Sterile gloves, gauze pads, and tape (for physician when catheter is removed)

## PROCEDURE

1. Assess pain, complete vital signs, level of consciousness, and neurovascular status following the surgery, and at intervals as ordered by the healthcare provider or as directed by facility guidelines.
   **RATIONALE:** *Baseline data will be needed for future comparison.*

2. Observe the wrapped local block site. Assess the extremity receiving the local nerve block for color, temperature, swelling, capillary refill, sensation, and solution leakage onto the dressing according to agency policy.

3. Monitor the infusion and maintain at the ordered infusion rate.

4. When the block is to be discontinued by the physician, provide sterile gloves, gauze pads, and tape.

5. Monitor the site several times daily until removed for drainage or discharge.
   **RATIONALE:** *Continued monitoring assists in identifying infection.*

6. Tingling felt in the fingers or toes of the affected extremity is the first sign that the nerve block is receding.

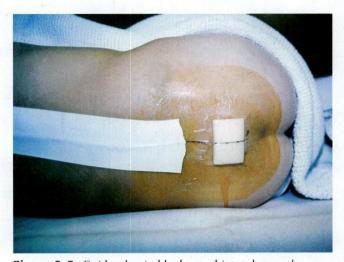

**Figure 8–5** *Epidural pain block taped into place and wrapped securely.*
Source: Courtesy of Shriners Hospital for Children, Spokane, WA.

### SAFETY ALERT

The dressing around a local pain block insertion site should NOT be removed to check the site. This could inadvertently dislodge the catheter. Check the skin that is visible and the dressing for drainage, but do not remove the dressing without specific healthcare provider orders.

# Chapter 9
# Positioning and Restraining Therapies

## ⌄ Skills

Guidelines for the use of mechanical and chemical immobilization for children should be established in all healthcare facilities. The Joint Commission provides specific standards with regard to the use of immobilization, and other organizations/agencies set guidelines to assist the healthcare provider (Box 9–1). Restraining procedures must be prescribed, staff must be trained to use them safely, guidelines for frequency of removal from and assessments should be stated in agency policy, the least restrictive choice for the type of restraint must be made, and restraints must be used only as long as needed. Examples of situations when restraining therapy may be necessary include immobilization to administer injections to children or to prevent violence to self or others. Ensure that all agencies where you are employed, such as emergency departments, acute care settings, mental health services, and schools, establish and implement guidelines on use of restraining therapies and educate staff to carry out the guidelines (Coin & Scott, 2014).

Immobilization can be accomplished by holding a child (human restraint), by wrapping with a blanket or other devices (mechanical restraint), or by sedation (chemical restraint). Occasionally, seclusion or isolation is needed, but should be rarely used for children. A preferred method of immobilization is to have a trained person be present with a child so that observation can replace mechanical or chemical measures whenever possible. For example, when a child must be held in position for a procedure, it is important to try to use an assistant rather than a mechanical device for this purpose.

Although some parents are comfortable holding their child for a procedure, most prefer to be close and act as a support person and allow healthcare providers to position and hold the child. This allows the parent to be free to provide comfort and to avoid the role of holding the child for a painful or stressful procedure. The child then can view the parent as a solace rather than as someone who brings pain. With the parent nearby, children are generally far less anxious and less likely to feel that they are being punished. Human and mechanical restraint techniques are described in this section.

## BOX 9–1  RECOMMENDATIONS FOR RESTRAINING THERAPIES

1. Create the least restrictive but safest environment to maintain dignity and comfort.
2. Use restraining therapies only in clinically appropriate situations and not as a routine component of therapy.
3. Determine if treatment of a condition would decrease the need for restraint. Consider alternatives to use of restraining therapies.
4. Use the least invasive option for restraining therapy to optimize patient safety, comfort, and dignity.
5. Document the rationale for restraint in the patient record.
6. Orders for restraint should not exceed 4 hours for those 18 years or older, 2 hours for those 9 to 17 years, and 1 hour for those under 9 years. Physical holding is limited to a maximum of 30 minutes (Joint Commission, 2015b). Frequently monitor patients for complications from restraining therapies. Assessments at least every 15 minutes are needed. Record findings in the patient record.
7. The patient and family should receive ongoing education about the need for and type of restraining therapies.
8. Medications to treat pain and psychiatric disturbance should be used as appropriate to treat conditions and mitigate the need for other restraining therapies, and not overused as a chemical restraint.
9. Use of a chemical restraint requires frequent assessment of actions and side effects. Documentation in the patient record must be performed.
10. All healthcare providers who prescribe, implement, or monitor restraining therapies should have complete and ongoing education in use for these therapies. Each agency must develop standards and guidelines for use of restraining therapies.

Note: Adapted from American Academy of Pediatrics, 2009; Joint Commission, 2015b.

# Human Restraint

## SKILL 9–1  Positioning a Child for Injections or Intravenous Access

### PREPARATION

1. Determine if the parent wants to be present during an uncomfortable procedure or to be available after the procedure to comfort the child.

2. When the parent wishes to be present, discuss the parent's role (e.g., holding the child or providing distraction or comfort during the procedure).

3. Make sure the person positioning and holding the child (parent or other assistant) clearly understands what body parts must be held still and how to do this safely.

### EQUIPMENT AND SUPPLIES

- Supplies for procedure to be performed
- Infection control supplies as needed

### PROCEDURE

*Supine Position*

1. Place the child in a supine position on a bed or stretcher.
   **RATIONALE:** *This position allows the child to see what is happening so that some of the child's fear is reduced.*

2. Have the nurse or an assistant restrain the child's body and extend the extremity to be used for access or injection. Have the parent perform this procedure if willing, and only if a healthcare provider is not available.
   **RATIONALE:** *The nurse provides a source of human contact as well as securing the child so that the procedure can be done quickly. Avoiding use of parents for restraint is advisable so that the child does not associate the parent with pain and discomfort in the situation, but rather a comforting presence.*

*Sitting Position*

1. Have the child sit on the parent's or assistant's lap with the child's legs held firmly between the assistant's legs.

2. The child's arm closest to the adult can be wrapped around the back of the parent's or assistant's waist.

3. Have the assistant hold the child firmly against the chest, wrapping arms around the child's upper body (Figure 9–1). Hold firmly but gently, ensuring that the child has chest expansion allowing for normal breathing.
   **RATIONALE:** *This hugging position adds comfort as well as security so the procedure can be done quickly.*

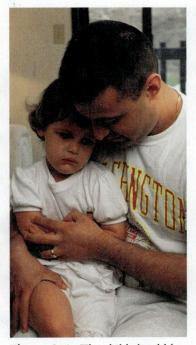

**Figure 9–1** *The child should be restrained by the assistant during intramuscular injections. Alternatively, the child's arm closest to the adult can be wrapped around the adult's waist, leaving the other arm in front to immobilize. The leg not used for the injection is securely located between the adult's legs. Be certain that the child can breathe freely during restraining procedures.*

## SKILL 9–2 Positioning a Child for Lumbar Puncture

### PREPARATION

1. Determine if the parent wants to be present during an uncomfortable procedure such as lumbar puncture or to be available after the procedure to comfort the child.

2. When the parent wishes to be present, discuss the parent's role (e.g., providing distraction or comfort during the procedure).

3. Make sure the person positioning and holding the child clearly understands what body parts must be held still and how to do this safely.

### EQUIPMENT AND SUPPLIES

- Supplies for procedure to be performed
- Infection control/protective gear as needed, generally clean gloves, gown, and mask

### PROCEDURE

1. Don protective gear. Place the child in the side-lying or sitting position that is preferred by the healthcare provider who will perform the lumbar puncture. The assistant can hold the child in position by wrapping one arm behind the knees and the other behind the neck, keeping the back curved.
   RATIONALE: *This position ensures the best possible access to spinal processes and disc spaces.*

2. The infant can be held in the desired position by holding the neck and thighs in your hands (Figure 9–2).

3. The older child can be quite strong, and someone with enough strength will be needed to hold the child in the side-lying position. Lean over the child with your entire body, using your forearms against the thighs and around the shoulders and head (Figure 9–3). Alternatively, the older child may be in a seated position, bending forward and supported by the assistant.

4. Be certain that the child has free air exchange. Another assistant may be assigned to monitor respirations and perform other assessments during the procedure.

### SAFETY ALERT

Lumbar puncture requires that the child be held still to prevent injury and to ensure success in obtaining fluid. It is advisable to have an experienced staff member hold the child in position for the procedure. Ensure that the child has free air exchange and receives no injuries. The healthcare provider performing the procedure may choose a variety of positions: side lying with or without flexion of the knees and hips or sitting upright.

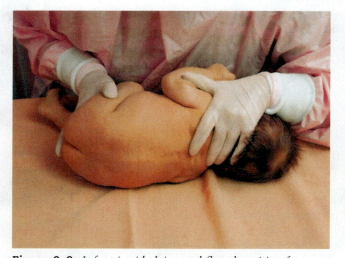

**Figure 9–2** *Infant in side-lying and flexed position for a lumbar puncture.*

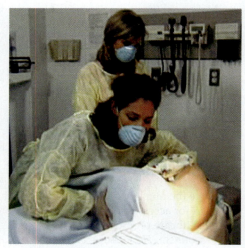

**Figure 9–3** *Child in side-lying and flexed position for a lumbar puncture.*

## SKILL 9–3 Positioning a Child for an Otoscopic Examination

### PREPARATION

1. If the parent is present, discuss the parent's role (e.g., holding the child or providing distraction or comfort during the procedure).

2. Make sure the person positioning and holding the child (parent or other assistant) clearly understands what body parts must be held still and how to do this safely.

## EQUIPMENT AND SUPPLIES

- Supplies for procedure to be performed
- Infection control/protective gear if needed

## PROCEDURE

### Supine Position

1. Place the child in a supine position on a bed or stretcher. Have the parent, a nurse, or an assistant lean over the child to position and hold the child's arms and body. The assistant may also assist with stabilizing the child's head.

2. Hold the otoscope in the hand closest to the child's face. When the child is cooperative, rest the back of your hand against the child's head.
   RATIONALE: *This action provides additional stabilization of the child's head to prevent pain and injury when the otoscope earpiece is inserted into the auditory canal.*

3. Use your other hand to pull the pinna toward the back of the head and either up or down (Figure 9–4).
   RATIONALE: *This action straightens the ear canal so that the tympanic membrane can be visualized.*

### Sitting Position

1. Have the child sit on the parent's or assistant's lap with the child's legs held firmly between the assistant's legs. The child's arms can be wrapped around the parent's or assistant's waist.

2. Have the parent or assistant hold the child's head firmly against the chest with one arm while the other arm holds the arms and upper chest.
   RATIONALE: *This position provides comfort to the child while securing the head.*

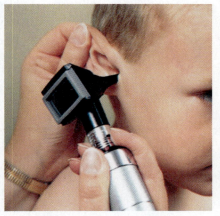

**Figure 9–4** *To straighten the auditory canal: pull the pinna back and up for children over 3 years of age; pull the pinna down and back for children under 3 years of age.*

# Mechanical Restraint

Temporary mechanical restraining therapies are used to decrease the child's movement and to allow the healthcare provider to carry out a procedure. They are effective when procedures are being performed on the head or on an extremity, as one limb can be left out for the procedure.

## SKILL 9–4 Applying a Papoose Board Immobilizer

The papoose consists of a board and cloth wrappings with Velcro fasteners at the chest, hips, and knees (Figure 9–5). Two sizes are available—one for infants and toddlers and one for larger children. Some papooses come with openings for arms. For example, if the child is positioned for a venipuncture, the arm can fit through the opening in the vest and then the remaining fabric pieces can be secured.

## PREPARATION

1. Gather equipment and supplies for the procedure.
   RATIONALE: *Having supplies prepared reduces the time the child spends in temporary restraint devices and reduces the anxiety felt by the child.*

2. Explain the reason for immobilization to the child and parent and how long it will be needed. Tell the child how the restraint will feel.
   RATIONALE: *Young children will be less anxious if the explanation about what they will feel is presented in nonthreatening, developmentally appropriate terms.*

3. Have an assistant (or the parent) available to help position and hold a body part if needed.
   RATIONALE: *The papoose is most often used when the healthcare provider does not have an assistant available or a parent willing to restrain the child for a procedure.*

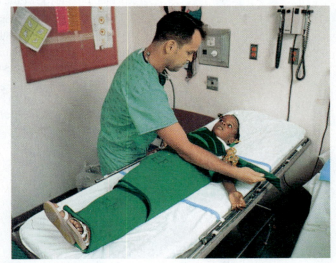

**Figure 9–5** *Child on a papoose board.*

### EQUIPMENT AND SUPPLIES

- Immobilization board (papoose) to fit the child's size
- Sheet
- Infection control supplies as needed

### PROCEDURE

1. Place a towel or sheet over the board.
2. Have the child lie supine on the board, with the head at the top of the board.
3. Place the fabric wrappings around the child, and secure the Velcro fasteners. To be most effective, the fabric wrappings should be secure over the elbows, hips, and knees to prevent flexion.
   **RATIONALE:** *This action prevents the child from pulling apart the wrappings and from kicking.*
4. After the procedure, release the child and allow the parents to provide comfort.

---

## SKILL 9–5 Applying a Mummy Immobilizer

Mummy immobilization consists of wrapping the child securely in a blanket or sheet.

### PREPARATION

1. Have all supplies and materials for the procedure collected and ready for use.
2. Explain the procedure to the child and parent.

### EQUIPMENT AND SUPPLIES

- Soft blanket or sheet 2 to 3 times larger than the child

### PROCEDURE

*Infant*

1. Put the blanket (or sheet) on the bed or examination table. Fold down one corner until it reaches the middle of the blanket.
2. Place the infant in a diagonal position with the neck on the folded edge.
3. Bring one side of the blanket over the infant's arm and then under the back. Tuck that edge under and over the other arm and around the back. It may be helpful to roll the infant on the side to smooth the blanket behind the back, and then roll the infant onto the back over the smoothed section of blanket.
4. Bring the other side of the blanket around the body and tuck underneath the body.
5. Bring the bottom corner of the blanket up and over the abdomen.

*Toddler and Older Child*

1. Put the blanket (or sheet) on the bed or examination table. Fold down one corner until it reaches the middle of the blanket.
2. Place the child on the blanket, positioning so that there is sufficient material to wrap the knees and lower legs. If necessary, fold down the top edges of the blanket to the shoulders.
3. Bring one side of the blanket over the arm, body, and legs, and tuck it under the other arm and around the back and legs (Figure 9–6A).
4. Bring the other side of the blanket up and around the body, and tuck underneath the back and legs (Figure 9–6B and C).
   **RATIONALE:** *The child should not be able to flex the knees and kick or it may be impossible to perform the procedure.*

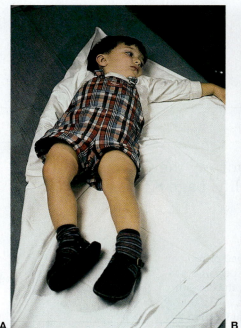
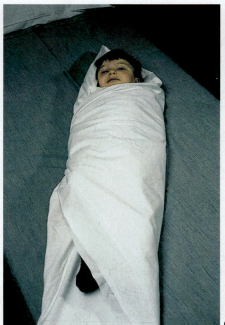
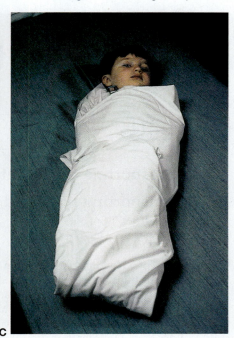

**A** **B** **C**

**Figure 9–6** *Steps in applying mummy immobilization.*

## SKILL 9–6 Applying Elbow Immobilizers

Elbow immobilizers (Figure 9–7) are used to prevent the infant or child from reaching the face or head, especially after surgery. Because these devices must be on the child for an extended period, a medical order is required and agency policy is followed for assessments and periodic removal of the devices.

### PREPARATION

1. Explain the need for the elbow immobilizers to the parent.
2. Verify the medical order for the device. Review the institution's policy for use of restraining therapies and plan the times when the child is released from them.

### EQUIPMENT AND SUPPLIES

- Ready-made elbow immobilizers are available commercially. Obtain them if available.

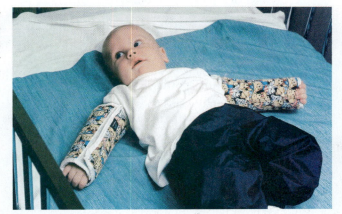

**Figure 9–7** *Infant with elbow immobilizers.*

- An elbow immobilizer can be devised from a piece of fabric that has vertical pockets sewn into it. Tongue depressors are inserted into the pockets.
- Pins or tape

### PROCEDURE

1. Wrap the elbow immobilizer around the arm from axilla to wrist and snug enough to prevent bending of the elbow.
2. The device may be secured with tape to the bedding or the child's clothing if needed. Such securing is more restrictive than simply using the immobilizers, should be used only if needed, and requires a written medical order.
3. Remove the elbow immobilizers at least every 2 hours (or the interval specified in the institution's guidelines).
   RATIONALE: *The immobilizer may cause skin abrasion or impair circulation if placed too snugly around the arm.*

# Chapter 10
# Transporting the Child

## ∨ Skills

Children must often be transported within the healthcare facility to have tests performed or receive treatments, or be transferred to home or another facility. Safety is the most important aspect of transporting infants and children. In determining the best method of transporting a child, the developmental stage must be taken into consideration. For short transports within the unit, an infant or young child may be carried in an adult's arms. However, for transports off the unit and when the child is older than a toddler, transport with cribs or other such equipment is used. For safety, the child should be visible to the transporting adult at all times. The child's comfort should also be considered, with measures taken to promote support and comfort. When parents are present, they may travel with the child to provide comfort. The nurse must learn and apply safe lifting procedures and use mechanical lifts when needed. Always verify the client identification and the order for movement to another site.

## SKILL 10–1  Transporting the Infant

### PREPARATION

1. Obtain necessary transporting equipment.
2. Securely fasten intravenous lines, feeding lines, ECG leads, and other equipment.
   RATIONALE: *Lines that are securely fastened are less likely to be dislodged during transport.*
3. Explain the transport plan to the family.
   RATIONALE: *Adequate explanation helps to decrease anxiety.*

### EQUIPMENT AND SUPPLIES

- Transporting vehicle (e.g., stretcher, crib, wheelchair)
- Wheeled poles for any necessary equipment
- Necessary supportive equipment such as oxygen tank or resuscitation bags/masks
- Blankets

### PROCEDURE

1. Perform an assessment of the infant.
   RATIONALE: *A baseline assessment provides for comparison with later findings. At times, transport may adversely affect the infant's condition. Initial assessment data provide necessary baseline information.*
2. The infant is placed in a bassinet or crib for transport. If the bassinet has a bottom shelf, it is used for carrying the IV pump or monitor.
3. Attach intravenous poles and other equipment to the crib. When this is not possible, adequate personnel are needed to push all of the equipment.
   RATIONALE: *Lines can be more easily kept intact if they are on one transport vehicle.*
4. Keep the infant covered with blankets.
   RATIONALE: *Adequate covers help to prevent hypothermia resulting from a cool environment, and they provide privacy.*
5. Allow parents to accompany the infant on the transport when possible.
   RATIONALE: *The presence of parents can provide a sense of security for the infant.*

## SKILL 10–2  Transporting the Child

### PREPARATION

1. Perform a baseline assessment of the child and obtain necessary transporting equipment.

2. Securely fasten intravenous lines, feeding lines, ECG leads, and other equipment.
   **RATIONALE:** *Lines that are securely fastened are less likely to be dislodged during transport.*

3. Explain the transport plan to the family and child.
   **RATIONALE:** *Adequate explanation helps to decrease anxiety.*

### EQUIPMENT AND SUPPLIES

- Transporting vehicle (e.g., stretcher, crib, wheelchair)
- Wheeled poles for any necessary equipment
- Necessary supportive equipment such as oxygen tank or resuscitation bags/masks
- Blankets

### PROCEDURE

1. Transport the toddler in a high-top crib (also used for infants, as shown in Figure 10–1), with the side rails up and the protective top in place. The child may be sitting or lying down. Alternatively, a child can be secured in a stroller or wheelchair of the proper size for the child's age.
   **RATIONALE:** *Stretchers should not be used for transport of toddlers because the mobile toddler may roll or fall off.*

2. Be sure to secure the child in the device with the seat safety strap (Figure 10–2).
   **RATIONALE:** *The child is secured to avoid falls and injury during transport.*

> **CLINICAL TIP**
>
> Specialized wheelchairs and other equipment are available to carry enteral feeding solutions, motors necessary for equipment, and other supplies. These transporters are helpful for the families when the child has a long-term disability, enabling them to take the child and equipment to school, stores, and other settings.

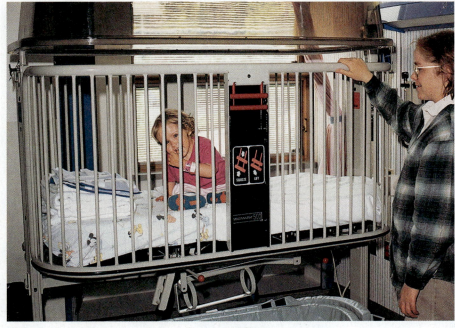

**Figure 10–1** *High-top crib for infant or toddler transport.*

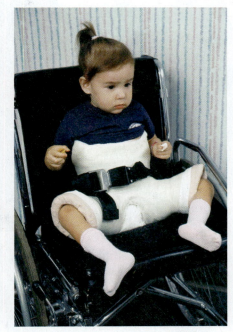

**Figure 10–2** *Toddler in a wheelchair with a safety strap.*

## SKILL 10–3  Transporting the Child With a Disability

### PREPARATION

1. Perform a baseline assessment and obtain necessary transporting equipment.

2. Securely fasten intravenous lines, feeding lines, ECG leads, and other equipment.
   **RATIONALE:** *Lines that are securely fastened are less likely to be dislodged during transport.*

3. Explain the transport plan to the family and child.
   **RATIONALE:** *Adequate explanation helps to decrease anxiety.*

## HOME AND COMMUNITY CARE CONSIDERATIONS

When the child with medical equipment or casts is going to be discharged, assist the family to plan for car seats and alteration of the home to facilitate the child's needs. Guidelines for transportation of preterm infants and children with disabilities are available (American Academy of Pediatrics, 2013; O'Neill, Bull, & Sobus, 2011). See your textbook for transport resources to offer parents and for information about car seat guidelines at each age.

### EQUIPMENT AND SUPPLIES

- Transporting vehicle (e.g., stretcher, crib, wheelchair)
- Wheeled poles for any necessary equipment
- Necessary supportive equipment such as oxygen tank or resuscitation bags/masks
- Blankets

### PROCEDURE

1. Use a wheelchair or stretcher for the older child who is unable to walk because of a disability or whose mobility must be restricted (Figure 10–3).
2. Secure safety belts and supervise the child closely.

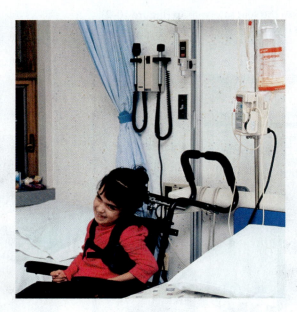

**Figure 10–3** *The child who is getting tube feedings or other infusions can easily and safely be transported in a wheelchair with the tube feeding or infusion on a pole. Pumps can also be attached to the pole when used to regulate infusion rates.*

# Chapter 11
# Specimen Collection

---

## ⌄ Skills

---

In the collection of any type of specimen, it is the nurse's responsibility to be sure that the specimen is collected accurately, labeled correctly, and sent to the laboratory using any special techniques or conditions needed, such as use of biohazard bags for specimen transport, immediate transport of specimen, or maintaining the specimen on ice. Be sure to review laboratory policy and procedures if you are not familiar with all of the guidelines for safely obtaining and transferring the specimen.

## Blood Samples

There are two methods of obtaining blood samples in children: capillary puncture and venipuncture.

A capillary puncture may be used to obtain a sample for complete blood count, reticulocyte count, platelet count, or blood chemistries such as electrolyte, glucose, or drug levels. Venipuncture is needed when the amount of blood required is larger than a capillary puncture can supply and for accuracy of certain laboratory tests.

## SKILL 11–1  Performing a Capillary Puncture

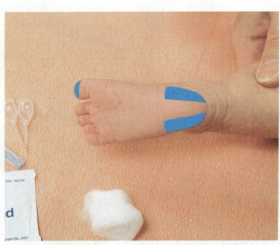

**Figure 11–1**  *Heel sites for capillary puncture.*

### CLINICAL TIP

If not contraindicated, newborns may be given 2 mL of 12% sucrose solution with a pacifier approximately 2 minutes prior to a capillary puncture as a pain-relief measure. Sucrose may provide natural pain relief by activating endogenous opioid systems in the body. The analgesic effect of sucrose lasts approximately 3 to 5 minutes, with a peak action in 2 minutes. Swaddling, shushing, swinging, and sucking are other methods to provide analgesia and comfort for minor pain during infant procedures (Harrington et al., 2012).

### PREPARATION

1. Explain to the child and parents what will be done and what the child is likely to feel.
2. Apply a hot pack to the collection site before the procedure to increase blood flow and improve results.
3. Have another nurse or an assistant ready to restrain the child.
4. Choose the appropriate site. Puncture sites include the plantar surface of the heel (Figure 11–1) (for newborns and children under the age of 1 year), the great toe (for children over 1 year), and the lateral surface of the tip of the third or fourth finger.

### EQUIPMENT AND SUPPLIES

- Chlorhexidine-based preparation or other approved skin preparation
- Lancet
- Gauze pads and adhesive bandage
- Appropriate microsize blood collection tubes and sealant
- Clean gloves

### PROCEDURE

1. Don gloves.
2. *Finger-stick.* Hold the child's hand with your nondominant hand (or have an assistant hold it), keeping the finger to be used extended and pointed down.
   *Heel-stick.* Hold the child's foot in your nondominant hand, supporting the dorsum of the foot with your thumb and the ankle with your other fingers.
   *Toe-stick.* Grasp the child's foot across the dorsum with your nondominant hand, supporting the toe with your thumb on the plantar surface.
3. Clean the site with the preferred skin preparation.
4. Using your dominant hand, pierce the skin quickly with the lancet.
5. Wipe the first drop of blood away with the dry gauze.
   **RATIONALE:** *The first drop may be contaminated by skin contact, and the blood cells may have been traumatized during the stick.*
6. Gently squeeze the site, hold the punctured site downward, and direct the blood into the appropriate tube by covering one end of the capillary tube with a finger and inserting the other end into sealant.
7. When collection is complete, have an assistant hold the gauze on the site until the bleeding has stopped. Apply an adhesive bandage.
8. Label the specimen and send to the laboratory. Document the specimen collected and time sent to the laboratory.

### HOME AND COMMUNITY CARE CONSIDERATIONS

When metabolic screening cards are completed in an office or clinic visit in the first days after birth, the specimen collected must be sent to the laboratory within 24 hours of collection.

## SKILL 11–2  Newborn Screening

Blood screening of the newborn is performed to evaluate blood sugar and to assess for phenylketonuria, hypothyroidism, sickle cell disease, and other inborn metabolic diseases. See your textbook for further information on newborn screening. A small amount of blood can usually be obtained by heel-stick for these tests. The timing of certain tests is important in the interpretation of results. Phenylketonuria testing must be done after 24 hours of age for accurate results; metabolic screening is collected before 72 hours of age.

## PREPARATION

1. Examine the newborn's record for results of any prior tests.

2. Verify the test and procedures for the specimen to be collected.

3. Explain the procedure to the parents.

4. Wrap a warm washcloth around the foot for a few moments to promote blood flow to the foot and improve blood collection.

## EQUIPMENT AND SUPPLIES

- Chlorhexidine-based preparation or other approved skin preparation
- Lancet
- Capillary tube and sealant
- Metabolic screening card
- Washcloth rinsed in warm water (optional)
- Clean gloves

## PROCEDURE

1. Don gloves.

2. Clean the site with the preferred skin preparation.

3. Flexing the infant's forefoot up toward the leg (dorsiflexion), use the lancet to puncture the heel, collecting one large drop of blood.

4. The blood may be placed in a capillary tube, onto a metabolic screening card, or onto a glucose reagent strip, depending on the test desired.

5. To place blood on a screening card, completely fill the indicated circles (see Figure 11–2). Insufficient coverage of the circles will result in the need to repeat the test.

6. Allow the paper to air dry in a horizontal position at room temperature on the screening form. Alternatively, if the blood is being sent to the laboratory in the capillary tube, seal the open end with sealant and transport according to agency policy.

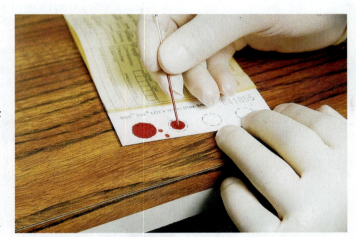

**Figure 11–2** *Collecting a blood sample from the newborn for neonatal metabolic screening.*

7. Clearly label the blood samples and cards with the newborn's identifying information. Record the day and time and the child's age in hours.

8. Document the specimen collection and time sent to the laboratory.

## SKILL 11–3 Blood Glucose Meters

Children with diabetes commonly perform capillary punctures several times daily to measure their blood glucose with a small instrument.

## PREPARATION

1. Verify the identity of the child. The procedure is explained to the child and family.

2. The nurse demonstrates the procedure as needed and observes the child or family on return demonstration.

3. The child with diabetes is taught over time how to safely perform repeated blood glucose tests and how to maintain materials.

## EQUIPMENT AND SUPPLIES

- Reagent strips
- Blood glucose meter
- Alcohol swab
- Lancet
- Clean gloves

---

### HOME AND COMMUNITY CARE CONSIDERATIONS

Children with diabetes who perform finger-sticks for blood glucose analysis should be taught about safe practices for cleaning blood from surfaces by using bleach solution. Safe storage is needed to prevent young children from having access to the lancets. Help the family plan with the pharmacy or healthcare office for safe disposal of lancets and other medical equipment. Identify a place in the school where the child can keep glucose-monitoring equipment and perform the procedure in private. Assist the school to plan for safe disposal of the medical equipment.

---

### PROCEDURE

1. Instruct the child and assistants to wash their hands.
   **RATIONALE:** *This removes surface contaminants from the child's hands to reduce the chance of infection or false readings (e.g., food residue on fingers).*

2. Don gloves and instruct the assistant to don gloves.

3. Clean the finger to be used with alcohol, if desired. For the diabetic client with repeated tests, soap and water is often used instead of alcohol (Figure 11–3).
   **RATIONALE:** *With repeated testing, alcohol can cause drying and cracking of the skin. Washing with soap and water removes most surface contaminants.*

4. Milk the finger gently or warm the hand if cold.
   **RATIONALE:** *This encourages blood circulation to the fingertip so that the sample can be easily obtained.*

5. Quickly puncture the side of the fingertip with the lancet.

6. Apply a drop of blood to the reagent strip.

7. Place the strip into the glucose meter and read the instrument as instructed (Figure 11–4).

8. Document the test results and time collected.

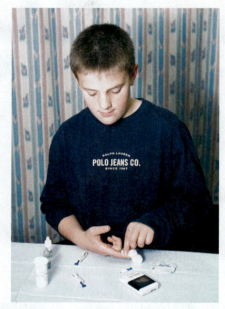

**Figure 11–3** *The child is cleaning his finger prior to piercing the skin for blood glucose monitoring.*

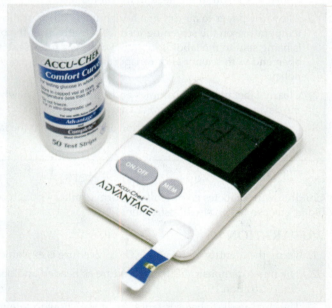

**Figure 11–4** *Blood glucose monitors are small and quickly analyze a drop of blood and display the blood glucose in milligrams per deciliter (mg/dL).*

---

## SKILL 11–4 Performing a Venipuncture

Venipuncture, or the puncturing of a vein, is used to obtain a sample for complete blood count, blood culture, sedimentation rate, blood type and cross-match, blood clotting times, drug screen, ammonia level, fibrinogen level, and other tests.

### CLINICAL TIP—VENIPUNCTURE

- Make sure the tourniquet is tight enough to restrict venous but not arterial blood flow.
- Keep the bevel of the needle up.
- Do not draw back too hard or rapidly on the syringe because the vein can collapse.
- If blood fails to enter the syringe, the needle may not be placed correctly in the vein. Advance it slightly.
- If a flash was seen initially but blood no longer appears, the needle may be located incorrectly in the vein. Gently draw back on the needle slightly.

## PREPARATION

1. Verify the identity of the child. Explain the procedure to the child and parent.
2. Choose the appropriate site. The veins of the antecubital fossa or forearm are usually the best choice because of their accessibility. However, the dorsum of the hand or foot also may be used. (See Figure 13–1B for venipuncture site locations.)

## EQUIPMENT AND SUPPLIES

- Chlorhexidine-based preparation or other approved skin preparation
- Tourniquet
- 20- to 27-gauge needle with attached syringe (slightly larger than volume of blood needed)
- Dry gauze pad and adhesive bandage
- Venous access device appropriate for child (a butterfly needle may be appropriate for smaller children)
- Appropriate blood collection tubes
- Clean gloves

## PROCEDURE

1. Don gloves.
2. Place a tourniquet proximal to the desired vein to distend it. If necessary, hold the extremity below heart level, gently rub or tap the vein, or apply a warm compress to promote dilation of the vein (Figure 11–5A).
3. Explain to the child that you are looking for the best vein to use to collect the blood.
4. Locate the vein by inspection (wiping with alcohol will make the vein shine) or by palpation.
5. Once the vein has been located, clean the skin with alcohol or the preferred skin preparation, using an outward circular motion (Figure 11–5B). Let dry. The skin will appear dull.
6. With your nondominant hand, hold the skin taut, gently pulling with your thumb just under the site of the puncture.
7. Puncture the skin with the needle, beveled up at a 15-degree angle and directed toward the vein. When blood appears in the tube, gently pull back on the syringe (Figure 11–5C).

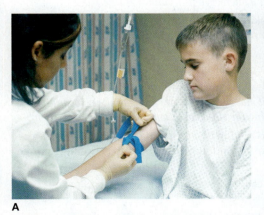
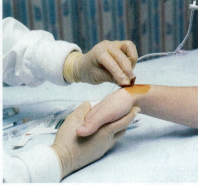
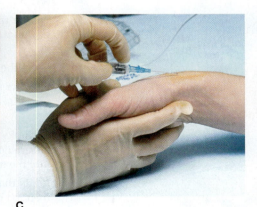

**A**                                   **B**                                   **C**

**Figure 11–5** *Venipuncture procedure:* **A,** *The tourniquet is applied to restrict venous blood flow.* **B,** *The area for venipuncture is cleaned by the nurse with the preferred skin preparation and dried with a cotton ball.* **C,** *The needle is placed with the bevel up and gently inserted into the identified vein.*

8. Release the tourniquet after all the blood has been collected. Remove the needle at the same angle used for entry, and apply pressure to the site with the dry gauze pad (alcohol will sting).

9. Recognize the child for his or her cooperation.

10. Have the assistant or parent maintain direct pressure over the site with a gloved hand for a few minutes until the bleeding has stopped, at which point an adhesive bandage can be placed. Meanwhile, discard the needle in a sharps container.

11. Attach the needle, and expel blood into the appropriate collection tubes as soon as possible. Sometimes a butterfly or other needle is attached to the vacuum container for collection so the blood is already in the desired collection container.

12. Document the blood collection and the time sent to the laboratory.

## SKILL 11–5 Blood Cultures

Cultures of blood samples may be performed to determine if a child has septicemia. Such samples are commonly drawn at two different times a few hours apart to assist in accurate diagnosis of causative microorganisms. Note that common errors in blood culture acquisition from a new intravenous line have been identified. Follow directions to allow the cleansing solution to dry, to sterilize the top of the blood culture bottle, to avoid palpating the site with a nonsterile finger, and to inject the sample directly into the blood culture tube without laying the sample down. In addition, an IV line inserted at another site may not be adequate for the blood culture procedure (Hall, Domenico, Self, et al., 2013). Check agency policy about personnel who are allowed to collect blood cultures. In some agencies and units, nurses perform the procedure, and in others, nurses assist laboratory or medical personnel in obtaining blood cultures.

### PREPARATION

1. Verify the identity of the child. Explain the procedure to the child and parents.

2. Choose the appropriate site. The veins of the antecubital fossa or forearm are usually the best choice because of their accessibility. However, the dorsum of the hand or foot also may be used. (See Figure 13–1B for venipuncture site locations.)

### EQUIPMENT AND SUPPLIES

- Iodine and alcohol or chlorhexidine for skin preparation
- Tourniquet
- 20- to 27-gauge needle with attached syringe (slightly larger than volume of blood needed)
- Dry gauze pad and adhesive bandage
- Venous access device appropriate for child (a butterfly needle may be appropriate for smaller children)
- Appropriate blood collection tubes
- Sterile gloves

### PROCEDURE

1. When infection is suspected, the first blood collection is performed before starting antibiotics.
   RATIONALE: *Antibiotics may alter the results so that a microorganism cannot be detected.*

2. Don sterile gloves, and thoroughly cleanse the skin according to agency policy. Allow to dry.
   RATIONALE: *Strict sterile technique reduces the chance that skin surface bacteria are found in the laboratory, leading to misdiagnosis.*

3. Use either venipuncture or an arterial line for samples as ordered.

4. Samples at the two different times are usually drawn from two different sites.
   RATIONALE: *Results can be compared to determine if microorganisms are present in the blood rather than just from skin contamination during the blood collection.*

5. Each blood collection specimen is divided and placed in two different culture tubes—one for anaerobic and one for aerobic bacteria. Place directly and immediately from collecting syringe into the tubes.

6. Verify that specimen labels match client identification; transport the specimens as recommended by the laboratory.

7. Document the specimen collection and time sent to the laboratory.

# SKILL 11–6  Arterial Blood Gases

Arterial blood gas (ABG) analysis is used to monitor the adequacy of ventilation and oxygenation, the oxygen-carrying capacity of the blood, and acid–base levels. ABG samples can be obtained from arterial puncture. At other times, the specimen may be collected from an indwelling arterial line. Check agency policy about personnel who are allowed to collect ABG samples. In some agencies and units, nurses perform the procedure, and in others, nurses assist other personnel in obtaining ABGs.

## PREPARATION

1. Explain the procedure to the family and to the child, as developmentally appropriate.

2. Use two methods of identification to determine you are with the correct child/family.

3. Choose the appropriate site. Arterial puncture can be performed on the radial, brachial, and femoral arteries. On newborns, samples are often obtained from the temporal or radial artery. Avoid using the femoral artery because use of this site increases the risk for aseptic necrosis of the femoral head. Arterial samples can also be obtained by deep heel puncture or from an indwelling arterial catheter.

4. Assess the collateral circulation of the extremity to be used for an arterial stick. The Allen test can be performed to assess collateral circulation of the radial, ulnar, and brachial arteries. Elevate and blanch the extremity distal to the planned puncture site. The two arteries providing blood flow to the limb are then occluded. The extremity is lowered and pressure from one artery is relieved. Color returning to the extremity in less than 5 seconds indicates adequate collateral circulation.

## EQUIPMENT

- ABG kit or heparinized syringe with 25- to 27-gauge needle and cap, specimen container
- Anesthetizing agent
- 2″ × 2″ gauze pads
- Adhesive bandage
- Chlorhexidine-based preparation or other approved skin preparation
- Label for specimen
- Ice for specimen transport
- Clean gloves

## PROCEDURE

1. Use developmentally appropriate nonpharmacologic methods to reduce pain and anxiety. If time allows, apply an anesthetizing agent such as EMLA (eutectic mixture of local anesthetics) (60 minutes before puncture). Alternatively, at the time of the procedure, a vapocoolant spray or intradermal injection of buffered lidocaine can be used to numb the skin.
   RATIONALE: *Arterial punctures are painful. Breath holding and crying can affect the accuracy of blood gas values.*

2. Don gloves and prepare the site for puncture with the preferred skin preparation.

3. Palpate the artery for puncture, and insert the needle at a 60- to 90-degree angle.

4. Watch for blood backflow into the syringe. Do not pull back on the plunger. Blood should automatically fill the syringe/container due to arterial pressure. Withdraw the required amount of blood into the syringe/container.

5. Withdraw the needle and apply pressure to the site with 2″ × 2″ sterile gauze pad for 5 to 10 minutes.
   RATIONALE: *Pressure must be applied to stop bleeding and prevent hematoma formation.*

6. Place the specimen in an appropriate container and check for air bubbles. Remove air bubbles.
   RATIONALE: *Air bubbles can affect the blood gas values.*

7. Verify that the specimen label matches the child's identification. Label with the child's temperature and percentage of oxygen administered, as both affect blood gas values. Place the specimen on ice and send to the laboratory immediately.
   RATIONALE: *Ice prevents red blood cell metabolism. Blood must be evaluated immediately for accurate results.*

8. Document the procedure, including site, results of Allen test (positive if adequate collateral circulation present), amount of blood withdrawn, time sent to the laboratory, and how the child tolerated the procedure.

# Urine Samples

A urine sample is obtained to assess for infection and to determine levels of blood, protein, glucose, acetone, bilirubin, drugs, hormones, metals, and electrolytes. Urine can also be evaluated for concentration/specific gravity, pH, and crystals or other substances.

A clean-catch or sterile catheter urine specimen is needed to evaluate the presence of microorganisms. The procedure varies according to the developmental level of the child. Infants and young children will have to be catheterized. Older children can often void and provide a midstream-voided specimen.

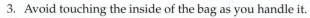

## SKILL 11–7  Applying a Urine Collection Bag (Infant)

### PREPARATION

1. Explain the procedure to the parents.

### EQUIPMENT AND SUPPLIES

- Urine collection bag (newborn or pediatric size as needed)
- Soap solution and water or packaged cleansing swabs for cleaning genitalia
- Urine specimen container
- Clean gloves

### PROCEDURE

1. Don gloves.
2. Remove the diaper and clean the skin well with soap and water, ensuring any skinfolds are opened for access to cleaning.

> **CLINICAL TIP**
>
> When applying the urine bag on girls, begin by placing the bag below the vaginal opening and then allow it to adhere to the labia. For boys, be sure the bag is adhered on the scrotum and that the scrotum is not inside the bag's opening. Cutting a hole in the disposable diaper so the end of the bag can pass through makes it easier to visualize when the infant has urinated.

3. Avoid touching the inside of the bag as you handle it.
4. Remove the covering from the adhesive strips. Attach the bag with the adhesive tabs (Figure 11–6): for girls, around the labia; for boys, around the penis.
5. Make sure the seal is tight to prevent leakage.
6. Reapply a diaper and check the bag frequently for urine.

### To Remove a Bag Containing Urine

7. Don gloves.
8. Gently pull the bag away from the skin. Fold the opening over and place the urine bag into the specimen container.
9. Cap the container tightly.
10. Label with name, date, time, and test ordered. Send promptly to the laboratory.
11. Document the specimen collection and time sent.

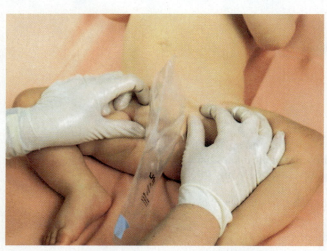

**Figure 11–6** *Attaching the urine collection bag.*

## SKILL 11–8  Routine Urine Collection (Older Child)

When a sterile sample is not required, the child may void into a container that is placed in the toilet to collect the sample. Don gloves. Pour the urine into the specimen collection cup.

## SKILL 11–9  Collecting a Clean-Catch Midstream Urine Specimen (Older Child)

### PREPARATION

1. Explain the procedure to the child and parents.

### EQUIPMENT AND SUPPLIES

- Towelettes
- Sterile urine specimen container
- Clean gloves

## PROCEDURE

### Male

1. The parent or nurse should instruct the older child to wash his hands well, and then clean the head of the penis (after pulling back the foreskin, if not circumcised) 3 times, each time using a different towelette, and moving from the urethral meatus outward. All ridges and skinfolds should be cleaned.

2. Don gloves.

3. Have the child begin to urinate a small amount into the toilet and then catch the flowing urine in the sterile container.

4. Cap the container tightly.

   RATIONALE: *Always wear gloves in case there are any urine spills on the container.*

5. Label with name, date, and time. Send promptly to the laboratory.

6. Document the specimen collection and time sent to the laboratory.

### Female

1. The parent or nurse should instruct the child to wash her hands well. The girl should sit back on the toilet as far as possible with her legs apart. After spreading the labia, wipe each side with a separate towelette using a front-to-back stroke. A third wipe is used to clean the meatus, repeating the front-to-back motion.

2. Don gloves.

3. Have the child urinate a small amount into the toilet and then catch the flow in the sterile container.

4. Cap the container tightly. Wear gloves in case of any urine spills on the container.

5. Label with name, date, and time. Send promptly to the laboratory.

6. Document the specimen collection and time sent to the laboratory.

## SKILL 11–10  Collecting a Sterile Urinary Catheter Specimen

### PREPARATION

1. Check the healthcare provider's orders to determine whether intermittent or indwelling catheterization is planned.

2. Determine the size of the catheter based on the child's size, age, and weight (Engorn & Elerlage, 2015). Sizes commonly vary from 4 to 5 French for infants, 6 to 10 French for children, and 8 to 14 French for adolescents.

3. Confirm the identity of the child and explain the procedure to the child and parent and why it is necessary.

### EQUIPMENT AND SUPPLIES

- Urinary catheter—size appropriate for the child's age, and one a size smaller
- Sterile urinary catheterization tray (containing drapes, sterile gloves, antiseptic solution, cotton swabs or balls, forceps, lubricant, and a sterile urine specimen container)
- Container for soiled cotton balls
- Syringe filled with normal saline if indwelling catheterization is prescribed
- Tape
- Drainage collection apparatus
- Absorbent pads
- Sterile gloves

### PROCEDURE

1. Have an assistant hold the child in position for the procedure. If the parents wish to stay with the child, have them stand at the child's head and try to distract the child.

2. Place absorbent pads under the child's perineum.

3. Open the tray, maintaining the sterile field. Open the lubricant and squeeze it onto the sterile field. Pour the antiseptic over the cotton swabs or balls.

4. Don sterile gloves. Lubricate the tip of the catheter and place the distal end in the tray.

### Female

1. Clean the perineum. Spread the labia apart with the nondominant hand. Pick up the antiseptic-soaked cotton balls with forceps using the dominant hand. Clean the meatus, using one ball for each wipe, in a front-to-back direction along each side of the labia minora, then along the sides of the urinary meatus, and finally straight down over the urethral opening. Discard each cotton ball away from the sterile field.

   RATIONALE: *Wiping in the direction from the urinary meatus toward the anus avoids contaminating the urinary meatus with fecal bacteria.*

2. Pick up the lubricated catheter tip with your dominant hand, keeping the distal end in the specimen container.

   RATIONALE: *The dominant hand remains sterile and should be the one to handle the catheter. Placing the distal end in a specimen container prevents contamination of the sterile field when urine flows.*

3. Gently insert the tip into the meatus (approximately 5 to 8 cm [2 to 3 in.] in the child) until there is a free flow of urine, and then 2.5 cm (1.0 in.) further. If resistance is felt, do not force the catheter. Gently try to rotate the catheter between your fingers and try to advance. If unsuccessful in advancing the catheter, try again with another sterile catheter, preferably one size smaller.

   RATIONALE: *A catheter should not be reused in order to prevent potential infection in the child.*

4. When the catheter is in place, collect the urine specimen and drain the bladder while holding the distal end of the catheter with the nondominant hand. Remove the tube.

5. Cap the container tightly. Always wear gloves in case there are any urine spills on the container.

6. Label with name, date, and time. Send promptly to the laboratory.

7. Document the specimen collection and time sent to the laboratory.

### Male

1. Clean the perineum. With the nondominant hand, hold the penis behind the glans and spread the meatus with your thumb and forefinger. Retract the foreskin if the child is uncircumcised.

2. Use the dominant hand to pick up the forceps and antiseptic-soaked cotton balls. Clean the tissue surrounding the meatus using one cotton ball for each wipe in an outward circular motion. Discard each cotton ball away from the sterile field.

3. Pick up the lubricated catheter tip with the dominant hand, and place the distal end in a specimen container. Lift the penis, exerting slight traction until it is perpendicular to the body. Insert the catheter steadily into the meatus until urine begins to flow, and then about 2.5 cm (1.0 in.) further (up to a total of 10 to 12 cm [5 to 6 in.] maximum) (Figure 11–7).

   RATIONALE: *The catheter is inserted an extra inch into the bladder to ensure proper placement for drainage when an indwelling catheter is planned.*

4. If resistance to the catheter is felt, have the child blow out to relax the perineal muscles, or rotate the catheter between your fingers and gently advance. Do not force the catheter. Another catheter, one size smaller, may be used if relaxation efforts are not successful.

5. Once the catheter is in place, lower the penis and collect the urine specimen while holding the distal end of the catheter with the nondominant hand. Remove the tube.

6. Cap the container tightly. Always wear gloves in case there are any urine spills on the container.

7. Label with name, date, and time. Send promptly to the laboratory.

8. Document the specimen collection and time sent to the laboratory.

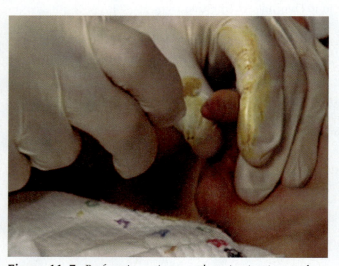

**Figure 11–7** *Performing urinary catheterization in a male infant.*

## SKILL 11–11 Collecting an Indwelling Catheter Urine Specimen

### PREPARATION

1. Explain the procedure to the child and parents if present.

### EQUIPMENT AND SUPPLIES

- Clamp
- Alcohol swab
- Syringe with needle
- Sterile specimen container
- Clean gloves

### PROCEDURE

1. Locate the self-sealing port on the urinary catheter tubing. The site is distal to the balloon that is inserted to keep the catheter in place.
   RATIONALE: *Self-sealing rubber catheters have a port that can be accessed with a syringe. This technique cannot be performed on plastic or silicone catheters. The port is distal to the balloon to avoid puncturing and dislodging the catheter.*

2. Wash hands and don gloves.

3. If there is no urine in the catheter, apply the clamp and wait for several minutes.

4. Clean the port with an alcohol swab.
   RATIONALE: *This minimizes the chance of transferring contaminants from the catheter surface into the urinary tract.*

5. Insert the needle on the syringe into the port at an angle. Release the clamp if it was applied.

6. Withdraw urine and transfer to a sterile specimen container. Discard the syringe in a sharps container.

7. Label with name, date, time, and test ordered. Send promptly to the laboratory.

8. Document the specimen collection and time sent to the laboratory.

---

## SKILL 11–12 Collecting a 24-Hour Urine Specimen

The 24-hour urine test is performed to measure the amount of a substance excreted in the urine over an entire day. Commonly, creatinine levels are measured to evaluate kidney function.

### PREPARATION

1. Confirm the identity of the client and explain the collection procedure to the family and child as developmentally appropriate. Assist the family members to choose a 24-hour time frame that is best for them and their child.

2. Document medications the client is taking and identify those that could affect the test results.

### EQUIPMENT AND SUPPLIES

- Labeled plastic container for urine collection
- Urine collection container for toilet or urinal
- Funnel
- Urine bags for infants
- Skin sealant such as Skin-Prep if not medically contraindicated (for infants wearing urine bags)
- Clean gloves

### PROCEDURE

1. Don gloves and assist the child to urinate at the beginning of the 24-hour collection period, and note the time. *Discard this urine.*

2. Record the start time on a labeled collection container.

3. For the next 24 hours, collect all urine in the agency-provided collection container, being sure to use clean gloves for each collection. Girls may void into the collection container in the toilet and use the funnel to pour urine into the plastic container. Boys may void directly into the collection container or other urine collection container. Urine should not be mixed with feces or toilet paper, as these may affect test results. Dark containers may be used for some collections,

or the specimen may need special handling, such as refrigeration; check the agency and laboratory procedure for the designated test. Care must be taken to obtain all of the urine.

**RATIONALE:** *The test evaluates protein levels or other substances in a 24-hour period to measure kidney function. Accuracy of the test depends on obtaining all urine within a 24-hour time frame.*

4. In anticipation of the end of the urine collection after 24 hours, let the child know when the final urine sample will be needed. At the end of the 24-hour period, ask the child to void and record the time the specimen was obtained. This is the stop time for specimen collection.

5. Verify that the specimen label matches the child's identification and test to be performed. Record the stop time on the urine collection container.

6. Send urine in the collection container promptly to the laboratory.

7. Document the procedure and time sent to the laboratory.

# Stool Culture

Stool cultures are used to detect the presence of bacteria and other organisms in the intestinal tract. A sample for culture can be obtained from stool collected in a cup, from a diaper, or from a swab that has been gently inserted into the child's rectum. A test for parasites requires larger-size samples and is usually submitted in a cuplike stool specimen container.

---

## SKILL 11–13  Obtaining a Stool Specimen

### PREPARATION

1. Gather supplies. The specimen may be obtained from a diaper or a device placed in the toilet to catch the stool and prevent it from falling into the toilet water.

2. Explain the procedure to the child and parents.

### EQUIPMENT AND SUPPLIES

- Two culturette swabs or a stool specimen container and two tongue blades
- Clean gloves

### PROCEDURE

1. Don gloves.

2. Open one culturette swab, holding it in your dominant hand while keeping the cover in your nondominant hand. If the swab is attached to the cover, hold the culturette tube in the nondominant hand and the swab and cover in the dominant hand.

3. Dip the swab into the stool. Replace the cover. Squeeze the bottom of the closed culturette to release the culture medium. Some laboratories will want the entire specimen sent in a sterile specimen collection cup.

4. Repeat with the second culturette.

5. Label with name, date, time, and test ordered. Promptly send to the laboratory.

### *For Parasitic and Other Specimens*

1. Don gloves.

2. Obtain the specimen from a diaper or toilet collection device by using tongue blades.

3. Place the specimen in a stool container.

4. Label the container with name, date, time, and test requested. Send to the laboratory immediately for parasite examination.

# Wound Culture

A culturette swab is used to obtain samples for microscopic examination from a wound or body site such as the eyes, ears, nose, throat, rectum, or vagina.

## SKILL 11–14  Obtaining a Sample for a Wound Culture

### PREPARATION

1. Gather supplies.
2. Explain the procedure to the child and parents.

### EQUIPMENT AND SUPPLIES

- One culturette swab
- Sterile gloves

### PROCEDURE

1. Don sterile gloves.
2. Open the culturette, holding it in the dominant hand while keeping the cover in the nondominant hand. If the swab is attached to the cover, hold the culturette tube in the nondominant hand and the swab and cover in the dominant hand.
3. Gently swab the infected area (Figure 11–8).
4. Place the swab into the culturette tube. Squeeze the tube to release the culture medium.
5. Label with name, date, time, site of culture, and test requested. Promptly send to the laboratory.
6. Document the specimen collected, site collected from, and time sent to the laboratory.

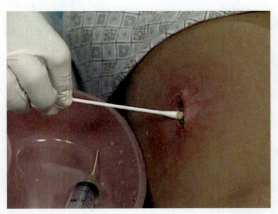

**Figure 11–8**  *Collecting a wound culture with a culturette swab.*

# Throat Culture

A culturette swab is used to obtain a sample from the throat for microscopic examination.

## SKILL 11–15  Obtaining a Sample for a Throat Culture

### PREPARATION

1. Verify the identity of the child. Explain the procedure to the child and parents.
2. Gather supplies.

### EQUIPMENT AND SUPPLIES

- Two culturette swabs
- Penlight
- Tongue blade
- Mask
- Clean gloves

### PROCEDURE

1. Don gloves and mask.
2. Open the culturette, holding it in the dominant hand while keeping the cover in the nondominant hand. If the swab is attached to the cover, hold the culturette tube in the nondominant hand and the swab and cover in the dominant hand.

---

### CLINICAL TIP

Throat cultures must be properly performed for accurate diagnosis. A sterile cotton-tip applicator is swabbed across the tonsils, posterior edge of the soft palate, and uvula. Cooperative children can be asked to put their hands under their buttocks, open the mouth, and laugh or pant like a dog. The throat is quickly swabbed. Uncooperative and young children are placed on their backs with their arms extended upward along the sides of the head and held by an assistant. The tongue is gently depressed with a tongue blade, and the throat is swabbed.

3. Use the penlight as needed to provide adequate views of the throat.

4. Gently swab the back of the throat along each tonsillar area with a separate culturette.

5. Place the swab into the culturette tube. Squeeze the tube to release the culture medium.

6. Label the specimen with name, date, and time. Promptly send to the laboratory.

7. Document the specimen collected and time obtained.

# Respiratory Secretions

Secretions are obtained to detect bacteria that cause respiratory infections. Different techniques are used for infants and older children. The infant will need suctioning. The older child can cooperate and cough into the provided container.

## SKILL 11–16  Collecting Respiratory Secretions From an Infant

### PREPARATION

1. Explain the procedure to the parents.

2. Gather supplies.

### EQUIPMENT AND SUPPLIES

- Sterile suction catheter
- Sterile normal saline
- Suction trap
- Personal protective equipment (mask, gown, eye protection)
- Sterile gloves

### PROCEDURE

1. According to the manufacturer's guidelines, attach the suction trap to low wall suction (60 mm Hg).

2. Don gown, mask, eye protection, and sterile gloves.

3. Suction the child's nose (refer to the description of suctioning in Chapter 15), using a small amount of sterile normal saline to clear the tubing.

4. Close the trap.

   NOTE:    *This will provide a specimen from the nasopharyngeal area. If a tracheal specimen is needed, the deep suctioning technique described in Chapter 15 should be consulted.*

5. Label the specimen with name, date, time, and test ordered. Promptly send to the laboratory.

**CLINICAL TIP**

A common respiratory infection in young children is caused by respiratory syncytial virus (RSV). In young children, the course of disease can be severe. Cultures may be taken to identify the disease in infants so that proper treatment can be instituted.

**CLINICAL TIP**

Some specimens require nasal washing that includes inserting saline into the nose before the specimen is collected. A nasopharyngeal swab is sometimes used instead of suction.

## SKILL 11–17  Collecting Respiratory Secretions From a Child

### PREPARATION

1. Verify the identity of the child. Explain the procedure to the child and parents.

2. Gather supplies.

### EQUIPMENT AND SUPPLIES

- Sterile specimen container
- Clean gloves
- Mask

### PROCEDURE

1. Don gloves and mask.

2. Encourage the child to take several deep breaths and then cough sputum up and spit it directly into the cup (Figure 11–9).

3. Have the child close the cup.

4. Label the specimen with the name, date, time, and test ordered. Promptly send to the laboratory.

5. Document the specimen collected and time sent.

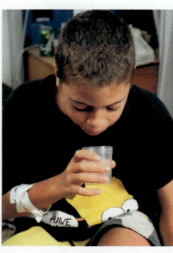

**Figure 11–9** *Child supplying a sputum specimen.*

# Bone Marrow Aspiration

The bone marrow is the tissue that manufactures the blood cells. The marrow should contain hematopoietic (blood-forming) cells, fat cells, and connective tissues. A bone marrow aspiration (and/or biopsy) is performed as a diagnostic procedure for the diagnosis and staging of hematologic disorders or cancers or to harvest bone marrow for transplant. Examination of the aspirate or biopsy specimen may also reveal infections. For a bone marrow aspiration, a thin needle is used to extract a small amount of liquid bone marrow. For a bone marrow biopsy, a small cylinder of bone and marrow is removed with a needle. Common pediatric sites for bone marrow aspiration are the posterior iliac crest, the anterior tibia, and the sternum.

A physician generally performs the aspiration, and the nurse assists with the procedure by positioning the child, preparing the child and family, and monitoring vital signs and response to the procedure prior to, during, and following the aspiration.

> **SAFETY ALERT**
>
> Absolute contraindications to bone marrow aspiration or biopsy include hemophilia and related coagulation disorders and infection of the biopsy area. Neither thrombocytopenia nor anemia is a contraindication.

## SKILL 11–18  Assisting With Bone Marrow Aspiration

### PREPARATION

1. Verify the identity of the child. Explain the procedure to the parents and child. Ensure that informed consent has been obtained.

2. Assess for any special medical problems or conditions that may complicate the procedure.

3. Gather proper specimen sample supplies, equipment, and pain/sedation medications (e.g., lidocaine hydrochloride and prescribed sedation medications).

4. Apply a local anesthetic agent (e.g., EMLA cream) well in advance of the procedure.

> **CLINICAL TIP**
>
> Bone marrow aspiration is a painful procedure. Effective sedation and pain management is important to reduce the child's anxiety and coping with this event and will facilitate management of future painful procedures.

### EQUIPMENT AND SUPPLIES

- Gown, sterile gloves, mask, eye shield worn by physician performing aspiration
- Sterile cotton balls or gauze
- Sterile forceps
- Sterile drape
- Stack of sterile 4″ × 4″ and 2″ × 2″ gauze pads
- Chlorhexidine-based, povidone-iodine, or other preferred skin preparation
- Sterile gloves, clean gloves for assistant
- Spinal needles
- Sheet or towel roll for client positioning
- #11 blade
- Bone marrow aspiration needles (16 gauge, 1 3/4 or 2 inch) or Jamshidi bone marrow biopsy needles (11 to 13 gauge)
- Sterile 10- and 20-mL syringes for sample procurement
- Specimen tubes, containers, and microscope slides with proper preservatives and fixatives, sealed container for biopsy
- Sodium heparin, injection, 1000 USP units/mL
- Lidocaine hydrochloride 1%, EMLA, pain and sedation medications
- Adhesive bandage or elastoplast tape for pressure dressing
- Pulse oximetry for monitoring the sedated child
- Oxygen, resuscitator bag, and emergency equipment and medications immediately available

## PROCEDURE

1. Assist with assembling the supplies and preparing the room.

2. Assist with the preparation, positioning, and immobilization of the client to provide optimal access to the aspiration site. Take baseline vital signs. Administer sedation and pain medication if prescribed.

3. Follow the guidelines for client monitoring before and throughout the procedure and until the child is fully responsive following the procedure. Monitor for signs of distress or excess pain. (See *Sedation Monitoring* in Chapter 8.)

   RATIONALE: *The child is often sedated for the procedure and needs to have vital signs carefully monitored.*

4. If the child is awake during the procedure, provide diversion or coping support.

5. After the site of the bone marrow aspiration is selected, personal protective equipment for physician and assistant are donned, the skin is cleansed and prepared, and the local anesthetic is applied or injected (the skin and periosteum are infiltrated with lidocaine 1%).

6. The skin is punctured at the insertion site with the #11 blade, and the bone marrow aspiration needle is inserted into the bone.

7. The stylette is removed and syringes are attached to withdraw marrow.

8. Samples are placed in the appropriate containers with labels, and needed preservatives are added.

9. After cleansing the site, apply a bandage.

10. Document the test performed, site used, vital signs and pulse oximetry readings, how the child tolerated the procedure, signs and symptoms of bleeding, and the time the specimen was sent to the laboratory.

# Chapter 12
# Administering Medications and Irrigations

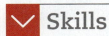
## Skills

# Administering Medications

Administering medications to children presents a number of challenges: deciding which drug forms to use, determining dosages, choosing methods and sites, and taking into account implications based on the child's development. See Table 12–1 for considerations needed when administering medications to children by various routes.

| TABLE 12–1 | Variations in Medication Administration to Children | |
|---|---|---|
| **Route** | **Developmental Considerations** | **Techniques** |
| Oral | Children under 5 years cannot generally swallow pills and capsules. | ■ Medications are usually given in liquid form (e.g., elixir, syrup, or suspension).<br>■ Sometimes tablets are crushed or capsules are opened and mixed with a small amount of food. Check with pharmacy to be sure this does not inactivate the drug. Never crush enteric-coated or timed-release medicine.<br>■ When choosing a vehicle for crushed tablets, use only 1 spoonful of applesauce, pudding, jelly, or similar food, or 1–2 mL of liquid so that it is easier to ensure that the entire dose will be taken. Do not use milk or other essential food as a vehicle for administration so that an adverse taste does not lead to the child refusing the food in the future.<br>■ Use an oral syringe when administering a liquid medication to increase accuracy. |
| | Children may not want to take medicine. | ■ Position young children upright to avoid choking and aspiration.<br>■ Give liquid medicines slowly by oral syringe (for infants) aimed at the inside of the cheek or by medicine cup (for toddler and preschooler) for drinking.<br>■ Communicate with the child that you expect that the medicine will be taken. Let children choose the type of fluid to drink after but do not ask if they will take their medicine now. |
| Rectal | Colon is small in size. | ■ Lubricate the tip of the suppository before placement.<br>■ Place the suppository at the rectal opening and advance past the sphincter.<br>■ For children under 3 years, the nurse's gloved fifth finger is used for insertion. After age 3 years, the index finger can usually be used. |
| Ophthalmic and otic | Young children may be fearful of medicines placed in the eyes or ears. | ■ Adequate immobilization is needed to avoid injury.<br>■ The nurse's hand can be stabilized by resting the wrist on the child's head.<br>■ Explanations and therapeutic play can be used with children old enough to explain the process of administration.<br>■ Have medication at room temperature. |
| Topical | Skin of infants is thin and fragile. | ■ Only prescribed doses and medicines appropriate for young children should be used on the skin.<br>■ Covering the area or keeping the child's hands occupied may be necessary to ensure adequate contact of medication with the skin. |
| Intramuscular | Anatomy and physiology of children differs from that of adults. | ■ The gluteus maximus muscle (dorsal gluteal site) is not recommended in children due to danger of injury to the sciatic nerve (Engorn & Flerlage, 2015).<br>■ The vastus lateralis site is preferred for children.<br>■ The deltoid muscle is rarely used in young children except for the small amounts injected in some vaccines.<br>■ Amounts to be administered should be limited to no more than 1–2 mL for ventrogluteal and vastus lateralis sites and 0.5 mL for deltoid, depending on muscle size.<br>■ Z-track technique (retracting tissue to the side and releasing it after injection to prevent seepage into tissue) is often used. |
| Intravenous | Veins are small and fragile. | ■ Careful maintenance of sites is needed.<br>■ Common infusion sites include hands and feet, although scalp veins are sometimes used in infants. |
| | Fluid balance is critical. | ■ Infusion pumps require frequent monitoring.<br>■ Syringe pumps are often used to administer medications when minimal fluid is to be given.<br>■ Central lines are commonly used for long-term intravenous medication therapy. |

Source: Courtesy of Kay Cowen, RN-BC, MSN, CNE.

Although the drug and the dosage are determined by the prescriber, it is imperative that the nurse observe the "six rights" of medication administration before any medication is given (Table 12–2). Follow all administrations with accurate documentation and monitoring of the client.

| **TABLE 12–2** | "Six Rights" of Medication Administration |
|---|---|

1. Right medication
   - Compare the name and concentration of the drug on the medication sheet with the name and concentration of the drug on the label of the drug container 3 times: (1) when taking the drug from storage, (2) when opening and preparing the drug, and (3) when securing the container and replacing the drug.
   - Check the container's expiration date.
   - Know the action of the drug.
   - Identify the potential side effects of the drug.
   - Use the pharmacy, hospital, or other drug formulary as a reference for medications with which you are unfamiliar.

2. Right patient
   - Verify the name, medical record number, and date of birth on the medication sheet with these items on the child's identification band. When in a setting with no name band (e.g., clinic), verify the child's name and date of birth with the child and parent by asking them to state the child's name and date of birth.

3. Right time
   - When prescribed to be administered at a specific time, a medication should be given within 20–30 minutes of that time.
   - For prn medications, check the last time the dose was given as well as the total 24-hour dose the child has received to verify that the child can receive another dose at this time.

4. Right route of administration
   - Always use the prescribed route for administration of a medication. If a change is needed (such as a change from oral medication when a child is vomiting), check with the prescriber to get an order for a change in route.
   - If a verbal order must be taken, read back the order to the prescriber to verify accuracy.

5. Right dose
   - Match the dose and concentration with the order.
   - Calculate the prescribed dose based on the child's weight in kilograms.
   - If in doubt about what constitutes an appropriate dose, compare with the pharmacy, hospital, or other drug formulary guidelines for recommended dose.
   - Question any order for which the dose is outside of recommended amounts.

6. Right documentation
   - Accurately document on the correct patient record the name of the medication, dose, route, time administered, and patient's response.

## Preparation

- Explain all procedures or treatments to the child and parents, based on the child's developmental stage, cultural considerations, limited English proficiency (LEP), and the level of understanding of both parties.
- Confirm the medication prescription and the identity of the child.
- Answer all questions before giving the medication.
- Identify any known drug allergies and prior reactions to medication.
- Match the drug available to the medication prescribed and check the expiration date.
- Observe the medication for intactness (tablet/capsule), clarity, and color change; discard and seek new medication as needed.

## Documentation

- Once a medication is given, record the name of the drug, the route, the date and time, and, if appropriate, the site.
- Record the response to the medication, including desired effects and undesired side effects. Design observations to coincide with the drug's onset and peak action times.

  RATIONALE: *A record of response is especially important with medications for pain control and those for treatment of an acute problem such as respiratory difficulty.*

## Calculation

It is the nurse's responsibility to calculate the dosage of the medication prescribed to determine if the dosage is within the normal range for the child's height and weight.

Dosages can be calculated using the child's weight (written as milligrams/kilogram [mg/kg]) or milligrams per total body surface area in square meters (mg/$m^2$). This is determined by plotting the child's height and weight on a nomogram (see Appendix C). Draw a line connecting the two columns, and note the results at the point where the drawn lines cross the center column. The dosage is ordered as mg/$m^2$.

### Example 1

The physician prescribes morphine (10 mg/mL) for a 3-year-old child who weighs 15 kg. The recommended dose for children is 0.1 mg/kg. What dose is appropriate for the child's weight? How much volume should be drawn?

### Answer

Recommended dose × Weight = Dose for client

0.1 mg/kg = 1.5 mg

$$\frac{\text{Dose desired}}{\text{Dose on hand}} \times \text{Quantity in mL} = \text{Volume to be administered}$$

$$\frac{1.5\ \text{mg}}{10\ \text{mg}} \times 1\ \text{mL} = 0.15\ \text{mL to be administered}$$

### Example 2

The physician prescribes a loading dose of phenobarbital (65 mg/mL) for a 5-year-old child who weighs 20 kg. The recommended loading dose for the child is 10 to 20 mg/kg. The physician prescribes 250 mg to be infused over 30 minutes. Is this dose appropriate for the child's weight? How much volume should be drawn? How do you set the infusion pump to administer the dose in the prescribed time?

### Answer

Recommended dose × Weight = Desired dose

10 mg/kg × 20 kg = 200 mg

20 mg/kg × 20 kg = 400 mg

Dose of 250 mg is within recommended range.

$$\frac{\text{Dose desired}}{\text{Dose on hand}} \times \text{Quantity in mL} = \text{Volume to be administered}$$

250 mg/65 mg = 3.85 mL

### PUMP SETUP

Using recommendations from the manufacturer, the nurse determines that the volume for the setup is 50 mL.

50 mL/30 min × 60 min/1 hr = 100 mL/hr

Rate = 100 mL/hr

# Oral Medication

Children younger than 5 years of age usually have difficulty swallowing tablets and capsules. For this reason, most medications for pediatric use are also available in the form of elixirs, syrups, or suspensions. If a medication is available only in tablet or capsule form, it may need to be crushed before being administered. Be sure not to crush medications with enteric coating. Remember to wear clean gloves if your hands might come in contact with the child's saliva.

---

## SKILL 12–1  Administering an Oral Medication

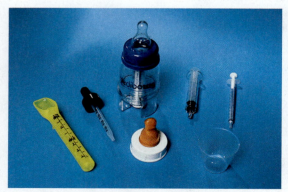

**Figure 12–1**  *Oral medications can be administered with various types of equipment, depending on the child's age and the volume of liquid to be administered.*

### PREPARATION

1. Verify concentration, dose, and route as described previously.

2. Measure the medication accurately to ensure that the dose is correct.

3. If the oral medication is liquid (especially if less than 5 mL), it should be measured in a syringe or dropper (Figure 12–1). A specially designed medication bottle may also be used.

4. If a tablet or pill needs to be crushed, place it in a mortar or between two paper medicine cups and crush it with a pestle. Once the tablet or pill has been pulverized, mix the powdered medication with a small amount of flavored substance such as juice, applesauce, or jelly to disguise any unpleasant flavor. Use only a small amount of the food since the child will need to consume all of it to receive the medication.

5. Verify identification of the child to receive the medication.

6. Explain the procedure to the parent. State the name of the drug to be given.

## EQUIPMENT AND SUPPLIES

- Medicine cup, oral syringe, or other device for administering medication
- Pestle and medicine cups
- Medication
- Mixing medium as needed, such as applesauce
- Clean gloves

## PROCEDURE

### Infant

1. Use a syringe or dropper to provide the best control.

2. Don gloves if needed.

3. Place small amounts of liquid along the inside of the infant's mouth between the cheek and the gum line. Wait for the infant to swallow before giving more.

   **RATIONALE:** *This helps to prevent aspiration and maximizes the chance that the infant will get all the medicine rather than spitting some out.*

   Alternative method: Have the infant suck the liquid through a nipple.

4. Document administration of the medication and both expected and side effects.

### Toddler or Young Child

1. Place the child firmly on your lap or the parent's lap in a sitting or modified supine position (Figure 12–2).

2. Don gloves if needed.

3. Administer the medication slowly with a syringe or small medicine cup. Allow cooperative children to self-administer if they wish to do so.

4. Document administration of the medication and both expected and side effects.

5. Instruct and demonstrate correct measurement and administration of medication that will be given at home.

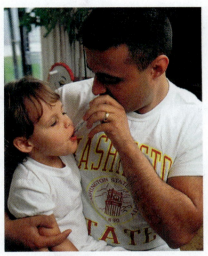

**Figure 12–2** *This father needs to administer a medication to his daughter at home. He has been instructed on how to hold her and administer the dose safely and effectively.*

---

### HOME AND COMMUNITY CARE CONSIDERATIONS

Parents who administer oral medications to children at home often use a variety of household devices. In a recent study, parents made measurement errors in about 40% of doses (Yin et al., 2014). These preventable errors should be addressed by using and demonstrating only milliliter (mL) dosing in prescribing and administering medications. Words such as teaspoon and tablespoon should not be used. Send the parents home with the proper measuring device, such as an oral syringe with metric markings (American Academy of Pediatrics Committee on Drugs, 2015).

---

# Intramuscular Injection

The site of the intramuscular (IM) injection (Figure 12–3) depends on the age of the child, the amount of muscle mass, and the density and volume of medication to be administered. Young infants may not tolerate volumes greater than 0.5 mL in a single site, whereas older infants or small children may be able to tolerate 1 mL per site. As the child grows, greater volumes can be administered.

The larger the volume of medication, the larger the muscle that will need to be used. Avoid areas that involve major blood vessels or nerves.

The preferred site for all children is the vastus lateralis muscle (Figure 12–4), which lies along the midanterior lateral aspect of the thigh. For the older child and adolescent, the sites are the same as for the adult: the vastus lateralis, deltoid (for small amounts only), and ventrogluteal muscles. The dorsal gluteal site is discouraged at all ages due to the risk of injuring the sciatic nerve.

As described in the "six rights" (see Table 12–2), carefully match the drug with the medication prescribed. If it will be reconstituted by

### SAFETY ALERT

Use of the dorsal gluteal site is discouraged at all ages due to the potential for damage to the sciatic nerve. The vastus lateralis site is recommended for children; the ventral gluteal site may be used when an alternate site is required.

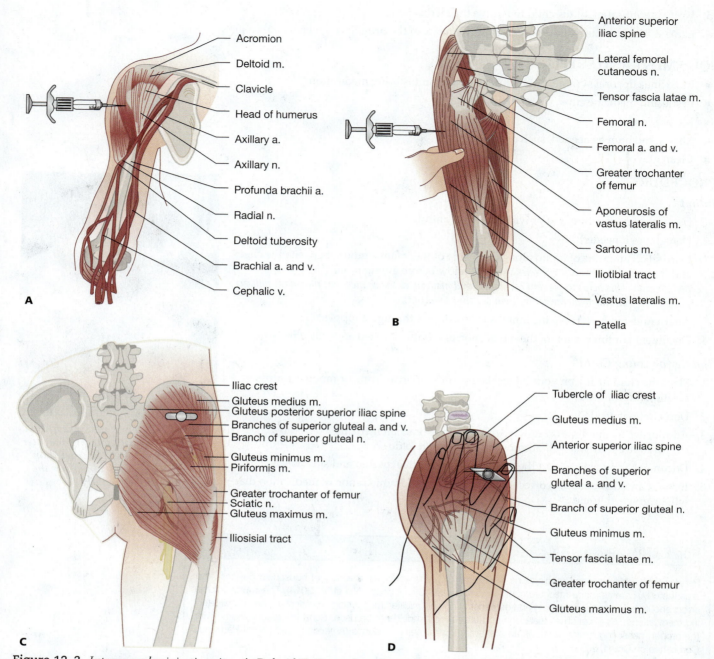

**Figure 12–3** *Intramuscular injection sites. A, Deltoid. B, Vastus lateralis. C, Dorsal gluteal. D, Ventrogluteal.*
Source: Redrawn and modified from Bindler, R., & Howry, L. (2005). *Pediatric drug guide with nursing implications* (pp. 41–44). Upper Saddle River, NJ: Prentice Hall Health.

Labels in A: Acromion; Deltoid m.; Clavicle; Head of humerus; Axillary a.; Axillary n.; Profunda brachii a.; Radial n.; Deltoid tuberosity; Brachial a. and v.; Cephalic v.

Labels in B: Anterior superior iliac spine; Lateral femoral cutaneous n.; Tensor fascia latae m.; Femoral n.; Femoral a. and v.; Greater trochanter of femur; Aponeurosis of vastus lateralis m.; Sartorius m.; Iliotibial tract; Vastus lateralis m.; Patella

Labels in C: Iliac crest; Gluteus medius m.; Gluteus posterior superior iliac spine; Branches of superior gluteal a. and v.; Branch of superior gluteal n.; Gluteus minimus m.; Piriformis m.; Greater trochanter of femur; Sciatic n.; Gluteus maximus m.; Iliosisial tract

Labels in D: Tubercle of iliac crest; Gluteus medius m.; Anterior superior iliac spine; Branches of superior gluteal a. and v.; Branch of superior gluteal n.; Gluteus minimus m.; Tensor fascia latae m.; Greater trochanter of femur; Gluteus maximus m.

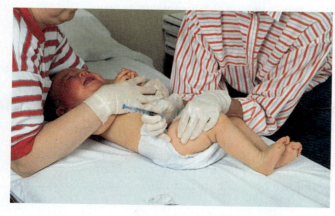

**Figure 12–4** *In children, the vastus lateralis muscle is preferred for intramuscular injections.*

adding liquid, follow the mixing and calculation instructions carefully. Follow sterile procedures and needle safety precautions. Record the procedure accurately.

## Growth and Development

Consider the child's age and developmental level when preparing for IM injections. Infants and toddlers will need to be held securely, with only minimal explanations understood. The preschooler and young school-age child can often understand the reason for the injection. Explain what it will feel like, such as, "I am going to clean your arm now with alcohol. This feels cold but does not hurt." And then, "You will feel the stick now and it's OK to tell me if it hurts." Children also can benefit from distractions that help them to manage the injection. "When I give the shot, let's count to 10 together. OK, it's in-one, two, three … ." And, finally, praise children for some part of their behavior. "I know you were scared but you held very still so we could do it fast."

---

## SKILL 12–2  Administering an Intramuscular Injection

### PREPARATION

1. Verify concentration, dose, and route as described previously.
2. Select the syringe size according to the volume and dose of medication to be delivered. The needle must be long enough to penetrate the subcutaneous tissue and enter the muscle. Needles with a length of 1.0 to 1.5 inches and 25 to 21 gauge are recommended for infants over 4 months and children. Infants under 4 months may require a 0.5-inch needle, depending on muscle mass. After drawing up the medication, the needle may be changed to prevent any medication from leaking into tissues during entry through the skin and subcutaneous layer.
3. Choose the appropriate site, as described previously.
4. Verify the identity of the child.
5. Explain the procedure to the parents and to the child if the child is old enough to understand. State the name of the drug to be given, and verify that the child has no allergy to the medication.

### EQUIPMENT AND SUPPLIES

- Labeled medication container
- Syringe filled with prepared medication
- Alcohol swab
- Gauze pad or cotton ball
- Small adhesive bandage
- Clean gloves

### PROCEDURE

1. Have another nurse, an assistant, or the parent position and hold the necessary body parts of the child during the injection (Figure 12–5).
   **RATIONALE:** *Adequate immobilization allows the procedure to be done safely and quickly and thereby minimizes trauma for the child.*
2. Don gloves.
3. Locate the site. Clean with alcohol using an outward circular motion and allow alcohol to dry.
4. Grasp the muscle between your thumb and fingers for stabilization. If using Z-track technique, move the tissue laterally and hold it in that position for the duration of the injection.

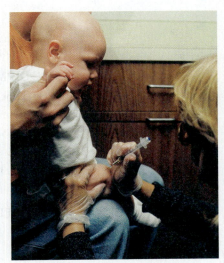

**Figure 12–5**  *The infant's legs and arms are controlled by the father and nurse so an injection can safely be administered.*

---

**CLINICAL TIP**

Aspiration (pulling back on plunger after inserting needle for injection) for 5–10 seconds has traditionally been recommended for intramuscular injections. The Centers for Disease Control and Prevention (CDC) has stated this is not needed for immunization administration. Evidence base for this practice is lacking and some agencies do not recommend aspiration for intramuscular injections (Greenway, 2014; Sisson, 2015; CDC, 2015). Check with your agency policy, and be alert for changes in guidelines.

---

5. Remove the cap from the syringe. Insert the needle quickly at a 90-degree angle. If using aspiration, pull back the plunger (aspirate) for 5–10 seconds with thumb or finger on the injecting hand.

   RATIONALE: *The 90-degree angle ensures entry into the muscle when the needle length is adequate. Pulling back of the plunger helps to rule out placement in a blood vessel.*

6. If blood is aspirated, do not inject and remove the entire syringe. Redraw the solution in a new syringe and administer.

7. If no blood is aspirated, inject the medication, wait about 10 seconds to assist with dissipation of the medication, withdraw the needle while releasing pressure on the skin, massage the area with a gauze pad or cotton ball (alcohol will sting), and return the child to a position of comfort. Apply a small adhesive bandage if there is a drop of blood visible.

8. Do not recap the needle. Discard it in a puncture-resistant container according to standard precaution recommendations.

9. Document the medication administration, site, and reactions of the child.

# Subcutaneous Injection

The site of the subcutaneous injection depends on the age of the child. Usually the dorsum of the upper arm or the anterior thigh is used in newborns, infants, and toddlers.

---

## SKILL 12–3 Administering a Subcutaneous Injection

### PREPARATION

1. Verify concentration, dose, and route as described previously.

2. Select the syringe size based on the volume or dose of medication to be delivered. The needle must be just long enough to penetrate the subcutaneous tissue, which lies below the skin and fat surface and above the muscle. Needles with a length of 3/8 to 5/8 inch (26 to 25 gauge) are recommended for infants and children.

3. Choose the appropriate site, as described earlier.

4. Verify the identity of the child.

5. Explain the procedure to the parents and to the child if the child is old enough to understand. State the name of the drug to be given, and verify that the child has no allergy to the medication.

### EQUIPMENT AND SUPPLIES

- Labeled medication container
- Syringe filled with medication
- Alcohol swab
- Gauze pad or cotton ball
- Small adhesive bandage
- Clean gloves

### PROCEDURE

1. Have another nurse, an assistant, or a parent position and hold the necessary body parts of the child while the injection is being given.

2. Don gloves.

3. Locate the site. Clean with alcohol using an outward circular motion and allow alcohol to dry.

4. Pinch the skin between your thumb and index finger.

5. Remove the cap from the syringe. Insert the needle quickly at about a 45-degree angle. Release the skin and pull back the plunger if aspiration is needed for the particular medication.
   RATIONALE: *A 45-degree angle is used to inject into the subcutaneous tissue rather than the underlying muscle.*

6. If blood is aspirated, do not inject, and remove the entire syringe. Redraw the solution in a new syringe and administer. Note that aspiration is not needed for immunizations because no major blood vessels or nerves are present in immunization administration sites (CDC, 2015).

7. If no blood is aspirated, inject the medication, withdraw the needle at the angle at which it was inserted, massage the area with a gauze pad or cotton ball (alcohol will sting), and return the child to a position of comfort. Apply an adhesive bandage if there is a drop of blood present.

8. Do not recap the needle. Discard it in a puncture-resistant container according to standard precaution recommendations.

9. Document the medication administration, site, and reactions of the child.

# Intravenous Medication

The principles of intravenous (IV) medication administration in children are the same as those in adults. Special considerations when administering IV medication are discussed in this section. Accessing lines when a medication lock is in place or a central line is used is discussed in Chapter 13.

Many drugs have specific dilution recommendations. Some medications are compatible with only specific fluids such as normal saline. Other medications must be given very slowly. Still other drugs can be administered quickly. Know your agency or pharmacy standards for IV push or bolus administration (less than 10 minutes) versus intermittent medication administration. Be sure you know which medications are incompatible with one another and with types of IV fluids.

## Special Considerations

It is recommended that IV medications for infants and children be put in a volume-control chamber such as a Soluset, Buretrol, or Metriset with the diluent and placed on an electronic pump for accurate administration. Alternatively, a syringe pump may be used, especially when fluid intake is closely regulated. Set the pump for the volume to be infused and the rate of infusion. Check the pump frequently in case of malfunction, and do not assume that the pump is functioning if it does not sound an alarm. Check frequently for signs of infiltration and extravasation. Flush the line after the infusion to ensure that all medication has been administered, as some medication will remain in the distal tubing. Consult agency policy for an acceptable flush solution.

---

## SKILL 12–4 Administering an Intravenous Medication

### PREPARATION

1. Review the medication, the administration recommendations, and the child's former responses and drug allergies.

2. Assess the IV line for patency.

3. If you are administering narcotics or benzodiazepines, have antagonists and ventilation equipment at the bedside.
   RATIONALE: *The effect of most IV medications is almost immediate.*

4. Prepare the drug according to the order, hospital protocols, and manufacturer guidelines. Reconstitution or withdrawal of solution from a vial or ampule may be needed.

5. Identify the child and explain the procedure to the child and family. State the name of the drug to be given, and verify that the child has no allergy to the medication.

### EQUIPMENT AND SUPPLIES

- Labeled medication container
- Syringe and needle or needleless system
- Prepared medication
- Dilution solutions
- Alcohol swabs
- Clean or sterile gloves

### SAFETY ALERT

It is recommended that needleless systems be used whenever available to decrease the chance of needle-stick injuries to clients and healthcare providers. Each agency should maintain policies and procedures for the specific types of needleless connectors used in that facility in order to decrease risk of infection or malfunction (Hadaway, 2012).

**PROCEDURE**

1. Assess IV line for patency, edema, redness, and pain. Report abnormalities before beginning injection. If the child has a medication lock in place, flush the line with 2 to 5 mL normal saline to check for patency or insert the IV line and allow to run for several minutes. Check the site again. See Chapter 13 for further details. Use only normal saline without preservatives for newborns.

2. Identify the port on the IV line to be used for push medications or for insertion of a syringe pump. Generally, a port proximal to the child is used, especially for intermittent infusion.
   RATIONALE: *A proximal port ensures that the medication will be delivered at the time administered. When an IV line is running slowly, it may take some time for the medication to travel from a distal port into the child.*

3. Identify the medication port on the volume-control chamber for intermittent infusion.

4. Don gloves.

5. Clean the port and surrounding tubing with an alcohol swab and allow to air dry.
   RATIONALE: *Cleansing minimizes the chance of instilling harmful organisms into the IV line.*

6. Insert the needle or needleless syringe for IV push medication. While watching the time, slowly insert the medication in the ordered time frame. Observe the child carefully during administration. Stop the infusion if the child suddenly becomes lethargic or hyperactive, demonstrates changes in respirations or color, or has other rapid changes in behavior or appearance.
   RATIONALE: *Because push medications travel quickly into the vein, side effects can appear rapidly. Close observation is needed to prevent and respond quickly to undesired effects.*

7. When using a syringe pump, insert the primed tubing into a port close to the child. Set the infusion time, as prescribed for the medication.

8. When using intermittent medication administration, insert the medication in the proper dilution in the volume-control chamber. Regulate the pump to administer the medication in the desired time.
   RATIONALE: *Medications should be administered in recommended time frames to ensure safety and effectiveness. Most antibiotics are administered over 20 to 60 minutes.*

9. Check on the child's condition several times during administration.
   RATIONALE: *Monitoring the child ensures that side effects are identified and that the IV infusion is patent and running on time.*

10. At the end of administration, flush the tubing with normal saline or by running IV fluid.
    RATIONALE: *Flushing ensures that the entire amount of medication is infused and not left in the tubing. Flushing also removes medication from the line so that it will not mix with other drugs administered.*

11. Document administration and effects observed. Assess the IV line and document findings.

# Ophthalmic Medication

The first ophthalmic medication is given as prophylaxis for sexually transmitted infection in the newborn. The procedure is described in Skill 12–5. Older children receive ophthalmic medication for treatment of infections and other eye conditions, and the technique for administration is described in Skill 12–6. Children usually fear having anything placed in their eyes, and special care is often needed to reduce the child's anxiety and promote cooperation during instillation of ophthalmic medications. An explanation of the procedure may help gain the child's cooperation. To prevent the transfer of pathogens to the eye, the medication and its dispensing port must be kept sterile.

### SKILL 12–5  Administering Neonatal Ophthalmic Ointment

*Neisseria gonorrhoeae* (the causative agent of gonorrhea), *Chlamydia*, and *Staphylococcus aureus* can colonize within the birth canal without causing symptoms in the mother. The infective agents can be transferred to the newborn during birth and lead to an eye infection, which is called *ophthalmia neonatorum*. Application of erythromycin ophthalmic ointment can prevent this infection and protect eyesight. It is easy to administer and causes few side effects. For this reason, the medication is applied soon after birth following drying of the newborn, attending to temperature, assessing initial adaptation, and ensuring adequate oxygenation. Eye prophylaxis is required by law in the United States and Canada; it can be declined in writing by parents in Canada.

## PREPARATION

1. Gather necessary supplies.
2. Verify the identity of the newborn.
3. Teach parents about the medication and the reason for administration.

## EQUIPMENT AND SUPPLIES

- Clean cotton pads
- Erythromycin ophthalmic ointment
- Sterile gloves (at least two sets)

## PROCEDURE

1. Perform hand hygiene. Swaddle the newborn and place in a supine position.
   RATIONALE: *Swaddling the baby will help to keep the newborn's hands from interfering with medication administration.*
2. Don sterile gloves.
3. Using a cotton pad, wipe excess fluid and vernix from one eye, working from the inner to outer canthus.
4. Repeat with the opposite eye using a clean cotton pad.
5. Remove gloves and perform hand hygiene. Open the medication.
6. Don a second set of sterile gloves.
7. Stand at the newborn's head.
8. Using the thumb and fingers of the nondominant hand, retract both the upper and lower eyelids so that the eye can be visualized.
9. Apply a 1- to 2-cm (half-inch) line of ointment into the lower conjunctival sac, working from the inner to outer canthus. Be careful not to touch the tube to the eye or mucous membrane.
10. Repeat on the opposite eye, maintaining sterile application technique.
11. Refrain from wiping the eyes after administration.
12. Remove gloves and perform hand hygiene. Document administration in the medical record.

---

### HOME AND COMMUNITY CARE CONSIDERATIONS

#### Instilling Eye Medications

It can be challenging to safely instill eye medication into young children. Give parents the following suggestions:

- Wash your hands well.
- Be sure the medicine is warmed to room temperature.
- Remove any drainage from the eye with a clean or sterile moist, warm cloth or gauze.
- Wash your hands again.
- Have the child lie on the back with eyes closed.
- Gently pull the lower lid down to form a small pocket.
- Apply a thin string (for ointment) or drops of the medicine.
- Allow the eyelid to return to the normal position.
- Have the child keep the eye closed for several seconds.
- Help prevent spread of the infection by keeping the child's hands clean.
- Enhance comfort by keeping the head elevated to decrease swelling and avoiding exposure to bright light.

---

## SKILL 12–6 Administering an Ophthalmic Medication

### PREPARATION

1. Gather supplies.
2. Verify the medication order with the available medication.
3. Identify the child and explain the procedure to the child and family. State the name of the drug to be given.

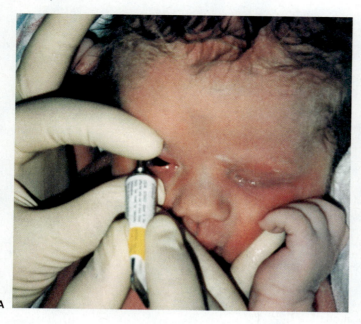

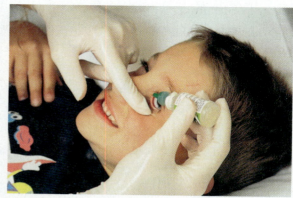

**B**

**Figure 12–6** *Administering an ophthalmic medication. A, Newborn prophylaxis. B, The child is instructed to close his eyes and pretend to look up toward his head. The nurse then gently retracts the lower lid and inserts the medication.*

### EQUIPMENT AND SUPPLIES

- Medication
- Sterile gloves
- Sterile gauze

### PROCEDURE

1. Have another nurse, an assistant, or a parent hold the child's upper body in a supine position with the child's head extended.

2. Don gloves.

3. Use your nondominant hand to pull the child's lower lid down while your other hand rests on the child's head (Figure 12–6).

4. Instill the drops or ointment into the conjunctival sac that has formed.

   Alternative method: Pull the lower lid out far enough to form a reservoir in which the medication can be instilled.

5. After the medication has been instilled, close the child's eyelids to prevent leakage.

6. Have the child lie quietly for a minimum of 30 seconds. Discourage the child from squeezing the eyes shut.

7. Dry the inner canthus of the eye with sterile gauze.

8. Keep the child's head in the midline position to prevent the medication from contaminating the other eye.

9. Document the medication administration and the child's response.

10. When the child requires ophthalmic medication at home, instruct parents in proper technique.

## Contact Lens Care

When children are hospitalized or receiving health care, healthcare providers should ask if contact lenses are used. Follow the prescriber's and family's directions for care of contact lenses. Encourage the child and family to care for lenses whenever possible. General guidelines include the following:

- Keep the lenses in the eyes for the recommended time only.
- Store each lens in the right or left containers as labeled.
- Wash hands carefully before contact with the child's eyes or lenses.
- Use a cleaning solution on the lens after its removal.
- Rinse the lens with the recommended rinsing solution.
- Keep the lenses in the case with the disinfecting storage solution.
- Note on the chart that the child wears contact lenses.

# Eye Irrigation

Irrigation of the eye is performed to flush out a foreign body or a chemical irritant (Figure 12–7). Children often close the injured eye tightly, so getting them to relax for this procedure is important. Care must be taken not to touch the cornea, which could cause further eye injury. Careful aseptic technique is needed to prevent infection. In community emergency situations caused by chemical burns, prompt irrigation with copious amounts of tap water is the best immediate treatment. If available, normal saline, normal saline with bicarbonate, lactated Ringer solution, BSS PLUS (balanced salt solution enriched with bicarbonate, dextrose, and glutathione), and diphoterine solution may all be used (Chau, Lee, & Lo, 2012).

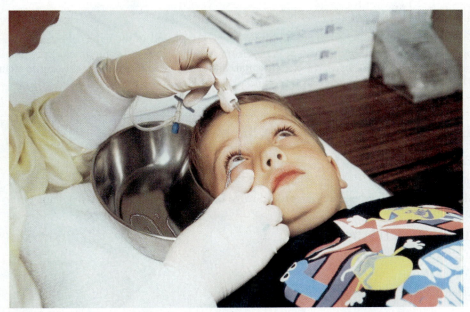

**Figure 12–7**  *Eye irrigation.*

## SKILL 12–7  Performing an Eye Irrigation

### PREPARATION

1. Check the prescriber's orders for the type of fluid and the volume to be used (most often sterile normal saline).

2. Identify the child and explain the procedure to the child and family.

3. The child will need to be held in position for this procedure. An assistant can hold the child supine, keeping the child's head turned slightly so that the eye to be irrigated is lower than the other eye, and being sure that the child has free exchange of air.
   **RATIONALE:** *This method is used to avoid cross-contamination of the eye not being irrigated.*

4. Attach the IV tubing to the bag of room-temperature normal saline. Purge the line, but keep the tip covered.

### EQUIPMENT AND SUPPLIES

- Absorbent pads
- Irrigation solution and tubing
- Basin
- Sterile gauze or cotton balls
- Sterile gloves

### PROCEDURE

1. Place absorbent pads under the child's head, neck, and shoulders, using towels for extra absorption. Place an emesis basin under the lower eye to catch drainage.

2. Don sterile gloves.

3. Using the thumb and forefinger of your dominant hand, gently separate the child's lids.

4. Remove the cover from the IV tubing. Open the clamp midway, pointing the stream of fluid into the lower conjunctival sac from the inner to the outer canthus. Periodically turn off the stream of solution and have the child close the eye.
   **RATIONALE:** *This allows the solution also to move into the upper conjunctival area.*

5. When the irrigation has been completed, dry the child's eye gently with gauze or a cotton ball from the inner to the outer canthus.

6. Assess the return for color, odor, and character. Observe the irrigation solution and eye for a foreign body.

7. Document the treatment, observations, and the child's response.

# Otic Medication

Otic medications, which are available in liquid form, are placed in the external ear canal using a dropper. They include antibiotics and pain medications. Otic drops are sometimes applied to soften cerumen, enabling it to be cleansed from the canal. The ear canal is not treated with sterile technique unless the tympanic membrane is ruptured and draining.

---

### SKILL 12–8 Administering an Otic Medication

#### PREPARATION

1. Gather supplies.
2. Identify the child and explain the procedure to the child and family. State the name of the drug to be given.

#### EQUIPMENT AND SUPPLIES

- Medication
- Cotton ball
- Clean gloves

#### PROCEDURE

1. Have another nurse, an assistant, or the parent hold the child in a supine position with the head turned as appropriate for administration, and ensuring free air exchange (Figure 12–8).

2. Don gloves.

3. For the child less than 3 years of age, gently pull the pinna straight back and downward to straighten the ear canal. For the older child, pull the pinna back and upward.
   **RATIONALE:** *These maneuvers straighten the ear canal.*

4. When the pinna is in the proper position, instill the drops into the ear.

5. Keep the child in the same position for a few minutes. Gently rub the area just anterior to the ear to facilitate drainage of the medication into the ear canal. If desired, a cotton ball may be loosely placed in the ear for about 5 minutes to promote retention of the medication.

6. Document the treatment and the child's response.

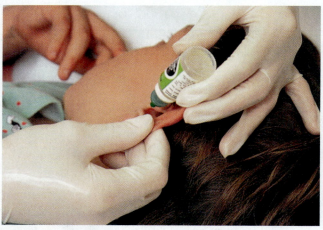

**Figure 12–8** *Administering an otic medication.*

# Ear Irrigation

Irrigation of the ear is performed to remove cerumen or a foreign body. Frequently, the child has symptoms of otitis media but the canal cannot be visualized. Always ask the parent if there has been any drainage from the ear and examine the ear with an otoscope (see your textbook for a description of proper use of the otoscope and normal ear landmarks). If there is drainage, contact the prescriber before irrigating the ear. Be sure to check the auditory canal with the otoscope after each 1 minute of irrigation to observe the effects of treatment.

## SKILL 12–9  Performing an Ear Irrigation

### PREPARATION

1. Check the prescriber's orders for the type of fluid to be used and the ear to be irrigated.

2. Identify the child and explain the procedure to the child and family.

### EQUIPMENT AND SUPPLIES

- Ordered solution, warmed to room temperature
- Irrigating syringe (bulb or Asepto) with tubing, ear irrigation machine, or Waterpik according to agency policy
- Clean gloves
- Absorbent pads
- Basin

### PROCEDURE

1. Examine the ear with an otoscope.
   **RATIONALE:** *The tympanic membrane should be intact before the irrigation is performed.*

2. Place the child in a supine position with the affected ear facing partially upward. Don gloves. For the child less than 3 years of age, gently pull the pinna straight back and slightly downward. For the older child, pull the pinna back and upward.
   **RATIONALE:** *These maneuvers straighten the ear canal.*

3. Place a waterproof pad on the bed under the head. Place an emesis basin under the ear to be irrigated (Figure 12–9).

4. Draw 20 mL of warm ordered solution into a syringe with the tubing attached.

5. Gently flush the solution into the ear canal, catching the draining fluid with the emesis basin. Gently turn the head toward the affected ear to facilitate drainage of the fluid.

6. Alternatively, use an ear irrigating machine or a Waterpik at the lowest setting to flush the ear.

7. Repeat according to the prescriber's orders.

8. Dry the child's ear, cheek, and neck.

9. Reexamine the ear with an otoscope and record changes noted. Document the treatment and the child's response.

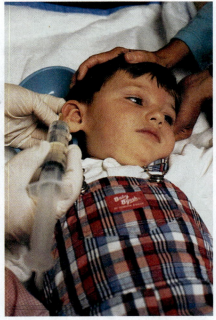

**Figure 12–9**  *Ear irrigation. Note that the affected ear is facing upward for the instillation of fluid; the head will be rotated toward the bed so that the fluid can drain out after the irrigation is completed.*

# Nasal Medication

Medications instilled into the nares drain into the back of the mouth and throat, and may cause sensations of difficulty in breathing, tickling, or bad taste. After instillation of the drops, the child should be observed for choking or vomiting. Saline nose drops are sometimes given to young infants who have respiratory disorders to clear the nasal passages. A preparation of influenza vaccine is available for nasal administration. The applicator is placed into the nares with one-half dose administered to each nostril (CDC, 2015).

## SKILL 12–10  Administering a Nasal Medication

### EQUIPMENT AND SUPPLIES

- Medication
- Clean gloves

### PROCEDURE

1. Verify the identity of the child and explain the procedure to the child and family. State the name of the drug to be given.

2. Place the child in a supine position with the head hyperextended over the parent's lap or over the edge of the examination table or bed.

3. Don gloves.

4. Instill the drops into the nostrils.

5. Keep the child in the same position for at least 5 minutes to allow the medication to contact the nasal mucosa.

6. Document the treatment and the child's response.

# Aerosol Therapy

Aerosol therapy is used when a medication needs to be deposited directly into the airway. Bronchodilators, steroids, and antibiotics can be administered to children in aerosol form. Several methods are used to provide aerosol therapy, including mist tents with medications added to a reservoir, intermittent positive-pressure breathing machines, and nebulizers. The most common aerosol therapy for children is the metered-dose inhaler (MDI) commonly used in the treatment of asthma (see your textbook for a description of this treatment for asthma).

---

### SKILL 12–11  Administering Nebulizer Aerosol Therapy

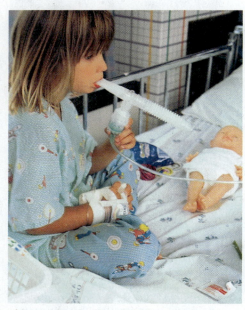

**Figure 12–10** *This child has been taught to use a nebulizer for treatment of her asthma in the hospital. After explanation and demonstration by the nurse, she now independently and effectively completes the treatment.*

#### PREPARATION

1. The dose of the medication is based on the child's weight. The medication is placed in the cup of the aerosol kit; 2 to 3 mL of normal saline can be added as a diluent if ordered.
2. Perform a baseline assessment, including heart and respiratory rates, peak flow, breath sounds, and respiratory effort.
3. Verify the identity of the child and review or explain the procedure to the parents and child.

#### EQUIPMENT AND SUPPLIES

- Reservoir
- Mouthpiece, mask, or blow-by tubing (depending on child's age)
- Portable nebulizing machine or tubing to hook to oxygen supply
- Clean gloves

#### PROCEDURE

1. Don gloves.
2. Place the mask on the child, have the child put the mouthpiece into the mouth (Figure 12–10), or provide an assistant or the parent the tubing for blow-by (used for infants or those unable to cooperate with mask or tubing).
3. Attach the oxygen tubing to the oxygen flow meter at 6 to 7 L/min or use a portable compressor.
4. Have the child take deep breaths during the treatment.
5. The aerosol administration should last about 10 minutes. Reassess the child's condition after the therapy.
6. Document the treatment and the child's response.

# Metered-Dose Inhaler (MDI)

MDIs are small canister devices with a mouthpiece used to treat asthma in the home setting. They may be used by children on a regular basis or during times of respiratory distress. MDIs may be attached to reservoirs, spacers, or extenders for young children who have difficulty holding their breath long enough or closing their mouths securely over the mouthpiece. These extenders maintain the medication near the mouth to facilitate inhalation.

---

### SKILL 12–12  Using a Metered-Dose Inhaler (MDI)

#### EQUIPMENT AND SUPPLIES

- Inhaler with medication
- Clean gloves

#### PROCEDURE

1. Verify the identity of the child and review or explain the procedure to the parent and child.
2. Don gloves.
3. Insert the canister into the mouthpiece.
4. Have the child take a deep breath of room air, inhaling and exhaling completely.

5. Ask the child to close the lips tightly over the MDI mouthpiece and then to inhale deeply and slowly through the mouth while simultaneously depressing the canister 1 time.

6. Have the child hold the breath for about 5 to 10 seconds to enable medication to reach the lungs.

7. Document the procedure and the child's condition and response.

# Topical Medication

Topical medications are available in gels, pastes, creams, lotions, and liquid forms. They are placed directly on the skin in the affected area to relieve or prevent a client's symptoms. Topical medications are easily absorbed through the skin of young children due to their thin skin and increased vascularity. Topical administration provides treatment to the affected area without wide systemic exposure to the medication, often avoiding broad side effects.

---

## SKILL 12–13  Administering Topical Medication

### PREPARATION

1. Verify the medical prescription.
2. Check the expiration date on the medication.
3. Identify the child and explain the procedure to the parents and child.
4. Assess the client's and family's developmental, cognitive, and cultural needs for education, as topical medications are often administered at home.
5. Review if the child has had complications with this or similar medications in the past.

### EQUIPMENT AND SUPPLIES (MAY BE CLEAN OR STERILE PROCEDURE)

- Medication
- Skin cleansing supplies: basin, warm water and soap or cleanser, cleansing cloth or sterile gauze
- Absorbent pad, if needed
- Appropriate applicator-sterile tongue blade or cotton swabs or the nurse's gloved hand may be indicated
- Container if small amount of medication to be given needs to be removed from larger, primary container
- Dressing (e.g., gauze, Tegaderm, tape) as needed
- Clean or sterile gloves, as needed due to skin condition

### PROCEDURE

1. Position the child to permit access to the affected area. Assistance may be needed to hold the child during the application.
2. Don gloves.
3. Assess the skin area or wound.
4. Using the basin, water, and cloth, gently cleanse the skin if intact. Use sterile gauze for open areas to remove debris from the affected areas, as ordered.
5. Dry the skin well, using gentle patting with gauze.
6. Apply the proper amount of medication with the appropriate applicator and spread over the skin as prescribed. Avoid an excess amount to prevent toxicity.
7. Apply a dressing over the site if indicated. Young children may need a dressing to cover and protect the site.
8. For transdermal patches, apply to a clean, dry, flat surface. Do not cut patches to adjust the dose. Rotate sites to ensure proper absorption.
9. Document the procedure and the child's response.

# Rectal Medication

Rectal administration is sometimes used when the oral route is contraindicated. Although absorption is less reliable than with oral preparations, many medications, such as acetaminophen, aspirin, antiemetics, analgesics, and sedatives, come in suppository form.

## SKILL 12–14 Administering Rectal Medication

### PREPARATION

1. If the suppository is to be halved, cut it lengthwise.
2. Verify the identity of the child and explain the procedure to the parent and child. State the name of the drug to be administered.

### EQUIPMENT AND SUPPLIES

- Water-soluble lubricant
- Suppository
- Clean gloves

### PROCEDURE

1. Have another nurse, an assistant, or the parent hold the child in a side-lying or (if small enough) a prone position on the parent's lap.
2. Don gloves.
3. Slightly lubricate the tapered tip of the suppository. Using either the index finger (in children over 3 years of age) or the little finger (in infants and toddlers), gently insert the suppository into the child's rectum, just beyond the internal sphincter.

   RATIONALE: *Lubrication provides for easy insertion and minimal trauma to the mucous membranes. The child's rectum is small in size. Insertion past the sphincter allows the medication to stay in place for absorption.*

4. Hold the buttocks together for 5 to 10 minutes, until the urge to expel the medication has passed.
5. Document the procedure and the child's response.

# Chapter 13
# Intravenous Access

## Peripheral Vascular Access

In both infants and children, veins of the extremities are used for venous access. Scalp veins may also be used in infants.

Over-the-needle catheters (19 to 27 gauge) are preferred for infants and children. The size of the catheter is determined by the size of the child and the size of the vein. For example, a 24-gauge catheter is commonly used for a newborn; a 20- to 22-gauge catheter is usually appropriate for an older infant, toddler, or school-age child. A butterfly needle (23 gauge) may be used in certain situations, such as when accessing a scalp vein in an infant or during an emergency for peripheral access in a toddler. Use of a butterfly needle should be considered a temporary measure, with continued effort made to achieve more stable and secure venous access.

### Choice of Site

#### SCALP

Scalp veins are used when other access cannot be obtained (Figure 13–1A). Protect the site by covering it with a commercial site protector or plastic medication cup secured with tape.

A

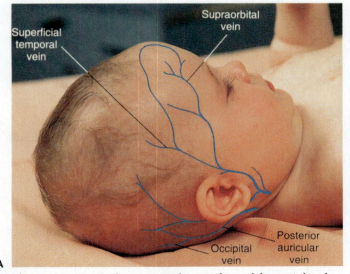

**Figure 13–1A** *Scalp veins are frequently used for peripheral vascular access in infants.*

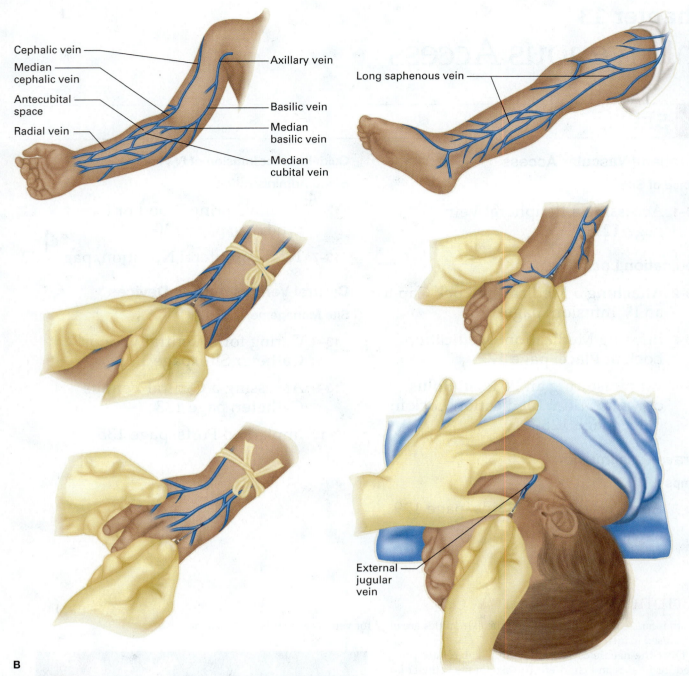

**B**

**Figure 13–1B** *Peripheral veins that may be accessed for intravenous administration of drugs and fluids are those of the arms, hands, legs, and feet plus the external jugular vein.*

## EXTREMITIES

Veins of the antecubital fossa or forearm are usually the best sites for venous access because they are highly visible; however, the dorsum of the hand and foot also may be used (Figure 13–1B).

*Special Considerations*

- Use foot veins as a last resort for sites in children who are walking.
- Avoid using the child's dominant hand or the hand used by an infant for finger sucking or blanket holding.
- If two sites are needed, do not use both antecubital veins because the child will be rendered unable to flex either arm.
- Use padded armboards as splints to decrease mobility of the extremity.
- Use gauze under tape or tape over tape to decrease skin contact with adhesive tape.

- Ensure that the line can always be visualized for inspection.
- Good hand hygiene and sterile procedures must be meticulously followed to prevent infections. Careful, frequent monitoring of the site for infiltration and extravasation as well as for signs of systemic infection is imperative.

## SKILL 13–1 Accessing a Peripheral Vein

### PREPARATION

1. Verify the order for intravenous start and solution, and gather supplies.
2. Place and maintain the child in a supine position with the help of an assistant, or have the child sit in a chair (or lap of assistant) with the arm on a padded table. Have the person assisting you extend the extremity to be used. An alternative to human immobilization is to use a papoose board (see Chapter 9).
3. Identify the child and explain the procedure to the child and parent.

### EQUIPMENT AND SUPPLIES

- Tourniquet
- Chlorhexidine or alcohol per agency policy
- Various sizes of armboards
- Over-the-needle IV catheter or butterfly needle (select appropriate gauge for size of vein)
- T connector that has been flushed and attached to a normal saline–filled syringe
- IV tubing and bag with solution
- Clean gloves

### PROCEDURE

1. If a scalp vein is to be used, place a rubber band around the infant's head to serve as a tourniquet to distend the veins. If the extremities are to be used, place the tourniquet proximal to the desired vein to distend it. If necessary, hold the extremity below heart level, gently rub or tap the vein, or apply a warm compress to promote dilation of the vein.
2. Don gloves.
3. Locate the vein by inspection (wiping with alcohol will make the vein shine) or by palpation.
4. If you are using an extremity, apply an armboard or footboard. Relocate the vein.
5. If using the antecubital fossa: Slightly hyperextend the child's elbow and pronate the arm. Secure the arm to the armboard by applying tape above the elbow and at the wrist.
6. If using the dorsum of the hand: Place the child's hand on the armboard, palmar side down, with the fingers wrapped around the distal edge (Figure 13–2). Apply tape over the fingers, then around the thumb separately. Next apply tape at the wrist. A gauze roll may be placed under the wrist to increase flexion.
   RATIONALE: *Positioning to avoid injury is an important nursing role.*
7. If using the foot: Apply the footboard to the child's foot, which is dorsiflexed. Apply tape across the toes, instep, and ankle. Use gauze as needed under the lateral malleolus.
8. Clean the skin with chlorhexidine or alcohol, per agency policy, using an outward circular motion. Let each area dry before continuing. Apply the tourniquet. Hold the skin taut, gently pulling with your thumb just distal to the site of the puncture.
9. Puncture the skin with the catheter, with the bevel side up, positioned at a 15-degree angle and aimed at the vein in the direction of the blood flow. When blood appears (called a "flash"), gently slide the catheter into the vein. Release the tourniquet. Remove the stylette.
10. Attach the normal saline–filled T connector and attempt to flush the catheter. If it flushes easily, apply a transparent dressing over the site, and wrap with gauze and stockinette to maintain the site. Alternatively, tape the catheter in place, using a V pattern around the catheter itself, and then secure the catheter with gauze and tape (taking care not to cover the area proximal to the site completely).

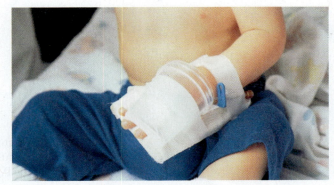

**Figure 13–2** *This intravenous site on the hand has been placed on an armboard, securely wrapped, and covered with a plastic protector to prevent the child from disrupting the line.*

**RATIONALE:** *Wrapping techniques promote intactness of the line and allow for visualization of the site for signs of infiltration or phlebitis.*

11. Write the date, time, catheter size, and your initials on a piece of tape and place it on the dressing.

    **RATIONALE:** *Agencies set policies about how long an IV line can be kept in place. Accurate documentation and labeling ensure changes on schedule to avoid infections.*

12. The T connector can be hooked up to a heparin or saline lock or used immediately for fluid or medication infusion.

13. Document the procedure and the child's response, as well as the present assessment of the intravenous site.

See Chapter 11 for further explanation of intravenous access to obtain a blood sample.

# Medication Lock

The medication lock is a small device placed on the IV catheter and taped in place. It maintains the IV site for future use when not hooked up to a running IV infusion. Some agencies use normal saline, whereas others use heparin solution, to maintain patency of medication. Know and follow your agency policy.

## SKILL 13–2 Attaching a Medication Lock Cap to an IV Infusion

### PREPARATION

1. Verify the order.

2. Verify the identity of the child and explain the procedure to the child and parents.

3. Record intake of intravenous fluid for documentation.

### EQUIPMENT AND SUPPLIES

- Syringe filled with 1 mL of prepackaged heparin flush solution (10 units/mL), if in agency protocol
- Syringe with 2 mL of sterile normal saline
- Luer-Lok male adapter
- Clean gloves

### PROCEDURE

1. Don gloves.

2. Prime the adapter (fill it, being sure to prevent air pockets) with the heparin or saline flush solution. Maintain sterility of the adapter tip that will be inserted into the intravenous line.

3. Save the rest of the flush solution to use when the lock is inserted into the IV tubing.

4. Be sure the IV line is securely taped in place (Figure 13–3*A*). Check the patency of the IV tubing by flushing with 2 mL of sterile normal saline. Be sure there is no redness, swelling, pallor, coolness, or pain at the IV site.

5. Clamp the T connector on the IV line to prevent outflow of blood.

6. Remove the IV tubing from the line and quickly place a primed catheter cap on the T connector.

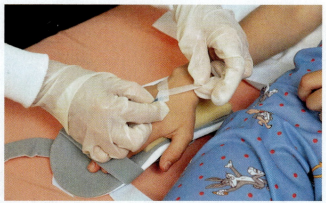
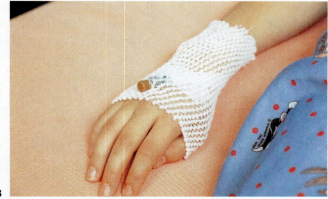

**A**    **B**

**Figure 13–3**  *A, Taping the IV line for placement of a medication lock. **B**, Medication lock in place.*

7. Open the clamp. Insert the flush solution or saline and slowly flush the adapter.

8. Remove the syringe and clamp the medication lock.

9. Secure the medication lock with tape and cover with an elastic bandage (Figure 13–3*B*). The tape is generally labeled with the date and time it was established.

10. Flush the line every 8 hours with heparin flush or saline solution as determined by agency policy.

11. Document the procedure and the child's response.

## SKILL 13–3  Infusing Medication: Medication Lock in Place

### PREPARATION

1. Check the order.

2. Calculate and verify the medication name, dosage, route, and concentration.

3. Verify the identity of the child and explain the procedure to the child and parent.

### EQUIPMENT AND SUPPLIES

- Alcohol swabs
- 19- to 27-gauge needle or needleless system
- Two syringes filled with 2 mL of normal saline with 19- to 27-gauge needles or needleless system
- Medication ordered
- Syringe with 1 mL of heparin flush solution (10 units/mL) or sterile normal saline (use only preservative-free saline for newborns)
- Clean gloves

### PROCEDURE

1. Prepare the medication to be administered.

2. Don gloves.

3. Clean the catheter cap with alcohol. Unclamp the medication lock.

4. Check the patency of the IV tubing by flushing it with normal saline. Check the catheter tip site for swelling.

5. If the IV line is patent and operating, apply the new syringe or needleless system on the distal end of the IV tubing through the cap after cleaning its surface.

    **RATIONALE:**  *Recessed needles or needleless systems are recommended whenever available to promote safety.*

6. Secure the IV tubing and connection area in place with tape.

7. Administer the infusion of medication according to the prescription.

8. Be sure to follow the infusion with 10 to 20 mL of IV fluid so no medication remains in the tubing.

9. After completion of the infusion, discard used equipment into a puncture-proof container according to standard precaution recommendations.

10. If the IV tubing is to be used again, cover it with a clean needle system to ensure sterility.

11. Clean the catheter cap with alcohol.

12. Flush first with 2 mL of normal saline and follow with the heparin flush solution if heparin is to be used (as in the preceding procedure). Clamp the medication lock and secure it in place.

13. Document the procedure and the child's response.

## SKILL 13–4  Administering an IV Push Bolus of Medication: Medication Lock in Place

### PREPARATION

1. Check the order.

2. Calculate and check the medication name, dosage, route, and concentration.

3. Verify the identity of the child and explain the procedure to the child and parents.

### EQUIPMENT AND SUPPLIES

- Alcohol swabs
- Two 1- to 2-mL syringes filled with normal saline with 19- to 25-gauge needles or a needleless system
- Syringe filled with 1 mL of heparin flush solution (10 units/mL) or sterile normal saline
- Medication in syringe covered with a 19- to 25-gauge needle or needleless system
- Clean gloves

### PROCEDURE

1. Don gloves.

2. Clean the catheter cap with alcohol. Unclamp the medication lock.

3. Pierce the catheter cap or attach a needleless system with a normal saline–filled syringe.

4. Flush the line with 2 mL of normal saline to check patency.

5. Remove the syringe and needle.

6. Insert the medication syringe through the catheter cap and give the medication according to the healthcare provider's orders. Check a medication resource book or contact your hospital pharmacy to determine the rate of administration. When all of the medication has been administered, remove the syringe.

7. Flush the line with the 2 mL of normal saline. Follow with heparin flush solution if heparin use is consistent with agency policy and not contraindicated in the patient. Clamp and secure the medication line.

8. Discard the equipment in a puncture-proof container according to standard precaution recommendations.

9. Document the procedure and the child's response.

## Intravenous Infusion

The amount of fluid to be administered to a child is based on the child's weight and pathophysiologic state. It is recommended that fluids be given to the infant or child through an infusion pump (Figure 13–4), as this device allows for a more accurate setting of flow rates than gravity does. Maintenance fluid requirements are based on the child's weight (see Table 13–1).

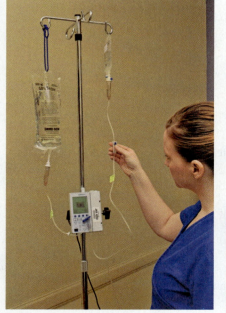

**Figure 13–4** *IV setup with infusion pump.*

| TABLE 13–1 | Pediatric Maintenance Fluid Requirements |
|---|---|
| **Weight (kg)** | **Fluid Requirements** |
| 0–10 | 100 mL/kg/24 hr |
| 10–20 | 1000 mL + 50 mL/kg/24 hr for each kg between 11 and 20 |
| 20–70 | 1500 mL + 20 mL/kg/24 hr for each kg between 21 and 70 |
| Over 70 | 2500 mL/24 hr (adult requirement) |

## Pumps

An infusion pump can be used to control the administration of small volumes of fluid, blood, medication, and total parenteral nutrition. A smaller syringe pump (Figure 13–5) can be attached directly to the lowest port on the IV tubing for immediate infusion of medication.

It is important to be familiar with the type of infusion pump used at your institution. Be sure to set controls for both the amount of fluid to be infused and the rate of infusion. Check the pump frequently to be certain it is programmed and working correctly. Realize that a pump can function even when an intravenous line is infiltrated; perform skin assessments at the site of the line frequently.

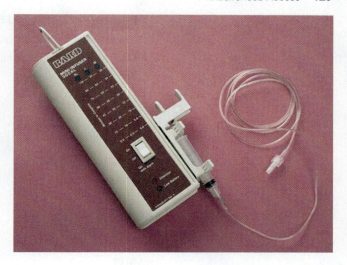

**Figure 13–5**  *Syringe pump.*

## SKILL 13–5  Administering IV Fluids

### PREPARATION

1. Check the fluid order for type of IV fluid and infusion rate. Compare with the fluid needs of the child (see your textbook for calculation of children's maintenance and replacement fluids).
2. Gather supplies.
3. Verify the identity of the child and explain the procedure to the child and parent.

### EQUIPMENT AND SUPPLIES

- Intravenous fluid
- Tubing
- Infusion pump
- Tape and labels
- Clean gloves

### PROCEDURE

1. Check the bag or bottle for leaks, expiration date, impurities, or color changes.
2. Open the tubing package. Make sure that the tubing is clamped off.
3. Remove the protective covering from the insertion piece (spike). Place the insertion piece into the entry port of the bag or bottle. Invert the bag or bottle and hang it on a pole.
4. Pinch the drip chamber (it should be no more than one half to three fourths full). Direct the distal end of the tubing into a clean receptacle, maintaining sterility of the end. Open the clamp and let the fluid run through the length of the tubing. Tap the tubing at each port to remove any trapped air.
5. Close the clamp, recap the sterile end, and check the entire length of tubing for air bubbles. The tubing is now primed and ready for use.
6. If a volume control chamber is used, first attach it to the bag or bottle. Close the clamp that is closest to the fluid and the one that is distal to the chamber. Open the top clamp.
7. Let about 50 mL into the chamber and then close the clamp. Pinch the drip chamber as in step 4. Open the distal clamp, and continue to purge the tubing (as described in step 5).
8. If you are using a pump, check the manufacturer's guidelines for purging the tubing.
9. Mark the bottle or bag with a label and tape that lists the child's identifying information, type of infusion, flow rate, and date and time of preparation.
10. Bring the primed intravenous infusion to the child.
11. Don gloves.
12. Check the IV site carefully for leakage, redness, pallor, swelling, and pain.
13. If replacing a bag that is finished, clamp the tubing on the venous line and on the existing tubing before removing the old tubing.
14. Remove the cover on the end of the IV tubing, maintaining sterility of the tip.
15. Place the tip into the existing IV line.

16. Unclamp the IV line and the tubing and begin the flow of fluid.
17. Check the site carefully as the infusion begins. Repeat assessments according to agency policy.
18. Document the application of a new bag and update the intake of the child considering the bag that has infused.

## Guidelines for Infusion of IV Fluids

Rules for determining flow rate for instilling IV fluids via gravity are based on the drip factor of the IV tubing being used.

### MICRODRIP TUBING

| Manufacturer | Drops/mL |
| --- | --- |
| All major manufacturers | 60 drops (gtt) = 1 mL |

### FORMULA

mL/hr = gtt/min

### EXAMPLE

1000 mL/8 hr = 125 mL/hr = 125 gtt/min

### MACRODRIP TUBING

| Manufacturer | Drops/mL |
| --- | --- |
| Abbot | 15 gtt = 1 mL |
| Baxter | 10 gtt = 1 mL |

### FORMULA

Total volume × Drop factor/Infusion time in minutes = Drops/minute

### EXAMPLE

1000 mL × 10(Baxter)/8 hr (480 min) = 21 gtt/min

## Blood Administration

To safely administer blood or blood products to the infant or child, be aware of the protocols followed at your agency. Check to be sure that an informed consent for blood administration has been obtained. Because hypersensitivity reactions can occur and other side effects can be severe, administration of blood is approached with many nursing cautions. Be sure to take vital signs and monitor the child closely. Follow instructions from the blood bank and other resources for correct administration of blood products, such as frozen plasma, cryoprecipitate, and clotting factors.

---

## SKILL 13–6 Administering Blood or Blood Products

### PREPARATION

1. Identify the bag to be used, and compare it with the requisition (type, Rh factor, patient number, blood donor number) and the child's identification bracelet. Do this step with another licensed nurse at the bedside. Both nurses are responsible for signing the slips as the transfusers.
   RATIONALE: *Administration of blood can potentially cause injury to the patient. Having two nurses check minimizes the opportunity for error.*

2. Check the blood for any bubbles, dark areas, or sediment.
   RATIONALE: *These discolorations can indicate that the blood is old or has not been properly maintained.*

3. Explain the procedure to the child and parents. Ask the child or family about previous transfusions, especially any history of allergic reactions.

4. Take the child's vital signs, including pulse, respiratory rate, temperature, and blood pressure.
   RATIONALE: *Baseline vital signs may be useful for comparison later in the procedure.*

**SAFETY ALERT**

Blood is administered according to the physician's orders. However, a bag should never remain hanging longer than 4 hours. Do not use the blood line for any other infusions. If a medication must be administered by that line, turn off the infusion, flush the line with normal saline, administer the medication, flush the line again with normal saline, and then restart the blood infusion.

5. When estimating preparation time, keep in mind that blood must be hung within 20 to 30 minutes after being removed from the blood bank refrigerator and administration must be completed in 4 hours. For trauma patients who need massive transfusions, the bag should be warmed to 37°C (99°F) (only an approved blood warmer should be used).

6. Use the correct tubing for the blood product being administered. A Y blood administration set is preferred. If a Y setup is used, hang normal saline at the extra connector.

## HOME AND COMMUNITY CARE CONSIDERATIONS

When a child receives a transfusion of blood or blood products, administration of live immunizations should be delayed for variable periods afterward. Live vaccines such as measles and varicella immunizations are most likely to be rendered ineffective by blood transfusions. Be sure to let parents know and provide in writing the type of product used (e.g., whole blood, packed red cells, frozen plasma) and the date of the infusion. Instruct them to take this with them when they next visit their regular healthcare provider so that adaptations in immunization administration may be implemented if needed (Centers for Disease Control and Prevention [CDC], 2015).

### EQUIPMENT AND SUPPLIES

- Blood product
- Blood warmer if needed
- Blood filter
- Y tubing and bag of normal saline
- Normal saline flush solution
- Sterile needle or needleless system
- Intravenous line in place with 18-gauge needle or larger
- Clean or sterile gloves

### PROCEDURE

1. Don gloves.
2. Attach the blood bag to one end of the Y tubing. Flush the line with normal saline attached to the other side of the Y tubing.
   RATIONALE: *Checking the line for patency and using normal saline to prevent incompatibilities contribute to safe infusion.*
3. Clamp off the tubing, keeping the distal end covered.
4. Disconnect it, covering the hub with a sterile needle or needleless system to keep it sterile. Flush the child's IV line with normal saline to ensure its patency.
5. Attach the blood tubing.
6. Slowly open the clamp on the tubing, adjusting the flow with the roller. Start the transfusion slowly. Instruct the child and/or parent to report any reactions immediately.
7. The flow rate may be increased if no reaction is noted.
   RATIONALE: *Most reactions occur within 20 minutes.*
8. Closely monitor the child's vital signs and response. Vital signs should be taken every 5 minutes for the first 15 minutes, every 15 minutes during the first hour, then hourly until the transfusion is complete (or follow your hospital's protocol).
9. If the child develops any sign of a transfusion reaction (Table 13–2), stop the transfusion, change the IV to normal saline, and notify the physician immediately.

| TABLE 13–2 | Transfusion Reactions | |
| --- | --- | --- |
| **Type of Reaction** | **Cause** | **Description** |
| Allergic | Caused by immune response to protein in blood | Signs and symptoms may include rash, itching, urticaria, wheezing, laryngospasm, edema, and/or anaphylaxis |
| Febrile or septic | Usually a result of contamination of blood; may also be caused by idiopathic conditions | Signs and symptoms include chills, fever, headache, decreased blood pressure, nausea and/or vomiting, and leg or back pain |
| Hemolytic | Caused by incompatibility of child's blood with donor blood, history of multiple transfusions, or infusion with a solution containing dextrose or other additives | Signs and symptoms include anxiety or restlessness, fever, chills, chest pain, cyanosis, change in vital signs with increased heart and respiratory rates or with decreased blood pressure and/or hematuria; can progress to shock and anuria if not treated promptly |
| Circulatory overload | Results from infusion of excessive amounts of fluid or too rapid administration | Signs and symptoms include labored breathing, chest or lower back pain, productive cough with rales heard on auscultation, and distended neck veins; central venous pressure may increase |

10. After the administration of blood, flush the line with normal saline and connect the IV fluid ordered by the physician. Place the used blood bag and tubing in a plastic bag, seal it, and return it to the blood bank with copies of the transfusion information sheet.
    **RATIONALE:** *This is a method of verification of the blood use and the patient data.*

11. Document blood administration, vital signs, responses, and interventions.

---

### HOME AND COMMUNITY CARE CONSIDERATIONS

Total parenteral nutrition (TPN) is increasingly administered in the home setting. It may run continuously or be started at night to enable the child needing extra dietary supplementation to have enhanced intake while sleeping. Be sure that parents understand infusion techniques, care of the line, and where to call with questions. Visit the home to be sure the setting can facilitate TPN treatment.

---

## SKILL 13–7 Total Parenteral Nutrition

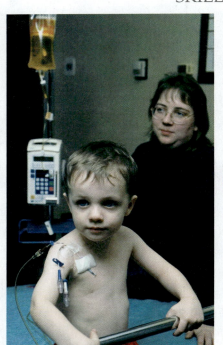

**Figure 13–6** *This child is receiving TPN.*

Total parenteral nutrition (TPN) is the administration of a nutritionally complete formula into a large central vein (see Figure 13–6). TPN is used for children who cannot tolerate gastrointestinal feeding. Children with disorders such as chronic intestinal obstruction, short bowel syndrome, chronic diarrhea, or tumors may require TPN.

Hyperalimentation solutions (TPN as well as lipid emulsions) are delivered by separate pumps and connector tubes. The child who is receiving TPN has a central venous catheter in place (see following skill). Solutions and tubes need to be changed every 24 hours using strict aseptic technique. Tips and connecting points need to be sterile. Nursing responsibilities when caring for a child receiving TPN are outlined in Table 13–3.

| TABLE 13–3 | Caring for the Child Receiving TPN |
|---|---|

- Monitor intake and output. Changes may indicate fluid and electrolyte disturbances.
- Weigh the child daily.
- Assess the infusion site. Watch for signs of redness, irritation, or infection. Change the dressing according to hospital protocol (see the procedure for managing a central venous catheter site in this chapter).
- Use the infusion site only for TPN solutions or keep the line open with normal saline. Do not use the line for medications or other infusions. The type of line required is related to the amount of glucose in solution. Work with the physician, pharmacist, and nutritionist to plan care and evaluation procedures.
- Make sure to set each pump correctly, noting the volume and rate of each infusion.
- Check laboratory values, especially glucose, minerals, electrolytes, liver function (bilirubin, alkaline phosphatase), proteins, and triglycerides.
- Note any change in glucose levels:
  1. During the first few days, the high concentration of glucose administration may lead to hyperglycemia. Inform the physician of high blood glucose levels. Insulin may be needed to help the body adjust to the formula.
  2. If hyperalimentation is discontinued abruptly, the child may become hypoglycemic, so taper the infusion gradually as prescribed to reduce this risk. Be aware of the signs and symptoms of hypoglycemia (see your textbook for a full description). Notify the physician if the child's blood glucose level is low.

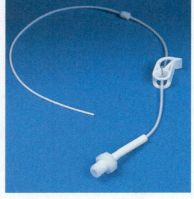

**Figure 13–7** *Broviac catheter.*

# Central Venous Access Devices

A central venous access device is surgically placed when long-term IV access is needed, such as for total parenteral nutrition, administration of antibiotics, or chemotherapy. Often the subclavian vein is accessed and the catheter is threaded into the right atrium.

A common catheter used for children is the Broviac catheter (Figure 13–7), which can have a single, double, or triple lumen. Other catheters such as the Hickman may be used with older children. Peripherally inserted central catheter lines (PICC lines) are also common in children.

Clear guidelines are available from the Centers for Disease Control and Prevention (CDC) and U.S. Department of Health and Human Services (USDHHS) for insertion of central lines and for their care (CDC, 2011; O'Grady et al., 2011). Catheter care and flushing must follow protocols to decrease the risk of central line–associated bloodstream infections (CLABSI) (CDC, 2011; Dumont & Nesselrodt, 2012). These procedures are described in the following skills.

## Site Management

The catheter site is covered with a transparent occlusive dressing that should be changed under sterile conditions according to national and agency protocol.

---

## SKILL 13–8  Caring for a Central Venous Catheter Site

### PREPARATION

1. Gather necessary supplies.
2. Evaluate the dressing and visible skin at the catheter site.
3. Verify the identity of the child and explain the procedure to the child and parents.
4. Assess the catheter location.

### EQUIPMENT AND SUPPLIES

- 2% chlorhexidine in 70% alcohol solution
- Central venous catheter kit (If not available, collect clean and sterile gloves, sterile gauze, and sterile occlusive dressing.)
- Sterile occlusive dressing
- Sterile chlorhexidine-impregnated patch if in agency protocol
- Clean gloves, sterile gloves, and mask

### PROCEDURE

1. Perform hand hygiene. Open the kit. Don the mask and clean gloves.
2. Remove the current dressing, working from the edges toward the center. Inspect the site. Discard the old dressing and gloves.
3. Perform hand hygiene, and don the sterile gloves.
4. Clean the catheter site with sterile 2% chlorhexidine in 70% alcohol or according to agency policy. Use back-and-forth scrubbing for 30 seconds.
5. Clean the catheter tubing from the exit site to the cap.
6. Let dry. Place chlorhexidine-impregnated patch if in agency protocol, or otherwise a small sterile gauze dressing over the catheter insertion site. Do not use antibiotic ointment or cream (except for hemodialysis insertion sites), as they may promote fungal infections and antibiotic resistance. Cover with a sterile occlusive dressing.
7. Write the date, time, and your initials on a piece of tape and place it on the dressing.
8. Document the procedure, the condition of the site, and the child's response.

---

## SKILL 13–9  Accessing a Central Venous Catheter

A central line may be accessed for the drawing of blood samples. The single-syringe method is described here. See Skill 11–5 in Chapter 11 for collection of blood cultures.

### PREPARATION

1. Check the physician's order for the blood tests to be done.
   **RATIONALE:** *It is recommended that the catheter be accessed no more than twice a day to minimize the chance of infection.*
2. Verify the identity of the child and explain the procedure to the child and parents.
3. Locate an assistant to open and close the clamps as necessary and put the blood in tubes while you are flushing the line.

### EQUIPMENT AND SUPPLIES

- Sterile 4″ × 4″ gauze pad
- Chlorhexidine or other solution per agency protocol

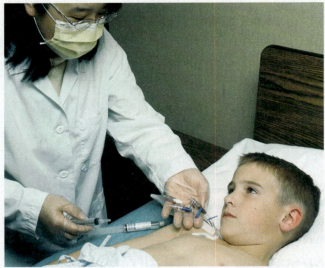

**Figure 13–8** *The nurse uses sterile technique and carefully examines the central line to plan access from the proper port.*

- Cotton-tipped swabs
- Appropriate blood collection tubes
- 19- to 27-gauge needles for transferring blood to tubes
- Padded clamp (if a clamp is not attached to tubing)
- Sterile gloves, mask

*For each port accessed:*
- Syringe filled with 5 to 6 mL of normal saline
- Syringe filled with 20 mL of normal saline
- Syringe filled with 2 to 3 mL of heparin flush solution (10 units/mL), if in agency protocol
- 10-mL empty syringe (to draw and discard initial blood)
- Syringes for blood samples
- Luer-Lok or Broviac catheter cap

**PROCEDURE**

1. Unpin the catheter from the child's clothes. Remove any tape. Open a sterile 4″ × 4″ gauze pad to serve as a clean work area. Don sterile gloves and mask. Place the gauze under the catheter connection. If the intravenous solution is infusing, turn it off (Figure 13–8).

2. Clean the connection site with chlorhexidine. Use three swabs, and clean for a total of 2 minutes. Let the connection site dry for an additional 20 seconds.

3. Make sure the catheter is clamped. Remove the catheter cap or infusion tubing (removal unnecessary if using needleless system), maintaining sterility. Flush the catheter with 2 to 5 mL of normal saline to ensure patency. Slowly aspirate 3 to 5 mL of blood (2 mL for infants less than 7.5 kg). Clamp the catheter and discard the syringe. Using another 10-mL syringe, aspirate the amount of blood necessary. Remove the blood-filled syringe, and cover with a 19-gauge needle or needleless system. Give that syringe to your assistant to fill the blood collection tubes. Meanwhile, attach the syringe filled with normal saline. Flush the line first with the 20 mL of normal saline, then, if used in agency, with the prepared heparin flush solution.

4. Clamp the catheter and remove the flush syringe. Connect the infusion solution, or cover the port with a sterile protector.

5. Secure the catheter to the child's clothing. Remove the gloves and wash your hands.

6. Ensure that blood specimens are labeled properly, kept at proper temperature, and transported to the laboratory.

7. Document the procedure, the condition of the catheter site, and the child's response, and note that the specimens were transported to the laboratory.

## SKILL 13–10  Implanted Ports

Implanted ports are used most often for children and adolescents who require long-term venous access. The stainless steel port has a self-sealing rubber septum and is surgically implanted under the skin over a bony prominence, most often the clavicle. The catheter is then inserted into the vein that leads to the right atrium. Entry is gained by piercing the skin directly over the port with a specially designed needle (Figure 13–9). Sterile gloves, mask, and gown are worn when accessing the site. Specially trained nurses may access the site to administer chemotherapy or other medications. Consult agency policy and advanced practice resources for more information about accessing implanted ports. The Port-a-Cath is used commonly in pediatrics.

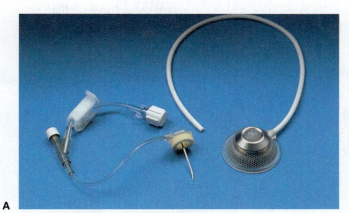
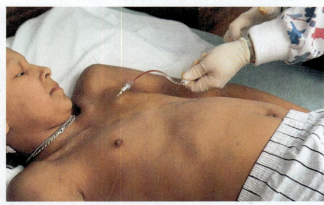

A    B

**Figure 13–9**  *A, Huber needle. B, Nurse drawing blood from an adolescent who has an implanted port.*

# Chapter 14
# Neurologic Assessment and Care

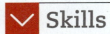 **Skills**

## Special Neurologic Assessments

### SKILL 14–1 Neurovascular Assessment

A neurovascular assessment of an extremity is performed frequently, such as when an extremity is injured, from a fracture or circumferential burn, or following surgery. The circulatory status and nerve function are both evaluated in the injured extremity and compared to the other extremity. See Chapter 18 regarding cast care for application of this assessment.

**PROCEDURE**

1. Assess the swelling in the extremity associated with the injury.
   **RATIONALE:** *The swelling associated with the injury may constrict blood flow to the distal extremity and pinch the nerves, especially when constriction is present, such as a cast.*

2. Assess the extremity distal to the injury for color and temperature and compare to the other extremity.

3. Assess the distal extremity for a pulse.

4. Assess the capillary refill time by pressing on a finger or toe for a couple of seconds, until the skin is blanched. Count how long it takes for blood or color to return to the area pressed. It should take 2 seconds or less.

5. Assess the extremity for pain and paresthesia (sensation of numbness, tingling, pins-and-needles sensation) and compare to the other extremity.

6. Assess the child's ability to move the fingers or toes of the affected extremity.

7. Consider all the findings simultaneously to complete the neurovascular assessment.

8. The presence of most or all of the five "Ps" indicates compartment syndrome (pressure that significantly impairs circulation and injures nerves) that needs urgent healthcare provider notification and emergency intervention:

   - Pallor or cyanosis, cool or cold temperature
   - Pain—moderate to severe
   - Paresthesia—numbness, tingling, or pins-and-needles sensation
   - Paralysis
   - Pulse is absent or capillary refill time is greater than 4 seconds
     **RATIONALE:** *If the circulatory and neurologic constriction is not detected and promptly relieved, permanent damage to the distal extremity may result.*

9. Document the assessment and repeat it frequently, especially if one or two findings are present.

## SKILL 14–2 Glasgow Coma Scale

The Glasgow Coma Scale is used to quantify the level of consciousness to compare with future scores and detect changes in the child's condition. Pediatric criteria, which take into account the child's developmental age for each category of the test, have been established to assess responses to eye opening, verbal response, and motor response (Table 14–1).

### PROCEDURE

1. When the child has an injury to the head or altered consciousness, assess the child using each of the three categories of the Glasgow Coma Scale according to the criteria in Table 14–1. In some cases, the child will need stimulation to obtain a response that can be scored. Initially, determine if all categories can be assessed (e.g., the child who is intubated cannot be assessed for verbal response).

2. Document the time performed, the score for each category, and the total score. The total for all three categories is the Glasgow Coma Scale score. See Table 14–1 for score interpretation.

3. Repeat the test at regular intervals for children defined in step 1.

   RATIONALE: *Because the test provides a numeric score for altered consciousness, regular measurements help detect subtle changes in the child's condition.*

| TABLE 14–1 | Glasgow Coma Scale for Assessment of Coma in Infants and Children | | |
|---|---|---|---|
| **Category** | **Score\*** | **Preverbal Child Criteria** | **Older Child and Adult Criteria** |
| Eye opening | 4 | Spontaneous opening | Spontaneous |
| | 3 | To voice or sound | To sound |
| | 2 | To pain | To pressure |
| | 1 | No response to painful stimuli | No response |
| Verbal response | 5 | Smiles, coos, cries to appropriate stimuli; words or sentences normal for age | Oriented; uses appropriate words and phrases |
| | 4 | Irritable; spontaneous crying | Confused |
| | 3 | Cries to pain | Words |
| | 2 | Moans to pain | Incomprehensible sounds |
| | 1 | No response | No response |
| Motor response | 6 | Spontaneous movement | Obeys commands |
| | 5 | Purposeful; localizes pain | Localizes pain |
| | 4 | Withdraws to pain | Normal flexion |
| | 3 | Flexion to pain | Abnormal flexion |
| | 2 | Extension to pain | Extension, extensor posturing |
| | 1 | No response; flaccid | No response; flaccid |

*Add the score from each category to get the total. The maximum score is 15, indicating the best level of neurologic functioning. The minimum is 3, indicating total neurologic unresponsiveness.

Source: Teasdale, G., & Jennett, B. (1974). Assessment of coma and impaired consciousness. *Lancet, 2,* 81–84; James, H. E. (1986). Neurologic evaluation and support in the child with acute brain insult. *Pediatric Annals, 15*(1), 16–22; Bethel, J. (2012). Emergency care of children and adults with head injury. *Nursing Standard, 26*(43), 49–56; Teasdale, G., Allan, D., Brennan, P., McElhinney, E., & Mackinnon, L. (2014). Forty years on: Updating the Glasgow Coma Scale. *Nursing Times, 110*(42), 12–16; Teasdale, G., Maas, A., Lecky, F., Manley, G., Stocchetti, N., & Murray, G. (2014). The Glasgow Coma Scale at 40 years: Standing the test of time. *Lancet Neurology, 13*(8), 844–854; Worrall, K. (2004). Use of the Glasgow Coma Scale in infants. *Paediatric Nursing, 16*(4), 45–47.

## SKILL 14–3 External Ventricular Drain Care

An intraventricular catheter may be inserted into the brain ventricle and attached to an external ventricular drain (EVD) to monitor intracranial pressure (ICP), to drain cerebrospinal fluid, and to instill medication. A surgeon inserts the intraventricular catheter using sterile technique, most often in the operating room or intensive care unit. Since the intraventricular catheter is inserted into the meninges and brain, the child is at risk for infection. Using sterile technique, the nurse primes the EVD system and then assists the physician to connect the EVD system and ICP monitoring equipment (see Skill 14–4). This skill describes maintenance care after the catheter has been inserted.

## PREPARATION

1. Review the child's electronic health record related to indications for the intraventricular catheter and EVD.

2. Review the physician's orders for care and drainage parameters.

3. Verify the identity of the child.

4. Provide explanations to the child and family about the care to be provided.

## EQUIPMENT AND SUPPLIES

- Sterile gloves, mask, and gown
- Sterile dressings (4″ × 4″ gauze)
- External ventricular drainage system
- ICP transducer system and monitor
- Sterile specimen cup

## PROCEDURE

1. Assess the child's neurologic status, vital signs, oxygen saturation level, and ICP level following the insertion procedure and hourly or at intervals according to hospital policy.

2. Ensure that the drainage system is attached to an IV pole at the correct height. Reassess the height of the system each time the child's position is changed.

3. Assess the drainage system every 4 hours or as directed by hospital policy. Inspect the entire drainage system for cracks or fluid leaking from the insertion site. Assess for kinks and any signs of blood or debris that could block the tubing.
   RATIONALE: *Any obstruction of the tubing will interfere with drainage and the ability to calculate the ICP.*

4. Describe the color and clarity of the cerebrospinal fluid (CSF). Measure the drainage from the tubing into the flow chamber at least every 4 hours or according to hospital protocol, and then empty the flow chamber into the drainage bag. CSF may initially be bloody after insertion of the catheter and then turn yellowish or clear. Notify the healthcare provider if CSF flow is obstructed.

5. Maintain the collection bag in an upright position to prevent the spread of bacteria toward the EVD. Empty the drainage bag when full through the injection site port into a container and discard the drainage in the toilet.

6. If an occlusive sterile dressing is placed over the EVD insertion site, remove and reapply a tight occlusive sterile dressing using sterile technique at the frequency directed by hospital policy. Take care to avoid pulling the catheter. Inspect the insertion site for leakage and signs of infection before reapplying the dressing.

7. Ensure that the tubing ports and stopcocks for the EVD system are clearly labeled.
   RATIONALE: *EVD lines must not be used for IV fluid or medication. Labeling the lines reduces this risk.*

8. If an EVD access port is to be accessed to instill medication or obtain a culture, scrub the access port with povidine-iodine or cleanser as recommended by hospital policy (American Association of Neuroscience Nurses [AANN], 2011).

9. Clamp the EVD, if directed by hospital policy, when the child has a response or procedure that may cause overdrainage of CSF, such as suctioning, vomiting, coughing, or repositioning (AANN, 2011). Remember to release the clamp when appropriate.

10. After removal of the EVD, assess the child's vital signs, oxygen saturation, and neurologic status. Monitor the site for a CSF leak to determine if an additional suture is needed to close the incision and prevent a potential infection.

---

## SKILL 14–4 Intracranial Pressure Monitoring

Intracranial pressure (ICP) is the force exerted by brain tissue, cerebrospinal fluid (CSF), and the blood within the cranial vault. Increased ICP can result from traumatic brain injury, brain tumors, or infection. Increased ICP results in decreased cerebral perfusion pressure (CPP), which is the amount of pressure needed to ensure that adequate oxygen and nutrients will be delivered to the brain.

ICP monitoring is often accomplished with intraventricular catheter placement, an EVD, or parenchymal monitors. CSF may also be drained from the EVD to lower the ICP.

## PREPARATION

1. Review the patient's chart related to indications for ICP monitoring.

2. Review the physician's orders for monitoring and CSF drainage parameters.

3. Verify the identity of the child.

4. Provide explanations to the child and family about the need for ICP monitoring.

## EQUIPMENT AND SUPPLIES

- ICP transducer system and monitor
- Sterile gloves, mask, and gown

## PROCEDURE

1. Ensure that the fluid-filled transducer system is placed and maintained at the level of the foramen of Monro. Balance the ICP transducer to zero for calibration (also called *leveling*) according to hospital guidelines, and rezero the transducer at each shift or when the child's position changes.

   **RATIONALE:** *This ensures the accuracy of pressure readings and waveforms by the transducer system.*

2. ICP monitoring is usually continuous. When an external ventricular drain is present, document the ICP and CPP at the frequency ordered by the physician or by hospital protocol. Turn the stopcock to the off position to the EVD, and the open position to the transducer to obtain the ICP reading and waveform. Document the ICP reading and print ICP waveforms. Waveforms provide information about brain compliance in relation to adaptation to increased ICP and decreases in CPP. See Table 14–2.

### CLINICAL TIP

Cerebral perfusion pressure (CPP) is calculated by subtracting the ICP from the mean arterial pressure. Normal CPP is 60 to 150 mmHg. Normal ICP is 5 to 15 mmHg.

### SAFETY ALERT

Use the agency guideline for placement of the transducer system (e.g., an anatomic landmark such as the tragus of the ear or the outer canthus of the eye). This increases accuracy in measuring ICP as all providers use the same reference point for leveling.

| TABLE 14–2 | ICP Waveforms and Implications | |
|---|---|---|
| **Waveform** | **Pressure (mmHg)** | **Implications** |
| A | 50–100 | Symptoms related to cerebral dysfunction; changes in vital signs, respiratory pattern, and motor function; headache; and emesis |
| B | 20–50 | Decreasing level of consciousness, agitation, varying respiratory pattern |
| C | 4–20 | No clinical significance |
| Normal | 4–15 | Normal |

| TABLE 14–3 | Signs of Increased Intracranial Pressure |
|---|---|
| **Timing of Signs** | **Signs** |
| Early signs | Headache<br>Visual disturbances, diplopia<br>Nausea and vomiting<br>Dizziness or vertigo<br>Slight change in vital signs<br>Pupils less reactive, may be unequal<br>Sunsetting eyes (cranial nerve IV palsy)<br>Seizures<br>Slight change in level of consciousness |
| Additional signs in infants | Bulging fontanelle<br>Wide sutures, increased head circumference<br>Dilated scalp veins<br>High-pitched, catlike cry |
| Late signs | Significant decrease in level of consciousness<br>Cushing's triad<br>  ■ Increased systolic blood pressure and widened pulse pressure<br>  ■ Bradycardia<br>  ■ Irregular respirations<br>Fixed and dilated pupils |

3. Assess the child's responsiveness, vital signs, and neurologic status. Assess for signs of increased ICP. See Table 14–3.

   RATIONALE: *Children with brain injuries or following neurosurgery are at risk for seizures and cerebral edema, which further compromise CPP.*

4. Assess pain and comfort level. Administer sedation and pain medication as prescribed.

   RATIONALE: *Patients may experience pain at the catheter insertion site and pain from increased ICP. Medications promote the child's comfort and help reduce elevations in ICP.*

5. Maintain the child's position with the head at midline with the remainder of the body and the head of the bed elevated 15 to 30 degrees or according to physician order.

   RATIONALE: *This position prevents compression of blood vessels in the neck and obstruction of venous blood flow from the brain to the heart.*

6. Monitor patient neurologic status during nursing care and continue or stop nursing interventions depending on patient response. Document care and patient response.

   RATIONALE: *Anxiety, agitation, pain, hypoxia, hypertension, head position out of neutral alignment, some environmental stimuli, and clustering nursing care procedures may elevate the ICP (Casey, 2013). Signs indicating poor patient response to interventions include deterioration in clinical signs, increase in ICP greater than 10 mmHg above baseline longer than 3 minutes, and wide-amplitude waveform and/or the appearance of plateau waves.*

7. Document the ICP reading, CPP, waveforms, and the child's neurologic status at intervals specified by hospital guidelines or physician order. Urgently notify the physician if the ICP reading increases beyond the parameter specified.

# Chapter 15
# Cardiorespiratory Care

# Administering Oxygen

When administering oxygen, the concentration ordered and the age of the child are important. Humidification is often necessary to prevent the nasal passages from drying out. Because oxygen is combustible, certain precautions must be taken during its use.

## Oxygen Delivery Systems

Several methods are used to provide supplemental oxygen to infants and children. Methods are often selected based on the desired concentration of oxygen. The amount of oxygen concentration delivered by the type of oxygen delivery system varies by the child's age, respiratory rate, and volume of air moved with each breath.

### MASKS

The size of the mask is important when administering oxygen. The mask should extend from the bridge of the nose to the cleft of the chin. It should fit snugly on the face but put no pressure on the eyes to avoid stimulating a vagal response. The following types of masks are available (Sarnaik, Clark, & Sarnaik, 2016):

■ The simple face mask (Figure 15–1A) can deliver from 30% to 65% oxygen when a flow rate of 5 to 10 L/min is used.

■ The partial nonrebreather mask has a reservoir bag and two open exhalation ports that also allow room air to enter during inspiration. It can deliver up to 60% oxygen with a flow rate high enough to keep the reservoir bag from collapsing (e.g., 5 to 10 L/min).

■ The nonrebreathing mask (Figure 15–1B) has a reservoir bag, exhalation ports, and valves that minimize the mixing of exhaled air and room air with oxygen. It can deliver up to 95% oxygen when a tight seal to the face is maintained.

### NASAL CANNULA

A nasal cannula is used to deliver low-flow, low-concentration oxygen. It does not provide humidified oxygen. A flow rate set higher than 5 L/min will irritate the nasopharynx without appreciably improving the child's oxygenation. The nasal cannula can deliver up to 23% to 40% oxygen with a flow rate of 1 to 5 L/min; however, the actual concentration varies by the child's respiratory rate and depth (Sarnaik et al., 2016).

The prongs of the cannula are placed in the anterior nares, and the elastic band is placed around the child's head (Figure 15–1C). Infants, preschoolers, and school-age children usually tolerate the cannula. Toddlers may pull the nasal cannula off. A face mask or blow-by oxygen is often a more appropriate method of oxygen administration for the toddler age group.

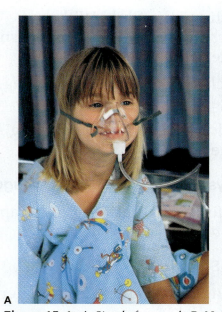
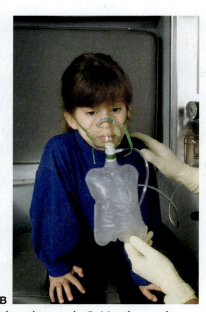
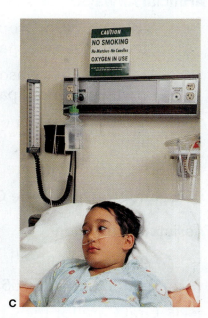

A　　　　　　　　　　　B　　　　　　　　　　　C

**Figure 15–1** *A, Simple face mask. B, Nonrebreather mask. C, Nasal cannula.*

## HOOD

An oxygen hood placed over the head or head and upper torso is used in neonates to provide a concentration of 30% to 60% oxygen, depending on how much room air is mixed in. This device provides good visibility of the head and greater access to the neonate without disturbing oxygen delivery.

## TENT

An oxygen tent, in theory, allows for delivery of 21% to 50% humidified oxygen at a flow rate of 10 to 15 L/min, but because of leakage, the higher concentration is rarely achieved. Concentration should be determined with an oxygen analyzer. To avoid air leakage, secure the edges of the tent with blankets. An oxygen tent reduces visibility of and access to the child for assessment and nursing care. The child may feel confined, isolated from parents, or claustrophobic. The child may respond more favorably to using a mask when awake and the tent while asleep.

## BLOW-BY CANNULA

A blow-by cannula may be either a narrow oxygen catheter with small perforations inserted through the bottom of a paper cup, or corrugated oxygen tubing. This method is used when the child will not tolerate other methods of oxygen therapy and when low oxygen concentrations with humidification are needed, such as in the emergency department. The concentration of oxygen delivered varies according to the flow rate and proximity to the face. The parent can hold the child in the lap and direct the tubing toward the child's face, moving it as the child moves. This technique reduces the child's anxiety and facilitates parental involvement in care.

---

## SKILL 15–1  Using Oxygen Delivery Systems

### PREPARATION

1. Review the healthcare provider's order for the oxygen delivery system.
2. Verify the identity of the child and explain the procedure to the child and parents.
3. Attach a sterile water-filled container to the oxygen or flow meter with a connecting tube.
4. Inform the child and parents about the need for oxygen, how it will be provided, and how they can assist with the procedure. Prepare the child for the sensation of air blowing on the face.

### EQUIPMENT AND SUPPLIES

- Oxygen canister or wall outlet, tubing, and flow meter
- Oxygen delivery system
- Sterile water-filled container
- Oximeter

### PROCEDURE

1. Perform a baseline assessment of vital signs, color, respiratory effort, pulse oximetry reading, and level of consciousness.
   RATIONALE: *The baseline assessment provides a comparison to measure the effectiveness of oxygen therapy.*
2. Turn on the oxygen to the ordered flow rate.
3. Place the oxygen delivery device on the child's face. If the child resists the device, check the fit, and try to improve the child's comfort. Use distraction while the child becomes accustomed to the device.
4. When an oxygen tent is used, secure the edges to prevent oxygen leakage. If the child resists the tent, try to have a parent reassure the child and provide activities that can be performed in the tent.
5. Monitor the child's response to the therapy with ongoing assessments compared to baseline.
6. Report and document the child's condition and changes related to oxygen therapy.

# Cardiorespiratory Monitoring

## SKILL 15–2 Oxygen Saturation: Pulse Oximetry

Pulse oximetry is a simple noninvasive method to measure the percentage of hemoglobin that is available to transport oxygen in the blood by emitting red and infrared light over a pulsating vascular bed and measuring the intensity of light transmitted through the tissue. Oxygenated hemoglobin absorbs more red and infrared light than deoxygenated hemoglobin. The red and infrared light is absorbed by hemoglobin in the arterial blood with each pulsation, and an estimate of hemoglobin saturation can then be calculated ($SpO_2$, the percentage of hemoglobin that is capable of transporting oxygen) (Chan, Chan, & Chan, 2013).

### PREPARATION

1. Verify the identity of the child.

2. Explain the procedure to the child and parent and why it is needed. Inform the child that pulse oximetry is a pain-free method of monitoring the oxygen level in the blood.

3. Select the appropriate sensor size for the child, either infant or pediatric size. Size is determined by the size of the child and/or the placement site.

4. Set the oximeter parameters for alarms according to healthcare provider directions or agency policy.

### EQUIPMENT AND SUPPLIES

- Pulse oximeter
- Appropriate-size sensor

### PROCEDURE

1. Perform a baseline assessment before attaching the sensor. Check respiratory status, including heart rate, respiratory rate, skin color, and respiratory effort.

2. Turn on the oximeter. Attach the sensor to the machine.

3. Place the sensor on the fingernail, toenail, or earlobe with the transducer on one side and the receiver opposite to it, separated by tissue with a pulsatile blood flow (Yönt, Korhanb, & Dizer, 2014) (Figure 15–2). It should be approximately at heart level.

   RATIONALE: *The earlobe is used when the child has poor perfusion. This site is considered a central location, especially because a large percentage of the blood goes to the head and brain.*

4. Position the sensor with the cord leading toward the child. Secure the cord to the child to stabilize the sensor for more reliable readings.

5. Watch for a readout of the pulse rate and oxygen saturation level.

6. Leave the oximeter on for continuous readouts. Remove the sensor from the extremity at least every 2 hours to check the condition of the skin.

7. If frequent but noncontinuous monitoring is ordered, leave the sensor on the child but disconnect it from the machine.

   RATIONALE: *Disconnecting the machine allows the child freedom to move and feel less confined.*

8. If the sensor is removed, place it on the plastic backing for further use. This maintains the adhesive so the sensor can be reused.

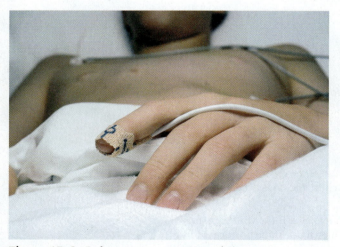

**Figure 15–2** *Pulse oximeter sensor on finger.*

## SKILL 15–3 Cardiorespiratory or Apnea Monitor

The standard cardiorespiratory monitor measures heart rate and respiratory rate when continuous assessments of the heart and respiratory rates are required. An apnea monitor is used to monitor for abnormal or irregular breathing in infants.

## PREPARATION

1. Verify the identity of the child. Explain the procedure to the child and parents, informing them that this is a pain-free method to monitor the child's condition.

2. The high and low limits are set according to the age of the child and the underlying condition. Usually a 15- to 20-second period of apnea will set off the alarm.

## EQUIPMENT AND SUPPLIES

- Cardiorespiratory monitor
- Electrodes (home apnea monitors may have straps to hold electrodes in place)
- Alcohol swabs

## PROCEDURE

1. Use alcohol swabs to clean the skin areas where the leads will be applied, and allow the skin to dry.
   RATIONALE: *Cleaning the skin will remove oils so the adhesive pads holding the electrodes have better adherence.*

2. Place the electrodes on the child's chest: one on the right side, one on the left, and one (ground) on the lateral side of the abdomen (Figure 15–3).

3. If the monitor alarm sounds, check the child immediately. Assess breathing and heart rate.

4. If the child is not breathing, stimulate the child, reposition the airway, and, if there is no response, initiate cardiopulmonary resuscitation (CPR) and call a code (see Skill 15–19).

5. If the child is not in distress, silence the alarm, check the connections and leads, and reset the alarm.
   RATIONALE: *Leads frequently become disconnected as the child moves and an alarm is triggered.*

6. Document the alarm, the nursing action, and the child's condition.

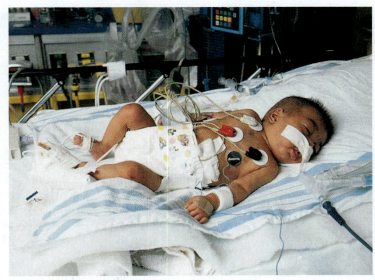

**Figure 15–3** *Placement of cardiorespiratory monitor electrodes.*

## SKILL 15–4 Placement of Electrocardiogram Electrodes

The electrocardiogram (ECG) is a graphic representation of the electricity produced by the heart muscle. Twelve leads are used to provide the optimal recording.

### PREPARATION

1. Verify the identity of the child.

2. Explain the procedure to the child and parents, and emphasize that it is a pain-free method to assess the heart. Discuss the need for the child to remain still briefly during the actual ECG.

### EQUIPMENT AND SUPPLIES

- Electrocardiogram recorder and lead wires
- Electrode patches
- Alcohol swabs

### PROCEDURE

1. Alcohol swabs may be used to clean the sites where the leads will be placed.

2. Electrodes are placed both on the chest and on the limbs in the locations described in Table 15–1. See Figure 15–4.
   RATIONALE: *Correct placement of the electrodes is important to ensure that the electrical impulses are accurately recorded.*

3. Turn on the electrocardiogram recorder and input client information. Collect the tracing.

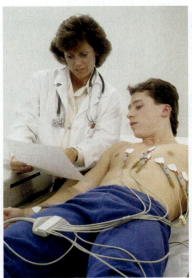

**Figure 15–4** *Position of electrodes on the chest for an electrocardiogram.*

4. When completed, remove the electrodes.

5. Ensure that the ECG tracing is labeled with the child's name, and place it in the designated section of the child's medical record or transmit it to the electronic health record.

| TABLE 15–1 | Placement of Electrocardiogram Electrodes |
|---|---|
| Chest electrodes | $V_1C$ fourth intercostal space to right of sternum<br>$V_2C$ fourth intercostal space to left of sternum<br>$V_3C$ midway between $V_2$ and $V_4$<br>$V_4C$ fifth left intercostal space at midclavicular line<br>$V_5C$ fifth left intercostal space at anterior axillary line (midway between $V_4$ and $V_6$)<br>$V_6C$ fifth left intercostal space at midaxillary line |
| Limb electrodes | One on each upper extremity slightly above the wrists<br>One on each lower extremity just above the ankles |

## SKILL 15–5  Peak Expiratory Flow Rate (PEFR) Monitoring

Peak expiratory flow meters are often recommended for home use to monitor pulmonary function in children with respiratory conditions such as asthma. Peak expiratory flow is the maximum speed of the air moving out of the lungs at the beginning of expiration, an indication of ventilatory capacity. The child's personal best average reading is determined by using the peak expiratory flow meter frequently over a 2- to 3-week period at several times of the day when the child's asthma is optimally treated (American Academy of Allergy, Asthma, and Immunology, 2014). This personal best average rate may then be used for comparison when the child has signs of breathing difficulty.

### PREPARATION

1. Verify the identity of the child. Explain the procedure to the child and parents and the reasons for its use. To help toddlers and preschoolers learn how to use a peak flow meter, have them practice by blowing into a noisemaker or party favor.

2. The indicator on the peak flow meter is placed at the bottom of the numbered scale.

3. The peak flow meter is then set to reflect the child's personal best score and "zones" indicating different levels of expiratory capacity (Table 15–2). These zones are used to guide the action plan for the child's medication management and adjustment.

| TABLE 15–2 | Peak Expiratory Flow Rate (PEFR) Readings and Action Plan for Medical Management |
|---|---|
| **Zone and PEFR Reading** | **Action Plan** |
| *Green*: The PEFR reading is between 80% and 100% of the child's personal best score. | Air is moving well in the child's lungs. The child has good asthma control and can continue daily activities. No modification of the treatment plan is needed. |
| *Yellow*: The PEFR reading is between 50% and 80% of the child's personal best score. | The child is developing breathing problems. The parents should follow directions in the child's asthma action plan that usually involves quick-relief medications. The child should feel better and the PEFR should improve over the next hour. If symptoms and the PEFR do not improve, contact the child's healthcare provider for additional treatment guidance. |
| *Red*: The PEFR is less than 50% of the child's personal best score. | The child has a severe asthma episode and needs urgent treatment with quick-relief medication. Call the child's healthcare provider for additional care guidelines or take the child to the emergency department. |

Source: Data from American Academy of Allergy, Asthma, and Immunology (AAAAI). (2014). *Peak flow meter.* Retrieved from http://www.aaaai.org/conditions-and-treatments/library/at-a-glance/peak-flow-meter.aspx; Johns Hopkins Medicine. (2012). *Peak flow measurement.* Retrieved from http://www.hopkinsmedicine.org/healthlibrary/test_procedures/pulmonary/peak_flow_measurement_92,P07755/; WebMD. (2012). *Asthma and the peak flow meter.* Retrieved from http://www.webmd.com/asthma/guide/peak-flow-meter

## EQUIPMENT AND SUPPLIES

- Peak expiratory flow meter
- Notebook to keep a log of PEFR readings

## PROCEDURE

1. Have the child stand and place the mouthpiece of the meter in the mouth (Figure 15–5). Advise the child not to cough or let the tongue block the mouthpiece. After taking a deep breath, the child should blow as hard and fast into the meter as possible. Read the number achieved.

2. Have the child repeat this procedure 2 or 3 more times. Use the highest number from all the readings to derive the PEFR.
   RATIONALE: *The child may need a couple of efforts to get the best reading.*

3. Compare the PEFR with the child's personal best, and interpret the level of respiratory distress and the appropriate intervention.

4. Document the child's PEFR and provide medication if needed.

5. Provide teaching for the parent and child on appropriate technique, recording results, and the action plan for responding to decreased PEFR readings when PEFR monitoring is performed on a regular basis at home.

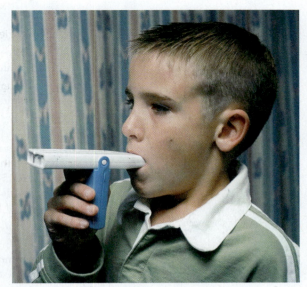

**Figure 15–5** *Child using a peak flow meter.*

## SKILL 15–6 Central Venous Pressure Monitoring

Central venous pressure (CVP) or right atrial pressure is the measurement used to assess the filling pressure or preload of the right ventricle of the heart in critically ill children. It is often used to monitor fluid balance. In a healthy child, the CVP closely resembles the left atrial pressure and is usually used to predict it. CVP can be monitored using catheters inserted into the right atrium by way of the internal jugular, subclavian, and femoral veins. An electronic transducer attached to the central venous catheter provides the pressure reading. *Central venous line insertion, site care, dressing change, and removal procedures are not discussed in this skill section.*

## PREPARATION

1. Verify the identity of the child.

2. Explain the procedure to the child and family. Clarify that the child will not feel any pain or changes once the central venous catheter has been inserted.

3. Assemble IV tubing, stopcocks, and high-pressure tubing.

4. Check all IV and stopcock connections to be certain they are tight. Connect the transducer to the monitor cable.

5. Prime all IV tubing, high-pressure tubing, and stopcocks with IV solution and ensure that the setup is free of air bubbles. Cover each port with a sterile cap.
   RATIONALE: *A smaller-than-usual waveform can be caused by air bubbles in the tubing (Burchell & Powers, 2011).*

6. A bag of IV fluid is pressurized to the prescribed level after the tubing has been flushed to prevent blood from entering the monitoring system, and the IV fluid flow rate is set to the rate specified by agency guidelines to constantly flush through the system.

## EQUIPMENT AND SUPPLIES

- IV pole, IV tubing, and stopcocks—appropriate for CVP monitor equipment
- Pressure monitor and cable
- Transducer set and mounting device
- Infusion pump or pressure bag
- IV solution ordered by healthcare provider
- T connector
- Level
- 10-mL syringe filled with normal saline
- Clean gloves

> **CLINICAL TIP**
>
> The CVP is often used to make estimates of circulatory function, in particular cardiac function and blood volume. The normal pediatric CVP value is 2 to 6 mmHg. A high pediatric CVP value is greater than 12 to 18 mmHg. A low CVP value suggests hypovolemia or decreased venous return. A high CVP value may indicate overhydration, increased venous return, or right-sided cardiac failure.

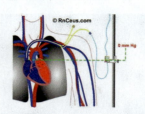

**Figure 15–6** *Level for setting the transducer to zero in the midaxillary axis. This position ensures alignment with the right atrium of the heart to give an accurate central venous pressure reading.*

Source: http://www.mceus.com

## PROCEDURE

1. Perform hand hygiene and don gloves.

2. The child should be supine for the procedure; however, the head of the bed may be elevated. Ensure that the child is in the same position each time the pressure reading is measured.

3. Verify correct placement of the catheter tip by observation of a change in pressure in different phases of respiration, free aspiration of blood through the catheter, and/or radiologic confirmation.

4. Use the level to verify that the transducer is aligned to the height of the child's right atrium, located at an imaginary line drawn down from the fourth intercostal space and a horizontal line midway between the anterior and posterior surfaces of the chest (phlebostatic axis) (Clores, 2014). See Figure 15–6.

   RATIONALE: *The child may have changed position between measurements. Inaccurate readings may occur if the transducer is not correctly aligned.*

5. Follow agency guidelines for the frequency for flushing the device to check for good flow through the tubing and confirming that the catheter is not obstructed.

6. Check that the transducer is calibrated to zero. Turn the three-way stopcock to be open to the transducer and the atmosphere and closed to the client. Press the monitor's zero function button to begin calibration. The transducer should recognize atmospheric pressure as zero.

7. Return the open stopcock position to the transducer and the client. A continuous CVP reading should then be seen.

8. Temporarily stop other IV infusions into the CVP port of the catheter (or as much as the child will tolerate to ensure an accurate reading). Other IVs and medications should infuse into other ports. Always restart any infusions temporarily stopped following the CVP reading.

   RATIONALE: *Infusion of large volumes into the CVP port can falsely elevate the reading.*

9. Observe the waveform on the monitor to ensure that all features of the wave are visible. If not, flush the device.

10. Document the CVP reading at the end of expiration. The CVP reading from an electronic monitor may be reported in millimeters of mercury (mmHg). The values may be converted to centimeters of water (cm $H_2O$) (10 cm $H_2O$ equals 7.5 mmHg). The reading is interpreted along with other clinical information such as peripheral perfusion, fluid balance, and vascular tone.

11. Notify the healthcare provider of any rapid changes in CVP readings.

## SKILL 15–7 Arterial Pressure Monitoring

Arterial pressure monitoring allows continuous monitoring of the systolic, diastolic, and mean arterial pressures and the pulse pressure. This type of monitoring is performed in critical care when the child has hemodynamic instability or a potential life-threatening complication from surgery or trauma. Sites available for arterial pressure monitoring include the radial, brachial, axillary, femoral, and dorsalis pedis arteries. The radial artery is most commonly used.

### PREPARATION

1. Verify the child's identity.

2. Explain the procedure to the child and family and the nursing care that will be provided. Describe the activity restrictions that are important to protect the arterial line.

3. Set up and calibrate the pressure-monitoring system prior to insertion of the arterial catheter.

4. A bag of IV fluid is pressurized to the prescribed level after the tubing has been flushed to prevent blood from entering the monitoring system, and the IV fluid infusion rate established by agency guidelines is used to constantly flush the system.

### EQUIPMENT AND SUPPLIES

- Arterial line placement set
- Local anesthetic
- High-pressure tubing; standard pump tubing may be utilized in a neonatal intensive care unit (NICU).
- IV solution and pump tubing
- T connector
- Chlorhexidine-based preparation or other approved skin preparation

- IV stand with transducer bar and cable
- Arterial blood pressure monitor
- Level
- Sterile gloves, gown, mask, eye shield

## PROCEDURE

1. Don sterile gloves, gown, mask, and eye shield.

2. Assist the physician with the skin-cleansing preparation, injection of local anesthetic, and insertion of the arterial line using sterile technique.

3. Protect the arterial line with a dressing, and secure the joints in neutral position to prevent movement. Maintain the arterial line and provide site care according to hospital guidelines. Provide a continuous infusion of flush solution ordered by the physician or per agency policy to maintain the catheter's patency.

4. Closely observe the extremity distal to the arterial line for temperature, color, pulsation, and capillary refill. Doppler may be used for pulses that are difficult to palpate. Observe for potential complications of arterial cannulation, such as infection and thrombosis with distal ischemia. Assess and document every 4 hours or according to agency policy.

5. Restrict client activities according to unit protocols and/or healthcare provider orders.

6. When attaching the pressure-monitoring device to the arterial catheter, every connection should be locked for safety.
   RATIONALE: *A disconnection could mean sudden hemorrhage from the arterial cannulation and could be fatal.*

7. The transducer should be aligned with the heart, using the level to set the transducer position at the imaginary point established by the intersection of the fourth intercostal space at the midclavicular line and the midaxillary line.

8. Ensure that the monitoring device is properly set to zero when the transducer is in the appropriate position. Verify or reset the monitoring device to zero every shift, when the transducer or the client's position changes, or when readings are questionable.

9. Check the pressure waveform on the monitor to make certain the catheter is patent and functional. A crisp waveform should appear. If dampened, the arterial reading is not accurate.

10. Obtain an auscultated blood pressure at least every shift using the same limb as the arterial catheter, unless contraindicated. Note the correlation between the arterial pressure and the auscultated blood pressure. Intra-arterial measurements are expected to be slightly higher than the auscultated blood pressure because the resistance of the distal vessels is higher, and the distance is slightly further.

11. Document the arterial pressure readings, pulsation waveform, auscultated blood pressure, and the limb temperature, capillary refill, and color.

# Artificial Airways

---

## SKILL 15–8 Assisting With Oropharyngeal Airway Insertion

The oropharyngeal airway is commonly used to maintain an airway in children who are unconscious. Pediatric sizes range from 4 to 10 cm in length. The oropharyngeal airway must be the correct size to keep the tongue of an unconscious child from falling into the posterior pharynx. An oropharyngeal airway is usually inserted by the physician or other healthcare provider.

## PREPARATION

1. Verify the identity of the child. Explain the procedure to the parents (the child is usually unconscious or not fully responsive when an oral airway is inserted).

2. Select the proper size (Figure 15–7). Select the airway that is the best fit for the child.
   RATIONALE: *If the airway is too large, it can obstruct the larynx. If it is too small, it will push the tongue into the posterior pharynx, causing it to obstruct the airway.*

## EQUIPMENT AND SUPPLIES

- Oropharyngeal airways of different sizes
- Airway suction equipment

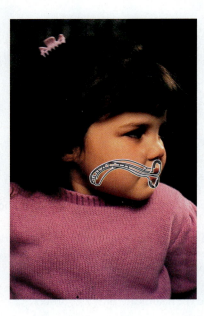

**Figure 15–7** *To determine the proper-size oral airway for the child, place an airway alongside the child's face with the bite block parallel to the hard palate and the flange at the level of the central incisors. The distal end of the airway should reach the angle of the jaw.*

### PROCEDURE

1. Carefully assess the child during the procedure.

2. Once the airway is in place, maintain the child's head and jaw in neutral position, neither flexed forward nor hyperextended.
   RATIONALE: *This position keeps the trachea from being crimped.*

3. If the child regains consciousness, remove the oropharyngeal airway.
   RATIONALE: *The airway will stimulate the gag reflex and vomiting, increasing the risk for aspiration.*

## SKILL 15–9  Assisting With Nasopharyngeal Airway Insertion

The nasopharyngeal airway provides a passage for air in situations when the tongue may fall back into the oropharynx and obstruct the airway. It is used for a conscious child with an obstructed airway, or for a child who potentially may lose consciousness and lose an open airway. The airway is made of soft plastic or rubber and comes in various sizes. The airway must be the correct size to maintain the airway. The physician or other healthcare provider usually inserts the airway in a posterior direction.

### PREPARATION

1. Verify the identity of the child. Explain the procedure to the child and parents. Explain that the airway should not be touched to prevent it from being dislodged.

2. Select the correct-size nasopharyngeal airway (Figure 15–8).

3. Lubricate the tip with water-soluble gel.

### EQUIPMENT AND SUPPLIES

- Nasopharyngeal airways of different sizes
- Water-soluble lubricant

### PROCEDURE

1. Assist the healthcare provider to insert the airway by positioning and holding the child's head at midline in a neutral position, neither flexed forward nor hyperextended.

2. Following insertion of the airway, observe for bleeding in the back of the throat. Blood may exacerbate the obstruction and further compromise airway management.
   RATIONALE: *Insertion of the tube may cause trauma to the nasopharyngeal airway passage.*

3. Assess the child's respiratory rate and effort.

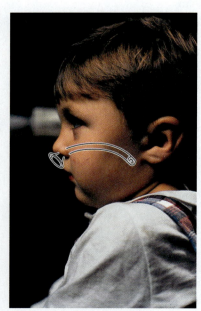

**Figure 15–8** *To select a nasopharyngeal airway of the correct size, measure the distance from the tip of the nose to the tragus of the ear for the tube length of the tube. The width must allow for passage through the naris.*

# SKILL 15–10  Tracheostomy General Guidelines

A tracheostomy is a surgical procedure to make an opening through the neck into the trachea and create an airway. It may be performed by a physician as an acute lifesaving procedure or for longer-term airway management.

A neonatal or pediatric tracheostomy tube is made of polyvinyl chloride and has an obturator used for insertion only. Tracheostomy tubes smaller than 5.0 have no inner cannula. The tube is held in place with twill tape tied around the child's neck or with Velcro straps. The child may be on a ventilator or wear a tracheostomy collar (mist collar) at the stoma site to keep the airway warm and moist (Figure 15–9). The collar may emit either oxygen or room air, depending on the healthcare provider's orders. The child with a permanent tracheostomy may alternatively wear a heat–moisture exchanger over the tracheostomy opening.

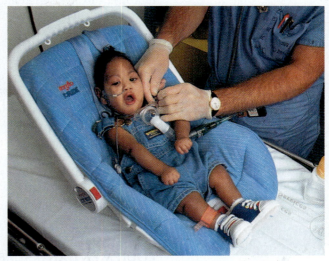

**Figure 15–9** *Infant with a tracheostomy collar.*

## PREPARATION

1. When a child with a tracheostomy is admitted, plan for close monitoring of the child's respiratory status.

2. Obtain equipment and supplies for any emergency intervention needed.

## EQUIPMENT AND SUPPLIES

- Resuscitation bag
- Oxygen
- Sterile suctioning equipment and catheters
- Preservative-free sterile saline and sterile water
- Water-soluble lubricant
- Tracheostomy tubes—one the size of the child's current tube and one a size smaller, an obturator to fit the current tracheostomy tube. The tube's inner diameter is imprinted on the flange.
- Twill tape or Velcro tracheostomy-securing straps
- Clean gloves

> **CLINICAL TIP**
>
> When the child is admitted with a tracheostomy, talk with the parents about the method used for tracheostomy management at home. Develop a nursing care plan for tracheostomy management that integrates home management as well as teaching to enhance home management techniques.

## PROCEDURE

1. Don gloves.

2. Observe the child with a tracheostomy carefully for signs of obstruction.

3. Vital signs and respiratory status, including breath sounds, respiratory effort, and airway patency, should be routinely checked. Be alert for changes in heart or respiratory rate, blood pressure, respiratory effort, breath sounds, color, or level of consciousness.

4. Watch for condensation in the oxygen tubing and empty it regularly.
   RATIONALE: *Fluid may drip into the tracheostomy tube, causing the child to aspirate if the oxygen tubing is not emptied regularly.*

5. When the child is in a crib, put the tubing through, rather than over, the bars.
   RATIONALE: *This prevents condensation fluid from entering the tracheostomy.*

6. Document findings about the tracheostomy and the child's condition.

> **CLINICAL TIP**
>
> Always keep two sterile tracheostomy tubes taped to the child's bed so that if the tube dislodges, a new one is available for immediate reintubation. One tube should be the size used by the child and the second should be one size smaller in case the airway narrows after decannulation.

## SKILL 15–11 Tracheostomy Care

Tracheostomy care is usually performed 2 or 3 times a day, according to agency policy. Follow agency guidelines for the frequency of tracheostomy tube replacement. A new sterile tracheostomy tube needs to be inserted immediately after removal of the old tube. Good stoma care is needed to maintain skin integrity and to help prevent infection.

### PREPARATION

1. Verify the identity of the child. Explain or review the procedure with the child and parents.

2. Have an assistant stand on the opposite side of the bed.
   **RATIONALE:** *For maximum safety, two persons should be present for the tracheostomy tube change.*

3. Have prepared tracheostomy tubes, oxygen, resuscitation bag, and suction tray with catheters at the bedside.

4. Prepare new ties for the tracheostomy tube. Cut two pieces of twill tape, about 12 in. each. Fold one end of each piece over lengthwise for approximately 1.0 to 1.5 in. Cut a small hole in the folded end. Alternatively, use commercial Velcro tracheostomy straps and secure them to the tracheostomy tube.

5. Place a towel roll under the child's neck to hyperextend it.
   **RATIONALE:** *This provides greater access to the neck, especially in infants and young children who have short necks.*

### EQUIPMENT AND SUPPLIES

- Resuscitation bag and oxygen
- Towel roll
- Precut twill tape or Velcro tracheostomy straps
- Cotton-tipped applicators or gauze saturated with normal saline or half-strength hydrogen peroxide
- Gauze pads
- Barrier cream and padding
- Scissors
- Sterile curved Kelly clamp
- Tracheostomy tube cleaning tray with sterile bowls, pipe cleaners, brush, and gauze pads
- Preferred tracheostomy tube cleanser or sterile hydrogen peroxide, preservative-free sterile normal saline, and sterile water
- Sterile suction tray and suction catheters sized to fit into tracheal tube
- Sterile gloves, mask, and eye shield

### PROCEDURE

1. Perform hand hygiene and don mask and eye shield.

2. Open sterile suction kit. Pour sterile saline into a sterile bowl and preferred tube cleanser or hydrogen peroxide into another bowl.

3. Preoxygenate the child or increase ventilatory support as needed.

4. Don the sterile gloves.

5. Unlock the inner cannula and place it into the bowl containing the preferred cleanser. Clean the cannula thoroughly with sterile applicators, pipe cleaners, or gauze pads, and rinse in normal saline. Replace the inner cannula and lock it into place.
   **RATIONALE:** *The inner cannula becomes obstructed with airway secretions and must be cleaned regularly to keep the airway open.*

6. Clean under the tracheostomy tube at the stoma site using cotton-tipped applicators or gauze saturated with a neutral-pH soap, normal saline, or other preferred solution. Start at the stoma and wipe outward with the applicators, making sure no dried or crusted secretions enter the stoma (Figure 15–10). With the tapes still tied, rinse the stoma with saline applicators and dry thoroughly. Wash the area behind the flanges of the tracheostomy and around the neck with damp gauze and dry. Observe for redness, drainage, and skin breakdown. Apply barrier cream to any area of redness.

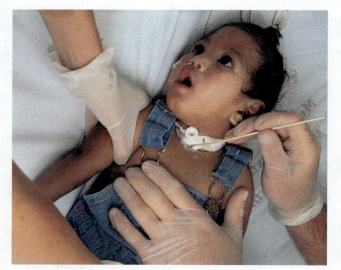

**Figure 15–10** *Cleaning the tracheostomy tube.*

7. Place a notched gauze pad or foam dressing under and around the tube to absorb secretions according to agency policy.

8. Have the assistant hold the tracheostomy tube in place to replace the ties for the tube. Cut the tapes and remove the old ties from the flange of the tube. Attach the prepared twill tape to the flange by first threading the end with the slit through the hold. Place the distal end of the twill tape through the slit and pull it securely. Alternatively, attach the Velcro strap to the flange. Repeat the process on the other side of the tube.

   RATIONALE: *Having an assistant ensures that the tube does not get expelled if the child coughs or moves unexpectedly.*

9. Tie the tape or secure the strap to hold the tracheostomy tube in place. The best fit is achieved when the child's neck is slightly flexed. The tape should be tied tightly enough to prevent dislodgment but should still be loose enough so that you can fit one finger between it and the child's neck. Padding may be placed under the tape to reduce skin irritation.

10. Triple-knot the twill tape for security. Place the knot at the side of the child's neck.

    RATIONALE: *This prevents skin irritation from the knot when the child is supine.*

11. Document the procedure, the condition of the tracheostomy opening and surrounding skin, and how the child tolerated the procedure.

### CLINICAL TIP

Remember that the child with an endotracheal tube or tracheostomy tube is unable to talk or cry. Implement other ways of communication. Picture boards with common activities or requests work for younger children. A tablet and pencil or computer notebook can be used by older children with normal cognitive and motor function.

## SKILL 15–12 Endotracheal Tube Care

An endotracheal (ET) tube is an emergency artificial airway used to maintain and secure an open airway in an unconscious child. ET tubes are sterile, disposable, and made of a translucent plastic or other synthetic material. The distal end is tapered and has an opening in the side wall (Murphy eye). The length of the tube is marked in centimeters to serve as a measurement reference point once it is in place. The tubes come in various sizes, both with and without cuffs (Figure 15–11). The ET tube must be just large enough to seal the airway to prevent air leaks. The uncuffed tube is often recommended for the child younger than 8 or 9 years old, as the airway is narrowest at the cricoid ring, sealing the airway effectively without a cuff. Intubation is usually performed by the healthcare provider or paramedic to maintain the child's airway.

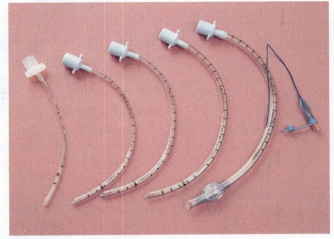

**Figure 15–11** *Endotracheal tubes of different sizes, cuffed and uncuffed.*

### PREPARATION

1. Verify the identity of the child and explain the procedure to the parents (the child will be unconscious or less than fully responsive).

2. Select the appropriate-size ET tube for the child from a length-based resuscitation tape, chart of ET tube size by age, or by formula.

3. Place the child in the supine position with the neck hyperextended (unless there is concern of cervical spine injury, in which case the neck is not hyperextended).

### EQUIPMENT AND SUPPLIES

- ET tubes of different sizes, cuffed and uncuffed
- Pediatric stylet
- Adhesive tape
- Laryngoscope with curved and straight blades of different sizes
- Water-soluble lubricant
- $CO_2$ detector
- Resuscitation bag and oxygen source
- Suction source and suction catheter (multiply the ET tube size by 2 to select the correct size French suction catheter)
- Stethoscope
- Clean gloves, gown, mask, and eye shield

### PROCEDURE

1. Don clean gloves, gown, mask, and eye shield. Assist the healthcare provider with intubation by positioning and holding the child's head at midline. The tube is held in position until taped securely.

### CLINICAL TIP

The ET tube size (uncuffed) recommended for infants under 1 year of age is 3.5 mm and for children 1 to 2 years is 4.0 mm. After 2 years, the formula for selecting the appropriate ET tube size is $(4 + age)/4$ (Chin-Sang, 2015). Since this is often an emergency procedure, many agencies use a length-based resuscitation tape or quick reference chart to select the appropriate ET tube size for the age of the child.

2. Once the tube has been placed by the healthcare provider, auscultate for equal breath sounds, and check for symmetry of chest movement and condensation in the tube. Attach a $CO_2$ detector to verify that the tube is in the trachea rather than the esophagus. The $CO_2$ detector should verify that carbon dioxide is being exhaled. Auscultate over the stomach for any bubbling or gurgling sounds that might indicate that the tube is in the esophagus. Listen at the trachea for air leaks.

   RATIONALE: *Correct placement of the tube in the trachea is critical for survival of the child. Verification of tracheal placement by multiple methods is essential.*

3. Once correct tube placement is verified, note the centimeter marking at the lip or tooth line and tape the tube in place.

   RATIONALE: *Identifying the level of tube placement provides one method of confirming placement of the tube during future assessments.*

4. Reassess tube placement after the tube is taped.

5. Continuously assess breath sounds, color, heart rate on the monitor, and pulse oximeter readout.

   RATIONALE: *The child with an ET tube needs constant assessment to ensure that the tube does not become dislodged from the trachea or move into the right bronchus mainstem.*

6. Initiate assisted ventilation with oxygen if spontaneous breathing is not present.

7. Document ET tube insertion, procedures for verification of correct placement, centimeter marking at the teeth or lips, tube size, and the client's response.

# Assisted Ventilation

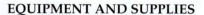

## SKILL 15–13 Bag-Mask Ventilation

Resuscitation bags and masks, such as a nonrebreather mask and bag, are used to perform assisted ventilation for children who are unable to breathe adequately on their own. This is an emergency procedure, performed until airway control is attained and a ventilator is provided.

### PREPARATION

1. Select the appropriate-size mask for the child. The mask should extend from the bridge of the nose to the cleft of the chin (Figure 15–12).

   RATIONALE: *The correct-size mask has a small volume that minimizes dead space and prevents rebreathing of expired carbon dioxide.*

2. Select the appropriate-size resuscitation bag for the child. The pediatric bag should have a volume of 450 to 750 mL. An adult bag (1200 mL) can be used with older children.

   RATIONALE: *Pediatric tidal volume is approximately 8 mL/kg. The bag size should be no smaller than the child's tidal volume.*

3. Connect the oxygen tubing to the resuscitation bag, and to the flow meter. Set the oxygen flow to 15 L/min.

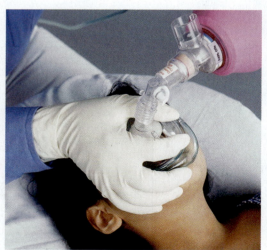

**Figure 15–12** *Bag-mask assisted ventilation. Note the position of the hand holding the mask in a C grasp, with fingers under the jaw and over the mask.*

### EQUIPMENT AND SUPPLIES

- Self-inflating resuscitation bag and appropriate-size mask for child
- Oxygen and tubing
- Appropriate-size suction catheters and suction source
- Pulse oximeter
- Oropharyngeal or nasopharyngeal airway
- Clean gloves

### PROCEDURE

1. Don gloves. Assess the child's respiratory status, and initiate assisted ventilation when the child is unable to breathe at an adequate rate or depth. Activate the emergency response system in the agency.

2. Position the infant or child to open the airway without hyperextending the neck. Place a towel roll under the infant's or toddler's shoulders to achieve a sniffing (neutral) position. The child older than 2 years may need a towel under the head.

   RATIONALE: *The head of the infant and toddler is large, and lifting the shoulders straightens the airway and places it in a neutral position.*

3. Open the child's airway with a head tilt–chin lift or jaw-thrust maneuver (see Skill 15–19). Use an oropharyngeal or nasopharyngeal airway if airway patency cannot be maintained (see Skills 15–8 and 15–9).

4. Apply the mask to the face and get an airtight seal. Pull the child's jaw into the mask rather than pushing the mask into the face. Use an assistant to maintain the seal.

   **RATIONALE:** *Failure to achieve a seal will result in a lower oxygen concentration or inadequate volume of air delivered to the lungs.*

5. Begin ventilation by squeezing the bag slowly over 1 second. Watch for chest rise. Squeeze the bag only until the chest rise is visible, then release. If the chest does not rise, reposition the child's airway and try again.

   **RATIONALE:** *Using more force than needed to make the chest rise will push air into the stomach and potentially cause the child to vomit, compromising the airway. Gastric distention compromises ventilation by elevating the diaphragm and decreasing lung size.*

6. With each ventilation, say "squeeze, release, release." The rate of ventilation should be 20 breaths a minute. When cardiopulmonary resuscitation is being performed, the rate of ventilation is 8 to 10 breaths a minute (Chameides, Samson, Schexnayder, et al., 2011, p. 149).

   **RATIONALE:** *The child needs a 1:2 inspiratory-to-expiratory ratio for gas exchange in the alveoli, and this phrase helps maintain that ratio. If CPR is performed, fewer breaths can be provided between the needed number of compressions.*

7. Assess the effectiveness of ventilations by observing for bilateral chest rise, auscultating lung sounds, and monitoring pulse oximeter level.

8. Document the procedure and the child's condition.

## SKILL 15–14  Ventilator

Ventilators are used for children who need assistance with breathing. These children may have a chronic condition, such as a neuromuscular disease or persistent lung pathology, or they may be acutely ill or injured and need emergency management of ventilation. The ventilator is usually attached to the child's endotracheal tube or tracheostomy tube.

### PREPARATION

1. Verify the physician's order.

2. Become familiar with the ventilator, and know the settings ordered by the physician (oxygen concentration, humidity, air temperature, pressure, tidal volume, and inspiratory/expiratory ratio and rate). Identify what the alarms mean, and know how to troubleshoot problems.

3. Verify the identity of the child, and explain the procedure to the child and parents.

### EQUIPMENT AND SUPPLIES

- Ventilator complete with tubing setup
- Cardiorespiratory monitor
- Pulse oximeter
- $CO_2$ detector
- Resuscitation bag and mask, appropriate size for child
- Appropriate-size suction catheters and suction source
- Sterile water for suctioning
- Oxygen source
- Orogastric or nasogastric tube
- Clean gloves

### PROCEDURE

1. Ensure that the child is attached to a cardiorespiratory monitor and pulse oximeter.

2. Don gloves. Obtain arterial blood gases as directed by healthcare provider order or agency guidelines.

3. Assess vital signs every hour, including heart and respiratory rates, blood pressure, temperature, and pulse oximeter reading. Auscultate the lungs in all fields to assess for equal breath sounds. Monitor the $CO_2$ detector waveform and reading for expected end-tidal partial pressure of exhaled carbon dioxide ($pCO_2$), which should be between 35 and 45 mmHg (Parker, 2012). Ensure that the child's respiratory rate is consistent with the ventilator setting.

4. An orogastric or nasogastric tube may be inserted (see Skills 16–1 and 16–2).
   RATIONALE: *The tube keeps the stomach decompressed to keep the child from vomiting and compromising the airway.*

5. Suction the endotracheal tube or tracheostomy tube as necessary. See Skills 15–24 and 15–25. Change the tracheostomy tube or the tracheostomy ties according to agency guidelines or when they become soiled. See Skill 15–11.

6. Protect the endotracheal tube by making sure it is securely positioned at the appropriate centimeter mark at lip level. Support the ventilator tubing to decrease traction on the endotracheal tube by attaching the tubing directly to the bed using a gauze roll and a safety pin.

7. Carefully monitor the child for decreased sedation and pain (e.g., a rise in heart rate and blood pressure or tearing suggests distress or pain). Acutely ill or injured children may be chemically paralyzed and sedated while on the ventilator. Provide additional sedation and pain medication as prescribed. Determine if elbow immobilizers are needed to prevent dislodgment of the endotracheal tube.

8. Listen and look for air leaks. Make sure that the ventilator is firmly attached to the endotracheal tube or tracheostomy tube.

9. Respond to ventilator alarms, which may indicate a kink in tubing, a need for suctioning, bronchospasm, pneumothorax, disconnected ventilator tubing, or a dislodged endotracheal tube or tracheostomy.

10. Provide oral care twice a day to reduce the risk for ventilator-associated pneumonia. See Skill 15–15.

11. Check the reservoir for humidification at least every 8 hours. Refill or replace water as needed. Watch for condensation in the tubing and empty it regularly.
    RATIONALE: *If fluid is not removed from the tubing, it may drip into the endotracheal tube, causing the child to aspirate.*

12. Tell the child what you are planning to do—for example, "I am going to wash your face," or "I am going to move your arms and legs." The child who is sedated or unresponsive may still be able to hear.

13. Support the family members by answering their questions. Encourage them to talk to the child and to bring in audiotapes of favorite music or of family members speaking to the child.

14. Document the child's condition frequently according to agency policy.

## SKILL 15–15  Oral Care for the Child on a Ventilator

Oral care is performed twice a day for children on a ventilator to reduce the development of plaque and bacterial colonization in the oropharynx that could lead to ventilator-associated pneumonia. The endotracheal tube provides a pathway for bacteria to travel to the lungs. An endotracheal tube causes the mouth to stay open and leads to dry mucous membranes.

### PREPARATION

1. Verify the identity of the child, and explain the procedure to the family and child as developmentally appropriate.

2. Elevate the head of the bed if possible.

### EQUIPMENT AND SUPPLIES

- Soft pediatric toothbrush
- Fluoride toothpaste
- Suction and suction catheter
- Foam swabs
- Chlorhexidine gluconate 0.12% mouth rinse
- Gloves

### PROCEDURE

1. Moisten the toothbrush and apply a small amount of toothpaste. Brush the teeth, gums, and tongue. Repeat tooth brushing every 12 hours.

2. Suction out excess toothpaste. Do not rinse the mouth to allow more of the fluoride to be absorbed.

3. Swab the oral mucosa with chlorhexidine gluconate 0.12% mouth rinse every 4 hours. Suction out excess, but do not rinse.

4. Moisten the mouth using foam swabs with clean water every 2 hours. Coat the lips with lip balm.

5. Document the oral care provided and the child's response.

# Chest Tubes

Chest tubes are inserted into the pleural or mediastinal space to drain fluid, blood, or air so the lung can reexpand. Chest tubes may be placed during surgery, postoperatively, or as an emergency. A chest tube may be attached to suction for negative pressure or sealed to prevent air from reentering the pleural space. Chest tubes are inserted by a physician.

## SKILL 15–16 Assisting With Placement of Chest Tubes

### PREPARATION

1. Verify the identity of the child, and explain the procedure to the family and child as developmentally appropriate.

2. Review the child's medical record related to the need for chest tube placement.
   **RATIONALE:** *Knowing the reason the chest tube is placed enables the nurse to respond appropriately if the tube is displaced.*

3. Assess the child's respiratory status to obtain the baseline respiratory rate, respiratory effort, breath sounds, and oxygen saturation level. Breath sounds may be diminished over an area of pneumothorax, hemothorax, or pleural effusion.

4. Assess the child's pain control. Prepare and administer pain medication as prescribed. Local anesthetic may also be used.

5. Prepare the chest tube drainage-collection system according to the manufacturer's recommendations. This may include filling the water-seal chamber to the 2-cm line with sterile water, and the suction-control chamber is filled with sterile water (often to a level of 20 cm of water). Tubing is then connected from the suction device to the chamber. See Figure 15–13.

### EQUIPMENT AND SUPPLIES

- Chest tube drainage system
- Sterile water for drainage-collection system plus a bottle at the bedside
- Continuous suction regulator
- Marking pen
- Chest tube insertion tray and supplies, including drapes, chest tubes, and suture material
- Chlorhexidine, povidone-iodine solution, or other preferred skin preparation
- Drainage catheter (size ordered, 10 to 24 French) and sterile connector
- Dressing preferred by physician (occlusive, nonocclusive, or transparent)
- Sterile gloves, gown, and eye shield
- Local anesthetic and syringe
- Banding gum and ties
- Occlusive tape and adhesive tape
- Sleeved Kelly clamps (two for each chest tube)
- Safety pins

### PROCEDURE

1. Attach the child to a cardiac monitor and pulse oximeter to monitor vital signs during the procedure.

2. Perform hand hygiene and don sterile gloves, gown, and eye shield. Set up the chest tube insertion tray using sterile technique.

3. Position and hold the child as directed by the physician.

4. Monitor the child's vital signs and respiratory status, and compare to baseline during the local anesthetic or sedation administration and also during chest tube insertion.

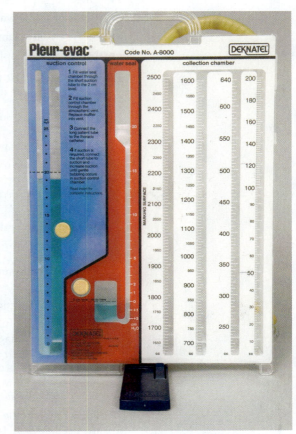

**Figure 15–13** *A three-chamber disposable chest drainage system with wet seal and wet suction.*

5. After the site is cleaned and the chest tube is inserted, maintain sterility while connecting the chest tube to the water-sealed drainage system or suction. Adjust suction to maintain a gentle bubbling in the chamber. A suture is usually placed to hold the chest tube in position.

6. Apply an occlusive dressing over the chest tube insertion site.
   RATIONALE: *Occlusive tape and dressing help prevent entry of air into the chest cavity.*

7. Band or secure all tubing connection sites.

8. Reposition the child. Obtain and assist with radiography, if ordered, to clarify placement and effectiveness of the chest tube.

9. Ensure that the drainage collection system stays upright for the seals to work correctly, but position it lower than the child's chest. Secure the chest tube to the bed with adhesive tape tabs and safety pin. Keep a bottle of sterile water or normal saline and sleeved Kelly clamps (two per chest tube) at the bedside or with the child at all times.
   RATIONALE: *Securing the chest tube drainage system reduces tension on the tubing and potential disconnection. In case of dislodgment, clamp the chest tube with a Kelly clamp or place the end of the tube in the sterile solution. This prevents air from entering the pleural space through the chest tube.*

10. Document the procedure, time, amount and color of drainage, and how the child tolerated the procedure.

---

## SKILL 15–17 Care of the Chest Tube

### PREPARATION

1. Verify the identity of the child.

2. Assess the child and family's knowledge related to the need for a chest tube. Explain care of the chest tube to the child and family.

3. Assess the child's pain level and management. Children may report pain at the insertion site.

### EQUIPMENT AND SUPPLIES

- Clean gloves
- Dressing supplies
- Bottle of sterile water or normal saline
- Sleeved Kelly clamps
- New drainage system (if being replaced)

### PROCEDURE FOR CHEST TUBE CARE

1. Don gloves.

2. Assess the child's respiratory status every hour or according to agency guidelines. Assess the respiratory rate, effort, breath sounds, and oxygen saturation level. Breath sounds over the chest tube site may be diminished.

3. Assess the chest tube insertion site. Inspect the dressing around the chest tube insertion site to make sure it is occlusive. If it is not occlusive, cover the site with sterile petrolatum gauze.
   RATIONALE: *An occlusive dressing helps prevent air leakage into the pleural space.*

4. Change chest tube dressings according to hospital policy. Document the amount of drainage and notify the healthcare provider if extensive. Palpate the area around the insertion site for crepitus, and document its presence and the size of the affected area. Notify the healthcare provider if crepitus is present when previously absent or the size of the area affected increases.
   RATIONALE: *Crepitus may indicate subcutaneous emphysema and a potential air leak. It may cause discomfort to the child.*

5. Check all connections and ensure that they are taped or banded securely.

6. Check drainage tubing to ensure that it is open and straight. If an occlusion is visible lift the tube to aid drainage by gravity or massage the tubing to loosen the clot. Do not milk or strip the tubing. The drainage-collection device must be positioned below the chest insertion site.
   RATIONALE: *Kinks or loops can prevent the tube from draining properly. Gravity enables drainage to flow to the drainage-collection device placed lower than the insertion site, and it prevents backflow of drainage to the child's chest.*

7. For safety, a bottle of sterile water or normal saline and sterile petrolatum gauze should be at the bedside at all times, and sleeved Kelly clamps (two per chest tube) should be with the child at all times.

8. If the chest tube is dislodged, cover the site with petrolatum gauze. If the tubing becomes disconnected, or the seal in the collection system is broken, clamp the chest tube with a Kelly clamp, crimp the tubing with your hand, or place the end of the tube in the bottle of sterile solution. These actions can prevent air from entering the pleural space through the disconnection or broken seal. Assess the child for signs of respiratory distress.

9. If the chest tube is connected to suction, compare the suction setting to the amount of suction ordered. Bubbling in the suction chamber should be intermittent with breathing rather than continuous. Continuous bubbling may indicate an air leak in the system, so check for loose connections.

10. Monitor the water levels in the drainage system and replace as needed to maintain the water seal and suction levels.

11. Check for the expected water movement called *tidaling*, the fall of water with inspiration and rise with expiration. If tidaling is not seen, check for kinked or clamped tubing or to see if a section of tubing is filled with fluid that needs to drain.

12. Document the type and amount of chest tube output as ordered or according to agency guidelines. Use a marking pen or tape to mark the fluid level, date, and time on the collection container for the running total. Report sudden increases in chest tube output. The drainage system is never emptied. Drainage systems are large enough to hold drainage from several days. When full, the system is replaced with a new one.
    RATIONALE: *The system would lose its negative pressure if it were opened.*

## PROCEDURE FOR CHANGING THE COLLECTION SYSTEM

1. Prepare the new drainage system as described in Skill 15–16.

2. Remove the tape and bands from the chest tube to the old drainage collection system.

3. Direct the child to blow out and then hold the breath. Then clamp the chest tube with a sleeved Kelly clamp about 3.5 to 6.0 cm (1.5 to 2.5 in.) from the insertion site.
   RATIONALE: *The clamp prevents air from entering the pleural space through the tube.*

4. Don gloves.

5. Disconnect the tubing from the old drainage-collection device and attach to the new device while keeping the end of the chest tube sterile.

6. Remove the Kelly clamp and tell the child to breathe.

7. Assess the new system for the amount of suction, continuous bubbling (may indicate an air leak), or the presence of tidaling.

8. Band or tape all connection sites, ensuring that the tubing is straight. Secure the tubing with adhesive tabs to the bed to reduce tension on the chest tube insertion site.

9. Assess the child's respiratory status.

10. Document the procedure, time, total drainage and character, and how the child tolerated the procedure.

## SKILL 15–18  Assisting With Chest Tube Removal

### PREPARATION

1. Verify the identity of the child. Assess client and family knowledge related to removal of the chest tube. Explain the procedure to the child and family.

2. The chest tube may be clamped for several hours prior to removal to evaluate the child's response.
   RATIONALE: *Clamping the chest tube provides information about how well the child will tolerate having no chest tube.*

3. Assess the client's baseline respiratory status, including the respiratory rate, effort, symmetric chest rise and fall, breath sounds, and oxygen saturation level.

4. The chest tube may be clamped 3.5 to 6.0 cm (1.5 to 2.5 in.) from the insertion site prior to removal, if not already clamped.

5. Assess the client's pain level and administer pain medication 10 to 15 minutes before the procedure.
   RATIONALE: *Removal of a chest tube will cause pain.*

6. Prepare the sterile dressing to be placed over the insertion site.

### EQUIPMENT AND SUPPLIES

- Clean gloves, sterile gloves
- Suture removal kit or tweezers and scissors
- Antibacterial petrolatum gauze, or occlusive dressing as preferred by healthcare provider
- Occlusive tape

### PROCEDURE

1. Position the child and have an assistant hold the child if necessary.

2. Don clean gloves and assist with removal and disposal of the dressing. Provide reassurance to the child as the dressing is removed.

3. Perform hand hygiene and don sterile gloves, mask, gown, and eye shield.

4. As the suture is cut, ask the child to take a deep breath and hold it. The chest tube is removed at maximum inspiration.
   RATIONALE: *At the end of inspiration, positive pressure in the thoracic cavity helps prevent air from entering the chest.*

5. Immediately cover the insertion site with an occlusive dressing and occlusive tape. Tell the child to begin breathing.

6. Reposition the child and assess breath sounds, respiratory effort, and oxygen saturation level to detect any respiratory distress. Assess pain. Repeat respiratory assessments every 15 minutes for the first hour, and if stable assess at the frequency as indicated by facility guidelines.

7. Document the procedure, time, child's respiratory status, and how the client tolerated the removal of chest tube procedure. Document total chest tube output.

8. Assist with the radiograph as ordered following chest tube removal to verify that the lung is still fully inflated.

# Cardiopulmonary Resuscitation

Cardiopulmonary resuscitation (CPR) is basic life support using techniques to maintain circulation, the airway, and breathing (the CABs). CPR guidelines have been specifically developed for infants and children up to the age of puberty onset. Healthcare providers should be skilled in both one- and two-person CPR.

---

## SKILL 15–19 Performing Cardiopulmonary Resuscitation

### PREPARATION

1. Become certified in basic life support and maintain certification.

2. Assess the child for unresponsiveness, lack of breathing, gasping, and no heart rate. Look, listen, and feel for breathing for about 5 to 10 seconds. Check for the rise and fall of the chest and abdomen, and listen and feel for the flow of expelled air at the mouth (Figure 15–14A). Simultaneously feel for a pulse. Use the brachial artery to assess for a pulse in an infant (Figure 15–14B). Use the carotid artery to assess for a pulse in a child (Figure 15–14C).

   - Infant: Determine unresponsiveness by gently tapping on the abdomen or soles of the feet. Use the brachial artery to assess for a pulse.
   - Child: Determine unresponsiveness by stimulating the child. Boldly ask, "Are you all right?" Use the carotid artery to assess for a pulse.

3. Call 9-1-1 on cell phone to activate the emergency response system, and turn on hands-free speaker for resuscitation guidance (Atkins et al., 2015).
   - If alone without cell phone, perform CPR for approximately 2 minutes before calling for help.
   - If assistance is available, have them call 9-1-1 and go for the automatic external defibrillator (AED).

4. If the infant or child is unresponsive and not breathing (or only gasping), but a pulse is felt within 10 seconds, begin rescue breathing. Send someone to get the AED, if available. If no pulse is felt, or it is uncertain whether a pulse is felt, begin compressions.

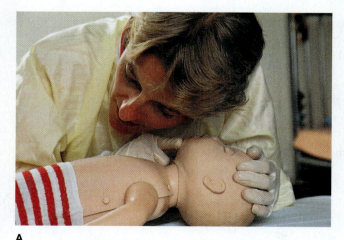

**A**

**Figure 15–14A** *Assessing breathing.*

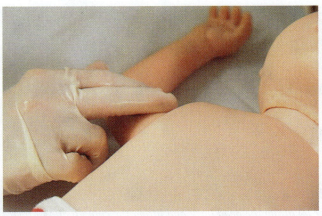
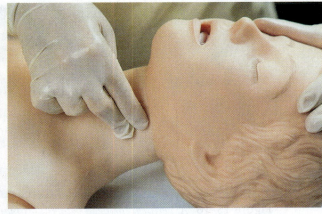

**Figure 15–14**  *B, Checking for the brachial pulse. C, Checking for the carotid pulse.*

5. For any child or adolescent with a sudden witnessed out-of-hospital collapse, assume the child has experienced a sudden ventricular fibrillation or cardiac arrest, and immediately begin compressions. Use AED as soon as it is available.

## EQUIPMENT AND SUPPLIES

- Resuscitation bag and mask
- Mouth-to-mouth-and-nose barrier device (may be used)
- Clean gloves

## PROCEDURE

### Infant or Child With a Pulse Less Than 60 Beats a Minute or No Pulse

1. Begin cycles of 30 rapid chest compressions (rate of 100 compressions per minute) and 2 rescue breaths if single rescuer. Two rescuers should initiate cycles of 15 rapid compressions and 2 rescue breaths (Atkins et al., 2015).

   RATIONALE:  *Bradycardia is a sign of impending cardiac arrest. Do not wait until the child is pulseless before beginning chest compressions.*

   - For newborns and small infants, place the two thumbs over the lower sternum and encircle the hands around the chest when two rescuers are present. The thumbs compress the sternum, and the fingers squeeze the thorax (Figure 15–15*A*). A single rescuer should use two fingers on the lower sternum, one finger's width below the nipple line. Avoid pressure on the xiphoid.

   - For children, position the heel of one or two hands (one hand over the other) at about the nipple line for compressions (Figure 15–15*B*).

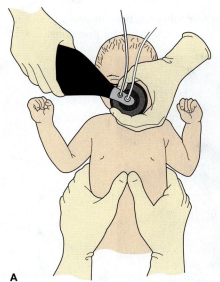
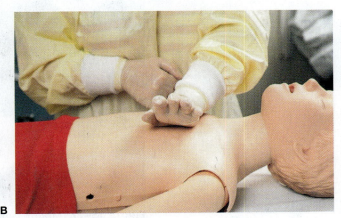

**Figure 15–15**  *Hand position for chest compressions. A, Infant. B, Child.*

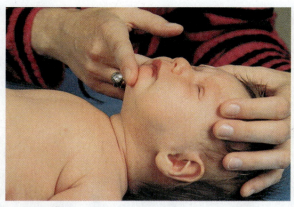
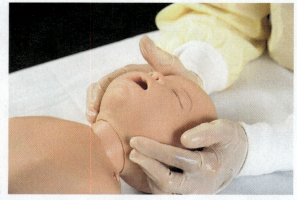

A    B

**Figure 15–16** *A, Perform the head tilt-chin lift maneuver by tilting the head back and lifting the chin up and outward.* *B, Perform the jaw-thrust maneuver by placing two or three fingers under each side of the jaw at its angle and lifting the jaw upward and outward.*

2. Perform chest compressions, pushing hard to depress the chest at least one third of its anterior-posterior diameter (4 cm [1.6 in.] in infants to 5 cm [2 in.] in children, and use adult compression depth of no more than 6 cm [2.4 in.] in adolescents) (Atkins et al., 2015). Allow the chest to fully recoil after each compression by lifting the fingers or heel of the hand slightly. Minimize interruptions during compressions.

   RATIONALE: *Blood return to the heart is improved if full chest recoil is permitted. Interruptions during compressions reduce blood flow to the brain and the chance for survival.*

3. Open the airway and have the second rescuer maintain the open airway position while providing rescue breaths.

   ▪ Position the infant or child on the back while supporting the head and neck. Open the airway by performing a chin lift—tilt the head back and lift the chin up and out (Figure 15–16*A*).

   ▪ If a child is suspected of having a cervical spine injury, open the airway by performing a jaw thrust—from a position behind the infant's head, place two or three fingers under each side of the jaw at its angle and lift the jaw upward and outward (Figure 15–16*B*).

   ▪ Observe for a visible chest rise with each ventilation. If the chest does not rise, reposition the child's head and try again. If the chest still does not rise, perform the procedure for choking (Skill 15–20).

4. Initiate ventilations after 30 compressions for a single rescuer (15 compressions for two rescuers). When one rescuer is present, the compression to ventilation ratio is 30:2 for infants and children. For two rescuers, the ratio is 15:2 (Atkins et al., 2015).

   ▪ Give rescue breaths, about 1 second each, making the chest visibly rise. Seal your lips and mouth to the barrier device around the child's mouth or around the infant's mouth and nose (Figure 15–17).

   ▪ Compressions should be paused for rescue breaths, but interruptions for rescue breaths should be minimized.

   ▪ When an advanced airway (endotracheal or tracheostomy tube) has been inserted, give 8 to 10 ventilations a minute with a resuscitation bag without interrupting compressions.

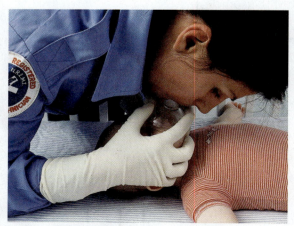

**Figure 15–17** *Mouth-to-mouth resuscitation using a barrier device.*

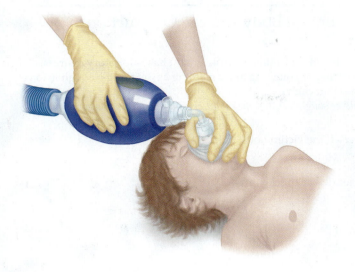

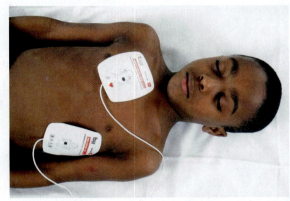

**Figure 15–19**  *Placement of pads for defibrillation of a child.*

**Figure 15–18**  *Assisted ventilation with a bag-mask resuscitator.*

- Begin using a bag-mask resuscitator hooked up to oxygen (flow rate of 10 to 15 L/min) as soon as possible (Figure 15–18). Ensure that the mask is the correct size, extending from the bridge of the nose to the cleft of the chin, and tightly sealed. See Skill 15–13. Avoid excessive ventilations. Give each breath slowly over 1 second using only enough force to make the chest rise.

  **RATIONALE:**  *Excessive ventilation increases pressure in the chest and may cause gastric distention or a pneumothorax. Intrathoracic pressure is increased, which reduces venous return, perfusion of the heart, and cardiac output (Chameides et al., 2011).*

5. Continue coordination of compressions and ventilations. Rescuers should rotate the compression role every 2 minutes, making the switch in about 5 seconds.

   **RATIONALE:**  *Rescuers performing compressions get fatigued and perform less-effective compressions.*

6. Use an AED or manual defibrillator as soon as available for the victim with a sudden witnessed collapse or no pulse.

   **RATIONALE:**  *A sudden collapse in a child or adolescent is likely to be caused by ventricular fibrillation or pulseless ventricular tachycardia, which may respond to defibrillation.*

   - Apply child pads or child paddles as directed by the equipment manual for any child between 1 and 8 years of age (Figure 15–19). Apply adult pads or paddles for any child over 8 years of age as directed by the equipment manual.

   - Minimize the time between compressions and defibrillation.

7. Apply 2 joules per kg for the first shock, and immediately follow with compressions and ventilations. The rhythm is then rechecked. A second shock of 4 joules per kg is given if needed. Continue CPR while assessing the infant or child.

8. If the infant or child has a return of both pulse and respirations and is not a trauma victim, place the child in the side-lying position.

   **RATIONALE:**  *This position is used to protect the airway in case of vomiting.*

### Inadequate Breathing Infant or Child With a Pulse Greater Than 60 Beats a Minute

1. If the infant or child is not breathing, or breathing inadequately, give rescue breaths at a rate of 12 to 20 breaths a minute (1 breath every 3 to 5 seconds). Continue until the child resumes spontaneous breathing. Reassess the child's pulse every 2 minutes.

   **RATIONALE:**  *Hypoxia develops from inadequate breathing and may lead to bradycardia if not treated.*

2. Initiate compressions and the CPR sequence if the heart rate falls below 60 per minute.

# Foreign Body Airway Obstruction

An airway obstruction may be caused by respiratory disorders (e.g., croup or epiglottitis) or a foreign body. Attempt to clear the airway in the following situations: a witnessed or strongly suspected aspiration of a foreign body (sudden onset of respiratory distress with coughing, gagging, or wheezing, and absence of fever or other respiratory symptoms) or the airway remains obstructed during attempts to provide rescue breathing.

# SKILL 15–20 Removing a Foreign Body Airway Obstruction

## PREPARATION

1. When the infant or child is suspected of aspirating or choking and has respiratory distress, encourage the child to continue crying or coughing and breathing as long as the cough is forceful. Call 9-1-1 and try to keep the child calm.

   RATIONALE: *Emergency care should be sought because the infant or child may develop a complete obstruction.*

2. Ask the child, "Are you choking?" If the victim nods, help is needed.

## EQUIPMENT AND SUPPLIES

- Mouth-to-mouth-and-nose barrier device (pocket mask)
- Bag-mask resuscitator
- Clean gloves

## PROCEDURE

### Infant

1. If the cough becomes ineffective and soundless, if increased respiratory difficulty or stridor is noted, or if the infant stops breathing, don gloves and attempt to remove the obstruction. Use the chin-lift position to open the airway.

2. Try to ventilate either by mouth-to-mouth-and-nose rescue breaths or with a bag-mask resuscitator bag (refer to Skill 15–19 for rescue breathing). If the airway is obstructed, reposition the infant's head and attempt to ventilate again.

3. Position the infant face down on your arm, supporting the head, if unable to ventilate.

4. Perform five back slaps with the heel of the hand between the infant's shoulder blades (Figure 15–20*A*).

5. Position the infant face up on your forearm. Place the fingers in the same position used for CPR (Figure 15–20*B*). Give five chest thrusts near the center of the breastbone.

6. Place your index finger on the bony prominence of the infant's chin and your thumb in the mouth on the tongue. Pull up and out to open the mouth. Look in the infant's mouth for the foreign body and remove it if seen. Do not perform a blind sweep.

   RATIONALE: *A blind sweep may actually push an object deeper into the trachea.*

7. If no object is found, try to ventilate the infant again. If the obstruction is still present, reposition the infant's head and attempt to ventilate once again.

8. If the obstruction remains, begin another series of back slaps and chest thrusts. Look in the mouth, try to ventilate, reposition the head, and attempt to ventilate again. Continue with this pattern until the airway is clear.

9. If the infant becomes unresponsive, begin CPR with compressions as described in Skill 15–19. Every time the rescuer opens the airway to deliver rescue breaths, look in the mouth and remove any object seen. Blind finger sweeps should not be performed (Chameides et al., 2011).

   RATIONALE: *Chest compressions during CPR increase thoracic pressure and may help push the foreign object into the mouth.*

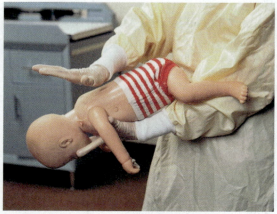 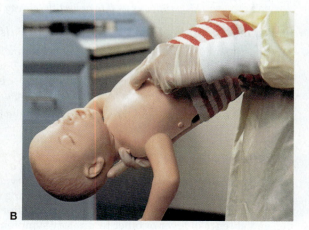

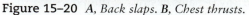

**Figure 15–20** *A, Back slaps. B, Chest thrusts.*

10. Once the airway is clear, give two slow, full breaths. Check for a pulse. At this point, provide whatever basic life support (BLS) maneuvers are necessary.

### Child

1. Perform subdiaphramatic abdominal thrusts (Heimlich maneuver) on the child in either a sitting or standing position (Figure 15–21).

2. Stand behind the child, with your arms under the child's axilla and around the chest. Place the thumb of one fist against the abdomen in the midline, below the xiphoid and above the navel. Grasp your fist with your other hand.
   RATIONALE: *The xiphoid is avoided to prevent injury to underlying organs.*

3. Deliver up to five quick, upward thrusts. Each thrust should be a distinct effort to remove the obstruction.

4. The series of five thrusts should be repeated until the obstruction is cleared or the child becomes unconscious.

5. If the child becomes unconscious, move the child to the floor and begin CPR as described in Skill 15–19. Every time the rescuer opens the airway to deliver rescue breaths, look in the mouth and remove any object seen. Blind finger sweeps should not be performed.
   RATIONALE: *Chest compressions during CPR increase the thoracic pressure as much as or more than abdominal thrusts.*

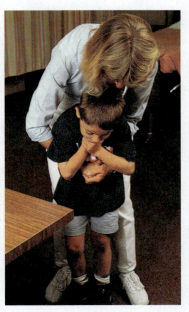

**Figure 15–21** *Abdominal thrusts (Heimlich maneuver).*

# Suctioning

The airway needs to be suctioned when excess secretions are present or when a decreased level of consciousness interferes with the child's ability to clear normal secretions. Suctioning of the nose, mouth, tracheostomy tube, or endotracheal tube may all be performed. The size of the suction catheter depends on the size, age, and weight of the child or on the internal diameter of the tube to be suctioned.

## SKILL 15–21 Performing Nasal/Oral Suctioning

A bulb syringe is used to remove secretions from an infant's nose or mouth. A tonsil tip or Yankauer catheter may be used for oral suctioning in children when copious, thick secretions or emesis needs to be removed.

### PREPARATION

1. Verify the identity of the child. Explain the procedure to the child and parents.

2. Assess the child's respiratory status, including breath sounds, respiratory effort, and airway patency. Observe for excess secretions that the child is unable to manage by swallowing them.

3. An assistant may be needed to gently position and hold the infant or child with the head in midline, and to keep the child's hands out of the way.

4. Turn on and set the wall suction to the pressure level ordered by the healthcare provider or suggested in the facility's procedure manual.

### EQUIPMENT AND SUPPLIES

- Bulb syringe
- Normal saline nose drops
- Large-bore rigid suction catheter
- Normal saline solution
- Clean gloves

### PROCEDURE

#### Bulb Syringe

1. Don gloves and place saline nose drops in a naris.
   RATIONALE: *The nose drops loosen dried secretions.*

2. Deflate the bulb. Insert the tip of the bulb syringe into the infant's naris (Figure 15–22*A*).
   RATIONALE: *Deflating the bulb first prevents pushing the secretions back into the nasopharynx.*

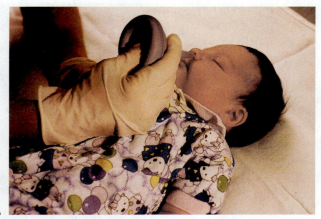 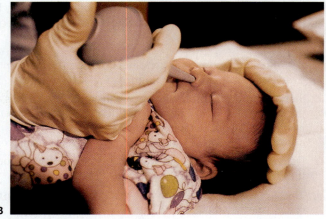

**Figure 15–22** *A, Insertion of a deflated bulb syringe. B, Removal of a reinflated bulb syringe.*

3. Release the bulb and remove the syringe from the naris (Figure 15–22*B*). Expel the secretions into the proper receptacle.

4. Repeat the procedure in the other naris. Assess the child's ability to breathe easily. Repeat the suctioning as necessary.

5. Document the procedure, the character of the secretions, and the infant's response.

### Large-Bore Rigid Suction Catheter

1. Don gloves. Insert the catheter tip into the mouth and turn on the suction.

2. Suction to remove secretions from the mouth and pharynx. Avoid causing a gag reflex.
   RATIONALE: *The gag reflex may stimulate vomiting and compromise the airway.*

3. Rinse the catheter with normal saline.

4. Assess the child's respiratory status. Repeat suctioning if needed.

5. Document the procedures, the character of the secretions, and the child's response.

## SKILL 15–22 Suctioning a Conscious (Awake and Alert) Child

A catheter is used to remove secretions from an older child's mouth or nose, a tracheostomy tube, or an endotracheal tube. The child with a decreased level of consciousness will likely require deep suctioning to remove secretions (see Skill 15–23).

### PREPARATION

1. Verify the identity of the child, and explain the procedure to the child and parents.

2. Have an assistant help you maintain the child's head in the midline position and hold the hands out of the way, as needed. Raise the head of the bed to 30 to 45 degrees.

3. Turn on and set the wall suction to the pressure level ordered by the healthcare provider or according to the agency guidelines.

4. Attach the proximal end of the catheter to the wall suction connecting tubing, making sure to keep the distal end sterile.

5. Encourage the child to cough secretions into the upper airway.

### EQUIPMENT AND SUPPLIES

- Appropriate-size suction catheter
- Sterile container with preservative-free sterile normal saline or distilled water
- Suction kit and suction source
- Water-soluble lubricant
- Sterile gloves

### PROCEDURE

1. Don gloves. Keep your dominant hand sterile and your nondominant hand clean for the procedure.

2. With your dominant hand, insert the suction catheter into the child's naris and suction for no more than 5 seconds, while gently rotating the catheter. (The depth of insertion depends on the size of the child.)

   NOTE:    *The mouth may also be suctioned for secretions, but care needs to be taken to avoid stimulating the gag reflex.*

   RATIONALE: *Suctioning longer than 5 seconds causes vagal stimulation and bradycardia.*

3. Remove and irrigate the catheter with sterile normal saline or distilled water between each pass of the catheter.

4. Assess the child's respiratory status and repeat as necessary.

5. Document the procedure, the character of the secretions, and how the child tolerated the procedure.

---

## SKILL 15–23  Suctioning a Child With a Decreased Level of Consciousness

Audible secretions, diminished breath sounds, and decreased oxygenation or coughing indicates a need for suctioning. The child with a decreased level of consciousness is often unable to cough secretions higher up into the airway. Deeper suction is often needed to clear the airway.

### PREPARATION

1. Have an assistant available as needed to keep the child's head in the midline position.

2. Verify the identity of the child, and explain the procedure to the child and parents.

3. Raise the head of the bed to 30 to 45 degrees.

4. Turn on and set the wall suction to the pressure level ordered by the healthcare provider or according to agency guidelines.

5. Attach the proximal end of the catheter to the wall suction connecting tubing, keeping the distal end sterile.

### EQUIPMENT AND SUPPLIES

- Appropriate-size suction catheter (e.g., size 8 French for infants, 10 French for children, and 12 French for adolescents)
- Suction source
- Sterile container with sterile normal saline or distilled water
- Bag-mask resuscitator
- Oxygen source, tubing, and mask or cannula
- Sterile gloves

### PROCEDURE

1. Assess the child's respiratory status. Place an oxygen mask or cannula on the child's face.

   RATIONALE: *Because suctioning potentially causes hypoxia, oxygenate the child prior to suctioning.*

2. If possible, encourage the child to cough to make the secretions pool in the hypopharynx.

   RATIONALE: *This may prevent the need for deep suctioning.*

3. Don gloves. Keep your dominant hand sterile and your nondominant hand clean for the procedure. Use only the dominant hand to manipulate the catheter.

4. Remove the protective sheath from the catheter, and test the suction by placing it in a cup of sterile saline.

5. Remove the child's oxygen mask or cannula.

6. For nasal/oral suctioning, use your dominant hand to insert the catheter into the child's naris or mouth without occluding the suction port.

   RATIONALE: *This decreases the time of suctioning and reduces the risk for hypoxia.*

7. Slowly advance the catheter only into the hypopharynx. Occlude the suction port and rotate the catheter, applying suction for 5 seconds.

8. Remove the catheter and clear the tubing with sterile saline. Repeat as necessary.

9. For deep suctioning, use your dominant hand to insert the catheter (without occluding the suction port) beyond the hypopharynx and into the trachea. Deep suctioning is defined as inserting the catheter until resistance is met at the carina and withdrawing it slightly before suction is applied (Boroughs & Dougherty, 2011).

   RATIONALE: *Suction pressure against bronchial tissue at the carina will cause mucosal trauma and inflammation.*

10. When the catheter is in place, gently rotate it as you remove the catheter, suctioning for no more than 5 seconds. Rotating the catheter ensures that the catheter eye has the greatest access to secretions.

11. Clear the catheter with sterile saline or water. Repeat as necessary.

12. Allow the child to breathe normally, and give supplemental oxygen between suctioning passes to reduce the risk for hypoxia and bradycardia.

13. Document the procedure, the character of the secretions, and the child's response and vital signs before and after the procedure.

---

### CLINICAL TIP

Obtain baseline vital signs before and after the procedure. When suctioning, watch for a decrease in pulse rate, an increase or decrease in respiratory rate, a change in skin color, or a change in the oxygen saturation reading. Bradycardia may be a sign of vagal stimulation. If any of these signs occur, stop immediately and give the child oxygen using blow-by, a face mask, or a resuscitation bag.

---

## SKILL 15–24 Tracheostomy Tube Suctioning

A tracheostomy is an opening through the neck directly into the trachea. It is used to provide adequate ventilation when the child is unable to breathe effectively alone. This is a surgical opening and must be treated carefully to maintain patency, ensure freedom from infection, and promote adequate oxygenation. Perform suctioning when the infant or child has signs of increased respiratory effort, diminished breath sounds, audible secretions, or is unable to cough up secretions.

### PREPARATION

1. Verify the identity of the child. Explain the procedure to the child and parents.

2. An assistant or parent may be needed to position and hold the child, to keep hands out of the way, and to oxygenate the child before and after suction passes.

3. Place the head of the bed at a 30-degree angle.

4. Turn on and set the wall suction to the pressure level ordered by the healthcare provider or suggested in the agency's procedure manual.

5. Turn on the oxygen source attached to the resuscitator bag to inflate the reservoir bag so it is ready to use. Have the assistant oxygenate the child with the resuscitator bag 5 to 6 times.

6. Attach the proximal end of the catheter to the wall suction connecting tubing, making sure to keep the distal end sterile.

7. Identify in advance the length of the tracheostomy tube and appropriate depth for catheter insertion.

### EQUIPMENT AND SUPPLIES

- Additional prepared tracheostomy tubes (see Skill 15–11 for tracheostomy care)
- Resuscitation bag with attached oxygen source
- Suction catheter with multiple holes at distal end (select the size closest to the internal diameter of the tracheostomy tube)
- Suction source
- Sterile container with preservative-free sterile normal saline or distilled water
- Sterile gloves

### PROCEDURE

1. Don gloves. Keep your dominant hand sterile and your nondominant hand clean for the procedure. Use only the dominant hand to manipulate the catheter. With your dominant hand, remove the catheter from the paper sheath, keeping it sterile.

2. Place the distal end of the catheter in a cup of sterile saline or water to test the suction.

3. With your nondominant hand, remove the humidity source from the child's tracheostomy tube. Have the assistant remove the resuscitator bag.

4. Using your dominant hand, place the suction catheter into the tube and advance the catheter no farther than 0.5 cm below the edge of the tracheostomy tube (Boroughs & Dougherty, 2011).

   RATIONALE: *Suctioning the full length of the tracheostomy tube is important to prevent a mucous plug. Going deeper into the trachea may stimulate a vagal response and damage the tracheal mucosa.*

### CLINICAL TIP

Choose a French suction catheter that has multiple holes at the distal end and is closest in size to the internal diameter of the tracheostomy tube. This improves the catheter's effectiveness in removing secretions from the walls of the tracheostomy tube (Boroughs & Dougherty, 2011).

5. Suction the tracheostomy tube while advancing and removing the suction catheter, limiting suction to 5 seconds (Boroughs & Dougherty, 2011). Rotate the catheter between the fingers and thumb to suction all areas of the tracheostomy tube wall (Figure 15–23).

6. Irrigate the catheter in a cup of sterile saline or water.

7. Repeat if necessary, oxygenating the child between suctioning passes.

8. Document the procedure, the character of the secretions, how the child tolerated the procedure, and vital signs.

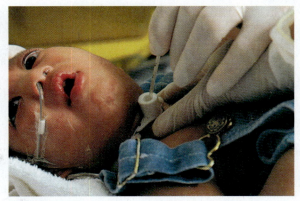

**Figure 15–23**  *Tracheostomy tube suctioning.*

## SKILL 15–25  Endotracheal Tube Suctioning

The child with an endotracheal tube is often sedated, so deep suctioning may be required to clear secretions that could obstruct the endotracheal tube. It must be performed with great care to keep the tube from being dislodged. Indications for endotracheal tube suctioning include any of the following signs: audible or visible secretions in the tube, coarse breath sounds on auscultation, coughing, and increased respiratory effort.

### PREPARATION

1. Verify the identity of the child. Explain the procedure to the parents, and to the child if alert.

2. Use an assistant to hold the endotracheal (ET) tube firmly in place whenever it is being manipulated: while the ventilator is being disconnected, when the resuscitator bag is being attached and removed for preoxygenation, and when suctioning. This prevents unintentional extubation.

3. Turn on and set the wall suction to the pressure level ordered by the healthcare provider or according to agency guidelines. Connect the proximal end of the catheter to the wall suction connecting tubing.

4. Turn on the oxygen source attached to the resuscitation bag to inflate the reservoir bag so it is ready for use.

5. Identify the length of the ET tube to determine how far the suction catheter will be advanced. Note the centimeter at the mouth and add 1.0 to 1.5 cm for the adapter.

### EQUIPMENT AND SUPPLIES

- Suction catheter sized 50% of the diameter of the ET tube for children and 70% of the diameter for infants (in general, double the size of the ET tube to identify the French catheter size)
- Sterile container with sterile preservative-free normal saline
- Resuscitator bag
- Oxygen source and tubing
- Sterile gloves

### PROCEDURE

1. Don gloves. Keep your dominant hand sterile and your nondominant hand clean for the procedure. Use only the dominant hand to manipulate the catheter.

2. With your dominant hand, remove the catheter from the paper sheath, keeping it sterile. Place the distal end of the catheter in a cup of sterile saline to test the suction pressure.

3. If the child is being ventilated, have an assistant disconnect the ventilator and manually ventilate and oxygenate the child with the resuscitator bag before suctioning. Give several breaths and then remove the resuscitation bag.

4. With your dominant hand, place the suction catheter into the ET tube and advance the catheter to a predetermined level, no farther than 0.5 cm below the bottom of the tube.
   **RATIONALE:** *Advancing the catheter beyond this distance causes damage to the tracheal mucosa.*

5. Cover the suction port and suction for 5 seconds while rotating and withdrawing the suction catheter (Boroughs & Dougherty, 2011).

6. Oxygenate the child.

7. Irrigate the suction catheter in a cup of sterile saline. Have the assistant oxygenate the child. Ensure that the ET tube is at the same position as before suctioning.

8. Repeat only if excessive secretions were noted. Assess the child's vital signs and preoxygenate the child between suctioning passes.

9. Document the procedure, the secretions cleared, their color and quality, how the child tolerated the procedure, and vital signs.

# Chest Physiotherapy/Postural Drainage

Chest physiotherapy is an airway clearance technique that combines positioning or postural drainage (allowing gravity to help drain secretions into central airways), rhythmic percussion of the chest wall (to help loosen secretions), and coughing and breathing. Chest physiotherapy is used in children who have excessive sputum production or retained bronchial secretions.

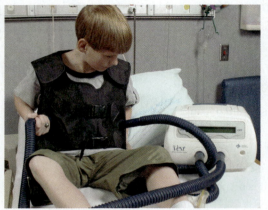

These procedures are usually done before the morning meal, and again at bedtime if the child is subject to nighttime mucus retention, plugging of airways, and/or coughing. Chest physiotherapy may be performed more frequently when an infection is present.

Aerosol hypertonic saline and bronchodilators are frequently administered before chest physiotherapy is performed.

Two maneuvers can be done to aid in postural drainage: percussion and vibration. Percussion produces chest vibrations that dislodge retained secretions, which are then drained by gravity to larger airways to be coughed up. Vibration is the application of a downward vibrating pressure with the flat part of the palm over the area that is being drained. Some children with cystic fibrosis use a vest airway clearance system (Figure 15–24). The vest provides high-frequency chest wall oscillation that increases airflow velocity to create repetitive coughlike shear forces that thin, loosen, and move secretions. The child stops the 20- to 30-minute treatment every 5 minutes to cough or huff to move secretions to be coughed up (Cystic Fibrosis Foundation, 2012).

**Figure 15–24** *Child with cystic fibrosis using a vest for chest physiotherapy.*

---

## SKILL 15–26 Performing Chest Physiotherapy/Postural Drainage

### SAFETY ALERT

Postural drainage positions may cause problems for children with gastroesophageal reflux. For example, in the positions with the head lower than the stomach, reflux can occur, causing discomfort, wheezing, and vomiting. Consider timing the postural drainage procedure to coincide with peak action for medication used to treat gastroesophageal reflux.

### PREPARATION

1. Verify the identity of the client, and review the procedure with the child and parents.

2. Ensure that several hours have passed since the child has eaten.
   **RATIONALE:** *Percussion stimulates coughing spells that can trigger vomiting. Vomiting is less likely if the stomach is empty.*

3. Perform a baseline respiratory assessment. Place the child on a pulse oximeter.
   **RATIONALE:** *Chest physiotherapy predisposes the child to arterial desaturation. A baseline assessment is performed to contrast with the child's responses during the procedure.*

4. Administer the aerosol hypertonic saline or bronchodilator, if prescribed, to hydrate secretions and relax the airway muscles.
   **RATIONALE:** *When the secretions are moistened and the airway muscles are more dilated, the secretions can drain easily.*

### EQUIPMENT AND SUPPLIES

- Commercial percussor, round oxygen mask, baby bottle nipple (for infants)
- Vibrator, vibration vest, or other airway clearance device
- Emesis basin or sputum cup
- Pulse oximeter
- Paper tissues
- Clean gloves

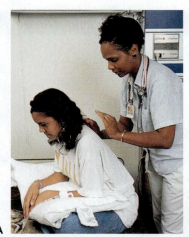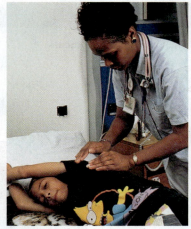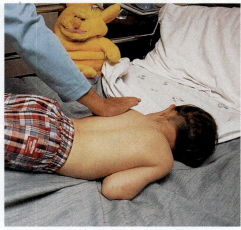

A    B    C

**Figure 15–25**  *A and B, Postural drainage can be achieved by clapping with a cupped hand on the chest wall over the segment to be drained to create vibrations that are transmitted to the bronchi to dislodge secretions. Various positions are used, depending on the location of the obstruction (see Table 15–3). C, Vibration technique of chest physiotherapy.*

## PROCEDURE

### Percussion

1. Place the child in the position to permit gravity drainage of secretions. If using the hands to percuss the chest, hold the hands cupped with fingers and thumb together. Keep the wrists loose and elbows partially flexed. Strike the chest, alternating the hands. Listen for a hollow sound (see Figure 15–25*A* and *B*).

2. Develop a rhythm with the alternate hands, and cover the targeted chest area in a circular pattern for 3 to 5 minutes.

3. Avoid tender areas, the breasts of an adolescent girl, and bony prominences such as the clavicles or vertebrae.

   RATIONALE: *Percussion should be focused over intercostal spaces to have the best effect in loosening secretions. Avoiding tender areas will minimize the child's discomfort.*

4. Have the child change position to drain another area of the lungs; percuss that area for 3 to 5 minutes. Continue this process until all areas of the chest have been percussed.

5. The positions used for each client are based on the location of mucous obstruction (see Table 15–3). In generalized obstructive lung disease, the lower lobes are drained first, followed by the middle lobes and lingula. The upper lobes are drained last. The various positions used for bronchial drainage in an infant are described in Table 15–4.

6. Encourage the child to take a few deep breaths and to cough or huff (taking a breath in and actively exhaling, as if to steam up a mirror) after percussion in each location. Have the child expectorate sputum into an emesis basin or cup.

   RATIONALE: *The deep breaths increase the velocity of the expired air and help to move the secretions toward the bronchial trees and trachea, where they can be coughed up.*

7. Monitor the child's cardiorespiratory status.

8. Document the procedures, the quality of expectorants, and how the child responded to the procedure.

### Vibration

1. Position one hand flat on the chest over the involved area and the other hand on top of the first. Alternatively, the hands may be placed side by side on the chest. Keep the arms and shoulders straight.

2. Tell the child to take a deep breath, inhaling through the nose and exhaling through the mouth.

   RATIONALE: *Vibration is performed only during exhalation.*

3. Vibrate the area by tensing and relaxing your arms for 10 to 15 seconds. Perform these tensing/relaxing actions for 3 to 5 minutes. Move to another area of the chest and repeat the process (Figure 15–25*C*).

4. Encourage coughing between vibrations and expectoration of sputum into a cup or emesis basin.

5. Document the procedures, the quality of expectorants, and how the child responded to the procedure.

| TABLE 15–3 | Positions Used for Postural Drainage in a Child |
|---|---|

**Bronchopulmonary segments**

| Location | No. | Color key |
|---|---|---|
| *Right Upper Lobe* | | |
| Apical | 1 | Red ▲ |
| Anterior | 2 | Light blue ▲ |
| Posterior | 3 | Green ▲ |
| *Right Middle Lobe* | | |
| Lateral | 4 | Purple ▲ |
| Medial | 5 | Orange ▲ |
| *Right Lower Lobe* | | |
| Superior | 6 | Lavender ▲ |
| Medial basal | 7 | Olive ▲ |
| Anterior basal | 8 | Yellow ▲ |
| Lateral basal | 9 | Red ▲ |
| Posterior basal | 10 | Turquoise ▲ |
| *Left Upper Lobe* | | |
| Upper apical— | | |
| Posterior | 1 | Red ▲ |
| Anterior | 2 | Light blue ▲ |
| Lower—lingular | | |
| Superior | 4 | Purple ▲ |
| Inferior | 5 | Orange ▲ |
| *Left Lower Lobe* | | |
| Superior | 6 | Lavender ▲ |
| Anteromedial | 8 | Yellow ▲ |
| Lateral basal | 9 | Red ▲ |
| Posterior | 10 | Turquoise ▲ |

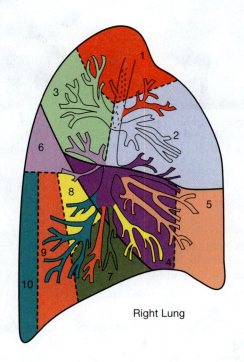

Right Lung

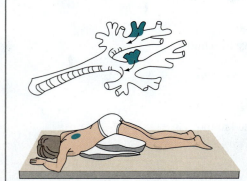

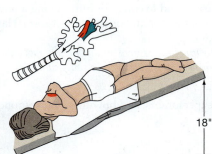

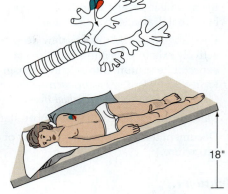

**Lower Lobes**

*Posterior Basal Segment (10)*
Elevate foot of table or bed 18 in. or 30 degrees. Have child lie prone, head down, with pillow under hips. Upper leg can be flexed over a pillow for support. (Percuss over lower ribs close to spine on each side of chest.)

*Lateral Basal Segment (9)*
Elevate foot of table or bed 18 in. or 30 degrees. Have child lie prone, then rotate 1/4 turn upward. Upper leg can be flexed over a pillow for support. (Percuss over uppermost portion of lower ribs.)

*Anterior Basal Segment (8)*
Elevate foot of table or bed 18 in. or 30 degrees. Have child lie on side, head down, pillow under knees. (Percuss over lower ribs just beneath axilla.)

| TABLE 15–3 | Positions Used for Postural Drainage in a Child (*continued*) |
| --- | --- |

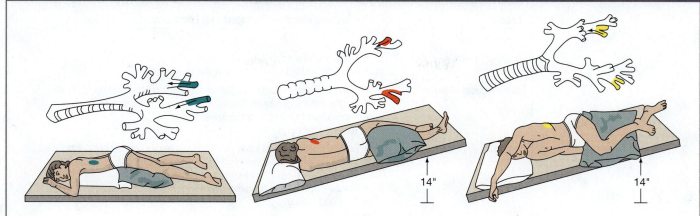

### Lower Lobes—cont'd

*Superior Segment (6)*
Place bed or table flat. Have child lie with pillows under hips. (Percuss over middle of back below tip of scapula on either side of spine.)

### Right Middle Lobe

*Lateral Segment (4)*
*Medial Segment (5)*
Elevate foot of table or bed 14 in. or about 15 degrees. Have child lie head down on left side and rotate 1/4 turn backward. Pillow may be placed behind child from shoulder to hip. Knees should be flexed. (Percuss over right nipple area.)

### Left Upper Lobe

*Lingular Segment—Superior (4)*
*Inferior (4)*
Elevate foot of table or bed 14 in. or about 15 degrees. Have child lie head down on right side and rotate 1/4 turn backward. Pillow may be placed behind child from shoulder to hip. Knees should be flexed. (Percuss over left nipple area.)

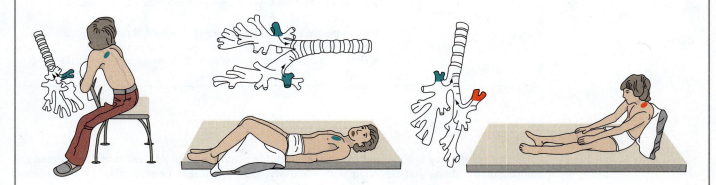

### Upper Lobes

*Posterior Segment (3)*
Have child sit up and lean over folded pillow at 30-degree angle. (Percuss over upper back on each side of chest.)

*Anterior Segment (2)*
Place bed or drainage table flat. Have child lie supine with pillow under knees. (Percuss between clavicle and nipple on each side of chest.)

*Apical Segment (1)*
Place bed or drainage table flat. Have child lean back on pillow at 30-degree angle. (Percuss over area between clavicle and top of scapula on each side of chest.)

Source: Modified from material provided by Datalizer Slide Charts, Addison, IL.

| TABLE 15–4 | Positions to Facilitate Bronchial Drainage in an Infant |
|---|---|
| **Lobes** | **Percussion/Vibration Positions and Locations** |
| *Lower Lobes* | |
| Posterior basal segment | ▪ Place the infant prone on a pillow on your lap.<br>▪ Percuss and vibrate the back at the lower ribs. |
| Lateral basal segment | ▪ Place the infant prone on a pillow on your lap at a 30-degree angle.<br>▪ Rotate the infant's body slightly so that one side is elevated.<br>▪ Percuss and vibrate over the lower ribs.<br>▪ Turn and repeat. |
| Anterior basal segment | ▪ Extend your legs and keep them slightly flexed (use a chair for support).<br>▪ Place the infant, supported on a pillow, in a side-lying position (30-degree angle) with the head down.<br>▪ Percuss and vibrate the area over the ribs under the axilla.<br>▪ Turn and repeat. |
| Superior segment | ▪ Place the infant prone on a pillow on your lap.<br>▪ Percuss and vibrate the back. |
| *Upper Lobes* | |
| Lateral and medial segments | ▪ Place the infant on your lap in the prone position.<br>▪ Rotate the infant slightly so that the right side is elevated.<br>▪ Percuss and vibrate the anterior chest at the nipple line.<br>▪ Turn the infant and repeat. |
| Posterior segment | ▪ Place the infant on your lap in a sitting position and leaning forward on a pillow at about a 30-degree angle.<br>▪ Percuss and vibrate both sides of the upper back. |
| Anterior segment | ▪ Place the infant supine on your lap.<br>▪ Percuss and vibrate the area between the clavicle and the midchest at the nipple line. |
| Apical segment | ▪ Place the infant on your lap in a sitting position. Lower the infant to a 30-degree reclining position, using a pillow for support.<br>▪ Percuss and vibrate the area between the clavicles and the scapulae. |

# Incentive Spirometry

Incentive spirometry is a method to encourage children to fully expand their lungs to prevent the pooling of secretions that can occur with inactivity. Although it may be prescribed by a healthcare provider, it can also be a nursing order. Children are often taught incentive spirometry preoperatively so they can effectively use the procedure after surgery.

## SKILL 15–27  Using the Incentive Spirometer

### PREPARATION

1. Verify the identity of the child. Explain the procedure to the child and parents and why it is important to take deep breaths.

2. Identify the incentive spirometer that matches the child's development.

3. If the child has had thoracic or abdominal surgery, show the child and parent how to splint the surgical site to reduce discomfort.
   RATIONALE: *Giving the child some control and a strategy to manage discomfort will lead to increased compliance with the procedure.*

### EQUIPMENT AND SUPPLIES

▪ Incentive spirometer
▪ Straw and cotton balls or plastic disk
▪ Pinwheel

## PROCEDURE

1. Assess the child's respiratory status before and after the procedure, including auscultation of the lungs.

2. With the incentive spirometer, have the child take a deep breath, close the lips around the tube, and blow forcefully but steadily into the tube to make the ball rise (see Figure 15–26). The blowing should be maintained for a few seconds to keep the ball suspended. Some spirometers require the child to close the lips around the tube and inhale to make the ball rise.

3. Repeat the procedure 2 to 3 times several times a day. Encourage the child to make the ball rise higher each time until the target level is reached. After the target level is reached, encourage the child to lengthen the time the ball is suspended.
   RATIONALE: *The forced, sustained exhalation helps move secretions to the central airway, making it easier to cough them up.*

4. An alternative method is to have the child use a straw to blow cotton balls or a plastic ball across a table. Make the procedure a game.
   RATIONALE: *Children respond to competitions and will work harder to perform the procedure successfully.*

5. Preschool children may respond to blowing a pinwheel. As the pinwheel's spinning slows, have the child take another deep breath and blow again. Encourage the child to stretch the expiration to make the pinwheel spin longer. When the child is able to blow more forcefully, slowly move the pinwheel farther away.

6. Document the procedure, the child's response, and respiratory status.

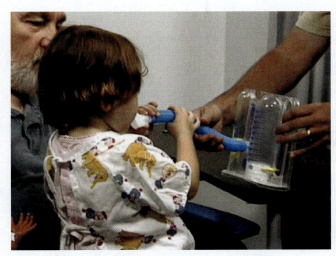

**Figure 15–26** *Child using an incentive spirometer.*

# Chapter 16
# Nutrition

 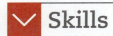
## Gastric Tubes

Gastric tubes are used in infants and children to provide a means of alimentation and to decompress or empty the stomach. The size of the nasogastric or orogastric tube is determined by the age, size, and weight of the child.

## Orogastric Tubes

Orogastric tubes are used in newborns and young infants who are obligate nose breathers, and in older children who are unconscious, unresponsive, or intubated.

### SKILL 16–1 Inserting and Removing an Orogastric Tube

**PREPARATION**

1. Verify the order and collect supplies.
2. Identify the child and explain the procedure to the child and parents.
3. Assess the child and document findings.

**EQUIPMENT AND SUPPLIES**

- Appropriate-size orogastric tube
- Suction catheter and equipment
- Water-soluble lubricant
- Stethoscope
- 10- to 20-mL syringe and pH paper to check tube placement
- Clean gloves

**PROCEDURE**

*Insertion*

1. Place the child supine with the head of the bed elevated, unless contraindicated.
2. Don gloves.
3. Use the tube to measure the distance from the mouth to the tragus of the ear and then to the xiphoid process to determine the distance to the stomach. (Alternatively, use a point midway between the xiphoid and the umbilicus.) Mark the tube with tape.
4. Have suction at hand. Apply a water-soluble lubricant to the orogastric tube.
   **RATIONALE:** *If the child vomits, it may be necessary to remove secretions.*

5. Position the child with the neck slightly hyperextended. Open the child's mouth and insert the tube toward the back of the throat. Continue advancing the tube slowly until you reach the mark. Coordinate advancement with swallowing if the child is able to cooperate.
   RATIONALE: *This position facilitates passage of the tube by opening the neck and mouth.*

6. Check the tube for appropriate placement.
   - Aspirate the stomach contents and check the pH of the aspirate on the unit or by the laboratory as determined by agency policy. A pH of 5 or below generally indicates stomach placement. However, respiratory secretions also can have a low pH, so the test is not definitive. In addition, some medications and tube feedings can alter the stomach pH. When verifying placement before future tube feedings, wait at least 1 hour after feedings and medications, flush the tube with about 30 mL of air, and then test pH. This will minimize the effect of feedings and medication on altering gastric pH. Visually evaluate the aspirate in addition to performing the pH test, as gastric contents are commonly clear or tan.
   - A radiograph may be used to verify correct placement.
   - Assess the child's respiratory status and color. A change in either or vomiting may indicate that the tube is located in the trachea rather than in the esophagus (American Association of Critical Care Nurses, 2010; Chan et al., 2012; Simons, 2012; Tho, Mordiffi, Ang, et al., 2011).

7. Once you have ensured that the tube is in place, mark the exit point from the body so it can be used in the future to confirm that the external length has not changed. Tape it securely to one side of the child's mouth, placing two pieces of tape in a V pattern around the tube at the lip; if necessary, use a third piece of tape over the other two. Clamp the end of the tube if it is not being used for feeding or suctioning. Repeat the assessment of the child at least every 4 hours.
   RATIONALE: *Measures must be taken to maintain the tube in the correct position so that it does not become dislodged.*

8. Document tube placement, length of tube inserted, the child's response, and results of the child's assessment.

### Removal

1. Verify the identity of the child and explain the procedure to the child and parents.

2. Have suction available.
   RATIONALE: *If the child vomits, it may be necessary to remove secretions.*

3. Instill approximately 10 to 20 mL of air into the tube to remove any secretions.

4. Untape the tube, pinch or fold it to prevent fluid leakage, and gently withdraw it.

## Nasogastric Tubes

Nasogastric tubes are used more frequently than orogastric tubes. They are inserted to provide alimentation, to decompress the stomach, or to empty the stomach of its contents in preparation for surgery or lavage.

---

## SKILL 16–2 Inserting and Removing a Nasogastric Tube

### PREPARATION

1. Verify the order and collect supplies.

2. Verify the identity of the child.

3. Assess the child and document findings.

4. Tell the preschool-age child what will happen in very simple terms. Give the school-age child and adolescent a rationale for the procedure. Because placement of the tube is uncomfortable, allow children to express their feelings and seek the support of family members.

### EQUIPMENT AND SUPPLIES

- Appropriate-size nasogastric tube (see Table 16–1)
- Suction catheter and equipment
- Water-soluble lubricant
- Stethoscope
- 10- to 20-mL syringe to check tube placement
- Clean gloves

| TABLE 16–1 | Recommended Sizes for Nasogastric Tubes |
|---|---|
| **Age** | **Nasogastric Tube Size (French Catheter)** |
| Preterm | 5 |
| Newborn and infant | 5–8 |
| 1–3 years | 10 |
| 4–6 years | 10–12 |
| 7–11 years | 12–14 |
| Adolescent | 14–16 |

Source: Adapted from Emergency Nurses Association. (2012). *Provider manual: Emergency nursing pediatric course.* Des Plains, IL: Author.

## PROCEDURE

### Insertion

1. Place the child supine, with the head of the bed elevated to the high Fowler position, if possible. Position and hold younger children because they will fight against the insertion of the tube. The child's body and arms can be held by an assistant, or the child can be put in a modified mummy immobilizer. The child's head will need to be held in the midline position.

2. Don gloves.

3. Use the tube to measure the distance from the tip of the nose to the tragus of the ear and then to the xiphoid process to determine the distance to the stomach (Figure 16–1). (Alternatively, use a point midway between the xiphoid and the umbilicus.) Mark the tube with tape.

4. Have suction at hand. Apply water-soluble lubricant to the distal end of the nasogastric tube.

5. With the child's neck slightly hyperextended, insert the tube into the child's naris, gently advancing it straight back along the floor of the nasal passages. If resistance is felt at the curve of the nasopharynx, use slight pressure or rotate the tube to continue advancing it.

6. If the child gags when the tube reaches beyond the oropharynx, flex the child's neck. If the child can take fluids by mouth, have the child sip water through a straw and swallow it to ease the passage of the tube over the glottis. If the child is not allowed anything by mouth, have the child swallow.

   RATIONALE: *Gagging is most common as the tube passes just beyond the back of the throat. Swallowing can decrease the gag reflex until the tube is advanced slightly beyond this point. This facilitates passage of the tube.*

7. After the gag reflex is suppressed, continue advancing the tube slowly until the marked location on the tube reaches the naris.

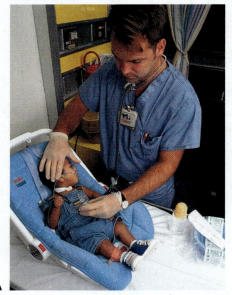
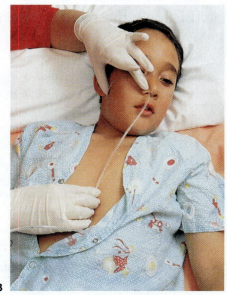

A           B

**Figure 16–1** *Measuring for nasogastric tube placement in A, an infant, and B, a child. (A similar technique is used in measuring for orogastric tube insertion. See the previous discussion.)*

8. Check the tube for appropriate placement.

   - Aspirate the stomach contents and check the pH of the aspirate; a pH of 5 or below generally indicates stomach placement. However, respiratory secretions also can have a low pH, so the test is not definitive. In addition, some medications and tube feedings can alter the stomach pH. When verifying placement before future tube feedings, wait at least 1 hour after feedings and medications, flush the tube with about 30 mL of air, and then test pH. This will minimize the effect of feedings and medication on altering gastric pH. Visually evaluate the aspirate in addition to performing the pH test, as gastric contents are commonly clear or tan.

   - A radiograph may be used to verify correct placement.

   - Assess the child's respiratory status and color. A change in either or vomiting may indicate that the tube is located in the trachea rather than in the esophagus (American Association of Critical Care Nurses, 2010; Chan et al., 2012; Simons, 2012; Tho et al., 2011).

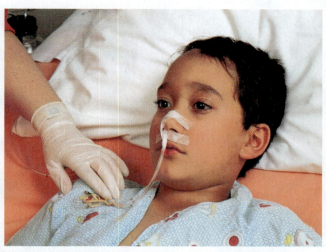

**Figure 16–2**  *Nasogastric tube taped securely in place.*

9. Once you are assured that the tube is in place, mark the exit point from the body so it can be used in the future to confirm that the external length has not changed. Tape it securely by placing two pieces of tape in a V pattern around the tube and attaching it to the nose or cheek (Figure 16–2). If necessary, use a second piece of tape over the first.

10. Document tube placement, length of tube inserted, the child's response, and results of the child's assessment. Assess tube and placement at least every 4 hours.

### Removal

1. Verify the identity of the child and explain the procedure to the parents and child.

2. Have suction available.

3. Place the child in a Fowler position.

4. Instill approximately 10 to 15 mL of air into the tube to remove any secretions.

5. Unfasten the tape, ask the child to hold his or her breath, pinch the tube, and gently pull it out.

6. Document tube removal and the child's response.

## Gastrostomy Tubes

Gastrostomy tubes are surgically placed in the stomach and are used primarily for gavage feeding. The tube should remain clamped when it is not being used for feeding or decompression.

Observe the site for skin breakdown. Keep the area clean and dry. Place a clean, dry dressing over the site at every shift. A 2″ × 2″ or 4″ × 4″ gauze pad can be used. A diagonal cut is made halfway into the square and placed around the tube, with tape used at the edges to secure it.

Keep the tube as immobile as possible to prevent unintentional removal or displacement. Tube placement can be checked by aspirating a small amount of gastric contents before each feeding.

The gastrostomy feeding button is a flexible silicone device that is often used for children who require long-term enteral feedings.

## Gavage/Tube Feeding

Infants and children require gavage or tube feeding to counteract absorption disorders, to provide supplemental feedings, and to conserve calories for growth. Feedings can be either continuous or bolus. They can be administered by gravity or by pump (Figure 16–3). A pump is preferred because it permits better regulation of the rate and volume of the feeding. Although feedings can be administered through orogastric or nasogastric tubes, an indwelling tube is usually surgically placed into the stomach when prolonged feedings will be needed. The tube is often placed by percutaneous endoscopic gastrostomy (and is then called a *PEG tube*); the tube may be placed in the stomach and be called a *gastrostomy tube* (G-tube), or into the jejunum or duodenum and be called a *jejunostomy tube* (J-tube). In these cases, a balloon or flared tip of the tube is anchored internally into the gastrointestinal system, and a small tube travels outside the body and is anchored on the skin, appearing like a "button" (Figure 16–4).

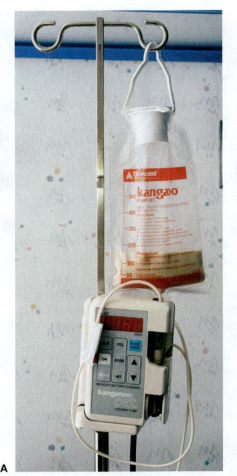

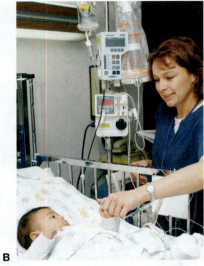

A                                                    B

**Figure 16–3** *A, Feeding pump. B, The pump helps regulate the rate and volume of feeding.*

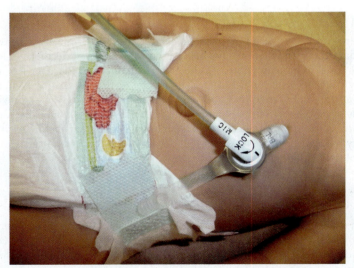

**Figure 16–4** *The gastrostomy tube can be implanted in the stomach, with a small "button" on the exterior of the body. It is opened to administer feedings when needed.*

# SKILL 16–3  Administering a Gavage/Tube Feeding

## PREPARATION

1. Verify the identity of the child. Review the feeding procedure with the child and family.

2. If the feeding is to be given by gravity, an IV pole may be used. If the feeding is to be given by pump, gather the necessary bag and tubing. Prime the appropriate tubing, keeping the distal end covered.

   **RATIONALE:** *The tubing is primed to eliminate air. If air is infused into the gastrointestinal tract, discomfort can occur.*

3. If possible, place the child in a semi-Fowler position. If not, a prone or side-lying position is preferred to the supine position.

   **RATIONALE:** *These positions decrease the risk of aspiration.*

## EQUIPMENT AND SUPPLIES

- Formula at room temperature (to prevent cramping)
- Water for irrigation of the tube
- Stethoscope
- 10- to 20-mL syringe to check tube placement
- Clean gloves

## PROCEDURE

1. Don gloves.

2. Check the placement of the tube before each feeding by aspirating the stomach contents or auscultating over the abdomen while a small amount of air (5 or 10 mL in older children) is injected through the tube into the stomach. See further methods of assessing for tube placement in previous skill sections.

3. Assess the child's respiratory status and color.

   **RATIONALE:** *Changes in either may indicate that the nasogastric or orogastric tube is located in the trachea instead of in the esophagus.*

4. Once you are assured that the tube is in place, check gastric residuals and proceed with the steps necessary for the feeding.

### Bolus Feeding

1. Aspirate the stomach contents to check the amount of residual. If the residual is less than half of the previous feeding, return the aspirated contents to the stomach. If the residual is greater, notify the physician.

   **RATIONALE:** *A large amount of residual indicates that the child is not absorbing the feeding. The type or amount may need adjustment.*

2. Attach the primed tubing from either the pump or the gravity set to the gastrostomy tube. Start the flow slowly while checking the patency of the tube. Set the rate and volume according to the physician's orders.

3. When the feeding has been completed, assess the child's condition. Clamp and disconnect the tubing. Flush the tubing with a small amount of water to clean it.

4. When families will carry out tube feedings at home, be sure that they understand the procedure and what to do for any problems (Table 16–2). Demonstrate a feeding and then actively involve family members in the second and subsequent feedings, until confident that all members who will administer medications and feedings can independently carry out the procedure.

5. Document the procedure, the gastric residuals, the child's response, and the teaching performed.

### Continuous Feeding

1. The procedure for continuous feeding is very similar to that for bolus feeding. However, the formula should hang no longer than 4 hours.

   **RATIONALE:** *Microorganisms can grow in warm formula, so it must be changed once left out for several hours.*

| TABLE 16–2 | Home Care Instructions for the Child Requiring Gastrostomy Tube Feedings and Care |
| --- | --- |

*Equipment*

Prepared, prescribed feeding

Enteral feeding pump

Long-nosed 20- to 60-mL syringe

*Procedure*

1. Wash hands with soap and water.

2. Warm prescribed formula to room temperature.

3. Pour formula to run through the feeding bag.

4. Allow formula to run through the tubing to remove air. Close clamp.

5. Attach an empty open syringe to the end of the gastrostomy tube. Unclamp the extension tube.

6. Note whether the formula from the previous feeding flows into the syringe. Check the amount of formula in the syringe. Follow specific guidelines from the healthcare provider if residual is noted.

7. Attach the feeding bag to the gastrostomy tube. Infuse at the prescribed rate. Alternatively, a bolus feeding may be given by syringe slowly rather than through a feeding bag.

8. Elevate the head of the child's bed or allow an older child to sit in a high chair or chair while feedings are infusing. Infants may be burped during and after feedings as necessary.

9. After feeding, flush the gastrostomy tube with 5 mL of water (or other prescribed amount) and clamp the tube.

*Psychosocial Needs*

Hold and rock the infant or child during feedings.

Give a pacifier to an infant or a bottle or cup to a child to meet developmental needs for oral stimulation.

*Medication Administration*

Use liquid medication when possible.

Avoid the use of tablets if possible.

If necessary, crush uncoated tablets to a fine powder and mix with water or juice.

Flush tubing with 3–5 mL of water after medication administration.

*Stoma Care*

Wash the area around the stoma daily with soap and water, and pat dry.

Look for signs of infection, such as redness, swelling, and discharge.

Notify the healthcare provider if any signs of infection or leakage, site irritation, or hypergranulation tissue are present.

*Problem Solving*

If the tube comes out, place a dressing over the site and call or visit the healthcare provider or emergency department.

If the formula will not flow, make sure the clamp is open. If the clamp is open, try flushing the tube with water. If this does not resolve the problem, call the number provided at discharge, unless more specific instructions were given at that time.

If skin irritation or breakdown occurs around the stoma site, call for advice before using any creams or ointments, unless specific instructions were given at discharge. Use only creams that the healthcare provider has prescribed.

Nurses should provide families with phone numbers to call when complications arise.

Source: Table compiled by Kay Cowen, MSN, RN-BC, CNE. Data from Correa, J. A., Fallon, S. C., Murphy, K. M., Victorian, V. A., Bisset, G. S., Vasudevan, S. A., . . . Lee, T. C. (2014). Resource utilization after gastrostomy tube placement: Defining areas of improvement for future quality improvement projects. *Journal of Pediatric Surgery, 49*, 1598–1601; Hannah, E., & John, R. M. (2013). Everything the nurse practitioner should know about pediatric feeding tubes. *Journal of the American Association of Nurse Practitioners, 25*, 567–577; Schweitzer, M., Aucoin, J., Docherty, S. L., Rice, H. E., Thompson, J., & Sullivan, D. T. (2014). Evaluation of a discharge education protocol for pediatric patients with gastrostomy tubes. *Journal of Pediatric Health Care, 28*(5), 420–428.

2. When the feeding bag is hung, label it with the time and date.

3. Change the feeding set every 24 hours or per agency policy.

4. Assess the child's condition and monitor respiratory status during the feeding.

5. Document the procedure and the child's response.

# Gastric Suctioning

Both orogastric and nasogastric tubes can be connected to a suctioning device (Figure 16–5) to provide either continuous or intermittent suction; these procedures are described next. They may also be allowed to drain by gravity.

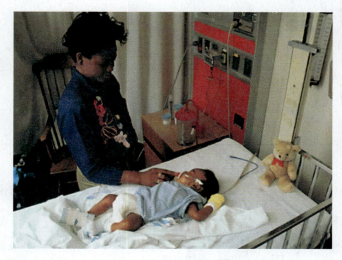

**Figure 16–5** *Nasogastric tube attached to a suctioning device.*

---

## SKILL 16–4 Performing Gastric Suctioning

### PREPARATION

1. Verify the identity of the child, and explain the procedure to the child and parents.
2. Check the suction equipment.

### EQUIPMENT AND SUPPLIES

- Suctioning equipment
- Stethoscope
- 10-mL syringe for air insertion
- Clean gloves

### PROCEDURE

1. Before making the connection, don gloves.
2. Check the tube for proper position by aspirating the stomach contents or auscultating over the abdomen while a small amount of air (5 or 10 mL in older children) is injected through the tube into the stomach.
3. Assess the child's respiratory status and color. Changes in either may indicate that the tube is located in the trachea instead of in the esophagus.
4. Attach the suction to the orogastric or nasogastric tube at its distal end. Tape the connection site.
5. Turn the suction to the setting ordered by the physician. Observe the color, amount, and character of the contents suctioned.
6. Document the child's response (vital signs, complaints of abdominal discomfort).
7. Monitor the child's condition frequently, and label the level of the contents collected.
   **RATIONALE:** *Contents can indicate difficulty absorbing nutrients or suggest problems with digestive processes. In the case of suction following poisoning, contents can indicate the amount of a poisonous substance that has been successfully removed.*
8. Document the procedure and the child's response.

# Chapter 17
# Elimination

## Urinary Catheterization

Urinary catheterization is performed to obtain sterile urine for diagnostic purposes, to measure the amount of urine in the bladder accurately, to empty the bladder, or to relieve bladder distention. In the hospital setting, it is performed as a sterile procedure. For children outside the hospital who need intermittent catheterization, it is done as a clean procedure.

### SKILL 17–1 Performing an Indwelling Urinary Catheterization

An indwelling urinary catheterization is performed when urine output needs to be carefully measured or the bladder needs to be continuously drained.

#### PREPARATION

1. Check the physician's orders to confirm that indwelling catheterization is planned.
2. Verify the identity of the child. Explain the procedure to the child and parents and why it is necessary.
3. Determine the size of the catheter based on the child's size, age, and weight.

#### EQUIPMENT AND SUPPLIES

- Urinary catheters—size appropriate for the child's age, and one a size smaller
- Sterile urinary catheterization tray (containing drapes, sterile gloves, antiseptic solution, cotton swabs or balls, forceps, lubricant, and a container for urine)
- Container for soiled cotton balls
- Syringe filled with normal saline
- Tape
- Drainage-collection apparatus
- Absorbent pads
- Sterile gloves

#### PROCEDURE

1. Have an assistant hold the child in position for the procedure. If the parents wish to stay with the child, have them stand at the child's head and offer distraction and comfort.
2. Place absorbent pads under the child's perineum.

3. Open the tray, maintaining the sterile field. Pour the antiseptic over the cotton swabs or balls.

4. Don sterile gloves. Open the lubricant and squeeze it onto the sterile field. Lubricate the tip of the catheter and place the distal end in the tray.

### Female

5. Clean the perineum. Spread the labia apart with the nondominant hand. Pick up the antiseptic-soaked cotton balls with forceps using the dominant hand. Clean the meatus, using one ball for each wipe, in a front-to-back direction along each side of the labia minora, then along the sides of the urinary meatus, and finally straight down over the urethral opening. Discard each cotton ball away from the sterile field.

   RATIONALE: *Wiping in the direction from the urinary meatus toward the anus avoids contaminating the urinary meatus with fecal bacteria.*

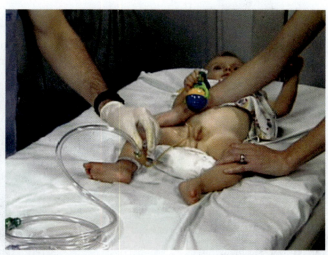

**Figure 17–1** *Attaching the catheter to the drainage apparatus, after performing an indwelling urinary catheterization.*

6. Pick up the lubricated catheter tip with your dominant hand, keeping the distal end in the specimen container.

   RATIONALE: *The dominant hand remains sterile and should be the one to handle the catheter. Placing the distal end in a specimen container prevents contamination of the sterile field when urine flows.*

7. Gently insert the tip into the meatus (approximately 5 to 8 cm [2 to 3 in.] in the child) until there is a free flow of urine, and then 2.5 cm (1.0 in.) further. If resistance is felt, do not force the catheter. Rotate the catheter gently between your fingers and gently advance. If unsuccessful, try again with another sterile catheter, preferably one size smaller.

   RATIONALE: *A catheter should not be used a second time to prevent potential infection in the child.*

8. When the catheter is in place, collect any needed urine specimen, as described in Chapter 11. Attach the tubing to the drainage apparatus (Figure 17–1). Tape the tubing to the leg to avoid pulling.

9. Use the syringe to inflate the balloon on the catheter to the recommended amount of normal saline.

10. Make sure the tubing has no kinks. Hang the drainage apparatus on the bed frame.

11. Document the procedure and how the child tolerated it.

### Male

5. Clean the perineum. Retract the foreskin if the child is uncircumcised. With the nondominant hand, hold the penis behind the glans and spread the meatus with your thumb and forefinger.

6. Use the dominant hand to pick up the forceps and antiseptic-soaked cotton balls. Clean the tissue surrounding the meatus using one cotton ball for each wipe in an outward circular motion. Discard each cotton ball away from the sterile field.

7. Pick up the lubricated catheter tip with the dominant hand, and place the distal end in a specimen container. Lift the penis, exerting slight traction until it is perpendicular to the body. Insert the catheter steadily into the meatus until urine begins to flow, and then about 2.5 cm (1 in.) further (up to a total of 10 to 12 cm [5 to 6 in.] maximum).

   RATIONALE: *The catheter is inserted an extra inch into the bladder to ensure proper placement for drainage when an indwelling catheter is planned.*

8. If resistance to the catheter is felt, have the child blow out to relax the perineal muscles, or rotate the tube between your fingers and gently advance. Do not force the catheter. Another catheter, one size smaller, may be used if relaxation efforts are not successful.

9. Once the catheter is in place, lower the penis and collect the urine specimen, as described in Chapter 11. Attach the tubing to the drainage apparatus. Tape the tubing to the leg to avoid pulling.

10. Use the syringe to inflate the balloon on the catheter to the recommended amount of normal saline.

11. Make sure the tubing has no kinks. Hang the drainage apparatus on the bed frame.

12. Document the procedure and how the child tolerated it.

### CLINICAL TIP

If catheterization is performed for bladder distention, rapid drainage can cause a vasovagal response. Take vital signs before beginning the procedure to establish a baseline. Monitor the child, and clamp the catheter if signs of decreased alertness or lethargy are noted. Once normal assessment findings are reached, slow drainage of urine can resume.

## SKILL 17–2 Double-Diapering With a Stent in Place

A double-diapering technique is used to protect the stent (small tube that drains urine) following surgical repair of hypospadias or epispadias.

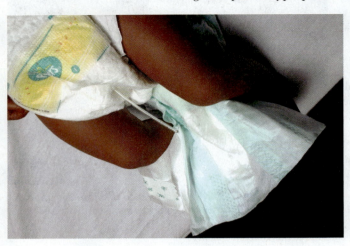

### PROCEDURE

1. Open two diapers and cut a small hole in the middle of one diaper for the stent. Place the diaper with the hole on top and place both diapers under the infant's perineum.

2. Insert the stent through the hole, and place the first diaper over the perineum. Position the stent to drain into the second diaper. Fold the second diaper into place (Figure 17–2).

   RATIONALE: *This process prevents contamination of the stent with feces. Urinary output and urine color can be assessed postsurgery.*

**Figure 17–2** *A double-diapering technique protects the urinary stent after surgery for hypospadias or epispadias repair. The inner diaper collects stool; the outer diaper collects urine.*

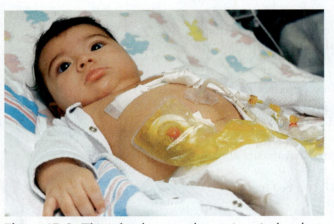

**Figure 17–3** *This infant has several gastrointestinal problems and requires ostomies both for gastric feedings and for drainage of fecal material. The care of the skin is challenging and important for this infant so that infection is prevented and adequate nutrition is provided.*

# Ostomy Care

Ostomies are performed when an infant or child requires fecal or urinary diversion (Figure 17–3). Infants and children may require an ostomy for several reasons, including necrotizing enterocolitis, Hirschsprung disease, imperforate anus, prune-belly syndrome, inflammatory bowel syndrome, spina bifida, tumor, and trauma. An ileostomy, colostomy, or urinary diversion is performed depending on the disorder and its location.

An adhesive appliance is usually applied just after surgery to measure drainage. If a dressing is applied instead of an adhesive appliance, the drainage can be measured by weighing the dressing both before and after saturation. For each 1-g increase in the weight of the dressing, approximately 1 mL of fluid has drained into it.

In children and infants, ostomies pose special problems because of the fragility of the skin. Care must be taken to prevent skin breakdown at the site.

## SKILL 17–3 Changing the Dressing for an Infant With an Ostomy

### PREPARATION

1. Explain the procedure to the child and parents.
2. Observe drainage on the dressing or in the ostomy bag carefully so it can be documented.

### EQUIPMENT AND SUPPLIES

- Gauze
- Tape or other supplies to hold gauze in place
- Clean gloves

### PROCEDURE

1. After each bowel movement, while using gloves, change the dressing, clean and dry the skin, and apply a nonporous substance.

   RATIONALE: *Fecal matter and intestinal fluids, which contain many enzymes, can cause skin breakdown. Measures must be taken to prevent this complication.*

2. Observe the stoma for complications.

   RATIONALE: *Common complications in children include prolapse, retraction, stenosis, and skin breakdown.*

**CLINICAL TIP**

Avoid adhesive enhancers on the skin of newborns and premature infants. Their skin is so thin that removal of the appliance can strip off the skin. Remember that adhesive contains latex, and it should not be used in those who are latex sensitive or allergic.

3. To absorb drainage, place gauze with slits cut to fit around the stoma. Use tape to hold the gauze in place. Alternatively, Montgomery straps, an Ace wrap, or a diaper can be used to hold the gauze in place.

   RATIONALE: *Tape sometimes irritates the fragile skin of infants, and other methods could be used to protect the skin.*

   NOTE: *Once the stoma has healed and the infant is large enough to wear a pouch, an appliance with a Stomahesive wafer will be used.*

## SKILL 17–4  Changing an Ostomy Pouch for an Infant or Child

### PREPARATION

1. Describe or review the procedure with the child and parents.
2. Ask the parents and child about the usual procedures used at home or preferences for changing the ostomy pouch if the child has had the ostomy for some time.

### EQUIPMENT AND SUPPLIES

- Pouch and clamp (one piece with adhesive wafer or two pieces with separate pouch and flange and an adhesive wafer). Some children have reusable clamps.
- Stoma measuring guide
- Stomahesive or other pectin wafer
- Water and washcloth or gauze and cotton balls
- Towel or gauze
- Scissors
- Pads for bed
- Bag for discarding used materials
- Clean gloves

### PROCEDURE

1. Don gloves.
2. Inspect for any signs of leakage around the pouch.
3. Place a pad on the bed to protect it from drainage.
4. Empty the pouch when it is one-third to one-half full.

   RATIONALE: *This prevents the bag from getting too heavy and pulling off, leading to leakage. This may reduce the frequency of pouch changes.*

5. Gently remove the pouch, and place it in a sealable plastic bag for disposal.
6. Children will commonly have Stomahesive around the stoma. Gently peel it from the skin if it needs to be changed.

   RATIONALE: *This is a wafer of protective material to which a pouch can be attached or from which the pouch can be removed, thus protecting the integrity of the skin. Most wafers need to be changed only once a week.*

7. Wash the skin and the stoma gently with water and soap without oil. Baby wipes contain lanolin or oil and should not be used. Slight bleeding from the ostomy skin may normally be seen. Note any skin breakdown or signs of infection. Dry the area.

   RATIONALE: *Lanolin or oil will reduce the effectiveness of the ostomy pouch adhesive.*

8. Apply skin barriers (e.g., liquid or powder) as needed to protect irritated skin.
9. Prepare the new pouch. Measure and cut the Stomahesive or wafer so that it is the same size as the stoma. Place it securely on the dried skin. Press the pouch firmly against the Stomahesive to form a tight seal. Be careful to avoid making any wrinkles. Close the opening of the pouch with the appropriate clamp.

   RATIONALE: *Measures are taken to prevent fecal matter from leaking onto the skin surface, where it could cause skin breakdown. During the immediate postoperative period, the size of the stoma can change, so careful measurement of the wafer to avoid skin damage by fecal material is needed.*

10. Document the procedure, the skin and stoma condition, and how the child tolerated the procedure.

# Enemas

There are three important considerations when giving an enema to an infant or a child: the type of fluid, the amount of fluid, and the appropriate distance to insert the tube into the rectum.

Generally, an isotonic fluid such as normal saline is used for children. However, a commercial hypertonic product, such as a pediatric Fleet enema, is sometimes used.

## SKILL 17–5 Administering an Enema

### PREPARATION

1. Explain the procedure to the child and parents.
2. Assure the child that a bedpan will be kept at the bedside.
3. If the child is toilet trained, place the child in a bed near a bathroom before giving the enema.
4. Ensure privacy.

### EQUIPMENT AND SUPPLIES

- Ordered solution (in container with attached tip) or enema bag and rectal tube (size 14 to 18 French for child; 12 French for infant)
- Solution container
- Enema solution (e.g., saline)
- Water-soluble lubricant
- Pads for bed
- Clean gloves

### PROCEDURE

1. Don gloves.
2. Place absorbent pads on the bed. Position the child on the left side, with the knees drawn up to the chest or the right leg flexed over the left leg. You may need an assistant to hold the child in position.
   RATIONALE: *When the child is on the left side, entry of the fluid into the colon is facilitated.*
3. If a rectal tube is being used, attach it to the solution container. Clamp the tube and add the solution. Loosen the clamp enough to fill the tubing with solution, and reclamp. Lubricate the tip. If a Fleet enema is being used, the tip is prelubricated.
4. Gently insert the tube the recommended distance (see Table 17–1). Allow the appropriate volume of fluid to run in slowly, for at least 10 to 15 minutes. Ask the child to try to retain the solution for as long as possible. If the child complains of cramping, stop the infusion to allow the child to rest, then continue.
   RATIONALE: *Giving the enema solution too quickly will cause cramping, and the child may be unable to retain the enema long enough for it to be effective.*
5. Infants and children may not be able to retain the fluid. Holding the buttocks together might help.
6. When the child is ready to expel the enema solution, escort the child to the bathroom or provide the bedpan. Provide privacy as requested. Assess for dizziness or weakness before leaving.
7. Clean the perineum. The child or parent may choose to perform this step.
8. Help the child resume a position of comfort.
9. Assess the enema return for amount and character.
10. Document the procedure, the amount and character of the enema return, and how the child tolerated the procedure.

| TABLE 17–1 | Guidelines for Administering an Enema to Children | |
| --- | --- | --- |
| **Age** | **Volume (mL)** | **Distance for Inserting Tube** |
| Infant | 40–100 | 2.5 cm (1 in.) |
| Toddler | 100–200 | 5.0 cm (2 in.) |
| Preschooler | 200–300 | 5.0 cm (2 in.) |
| School-age child | 300–500 | 7.5 cm (3 in.) |
| Adolescent | 500–700 | 10.0 cm (4 in.) |

# Chapter 18
# Skin and Musculoskeletal Care

## ⌄ Skills

### Skin

### Casts

### Crutches

### Braces

### Traction

## Skin

The skin of infants and young children is thin and prone to breakdown. Meticulous skin care is needed, particularly when the child is at risk for skin alterations. Newborns and infants may absorb certain materials readily through their thin skin, and so only products that are approved for this age group should be used to cleanse skin or administer treatments. Use these products only as directed. The newborn undergoing treatment for hyperbilirubinemia is prone to having loose stools and will need special perianal care (see Chapter 5 in this manual). The child with cancer may experience skin and mucous membrane deterioration and require skilled care. Intravenous therapy and ostomy care require frequent evaluation and care to prevent skin breakdown (see Chapters 13, 16, and 17 in this manual). These are just a few examples of the skin-care challenges in children.

## SKILL 18–1 Wound Irrigation

Wounds may be irrigated to clean away organisms and dead tissue and to promote healing. Irrigations may be done one time or repeated on a daily or more frequent basis.

### PREPARATION

1. Identify the child and explain the procedure to the child and parents.

2. Perform a pain assessment. See Chapter 8 in this manual.
   **RATIONALE:** *The child may need pain medication before the procedure begins to promote comfort.*

3. Place absorbent material under the area.

4. Don sterile gloves and remove any dressings from the wound.

5. Observe the type and amount of drainage for documentation after the procedure.

6. Discard gloves and wash hands.

### EQUIPMENT AND SUPPLIES

- Irrigation solution as ordered. Unless contraindicated, the solution should be at room temperature to promote client comfort.

- Irrigation set or sterile syringes with irrigating tip

- Sterile basin

- Method for protecting bed

- Clean linens

- New topical medications and sterile dressing as ordered
- Sterile gloves

## PROCEDURE

1. Check to be sure that pads and other absorbent materials are adequately positioned under the area to be irrigated.

2. Set up a sterile field and open supplies needed using sterile technique.

3. Don sterile gloves.

4. Withdraw sterile solution for irrigation.
   **RATIONALE:** *Solutions are ordered for the ability to clean the area or treat infection. Examples include isotonic saline, lactated Ringer solution, and dilute antibiotic solutions.*

5. Release the solution from the syringe, allowing it to flow over the wound. Collect it in a sterile basin under the wound.

6. Repeat several times until all the solution is used and/or the wound debris is cleansed.

7. Apply topical medications and dressing, as ordered.

8. Clean and dry the child.

9. Clean the area around the wound and the area that became moist during the procedure to discourage growth of microorganisms.

10. Document observations of the wound and the child's response to the irrigation.
    **RATIONALE:** *The condition of the wound and the child's pain level may indicate healing or infection of the wound.*

## SKILL 18–2  Burn Wound Care

Children with deep partial-thickness burns often have regular dressing changes and debridement during the healing process. A topical antibiotic cream such as Silvadene is used as a barrier to infectious organisms. Some children have a silver-based antimicrobial dressing such as Aquacel applied over debrided skin to collect exudate. Daily cleansing, debriding, and application of topical antibiotic cream is not performed on burns treated with a silver-based antimicrobial dressing.

### PREPARATION

1. Verify the identity of the child. Explain the procedure and why it is needed to the child and parents. Encourage the parents to provide a distracting activity, such as reading a story or watching a video, during the dressing change.

2. Check the physician's orders. Because burn care is a painful procedure, check for pain medication orders and administer medication at least 30 to 60 minutes before starting burn care. Sedation may be used for some debridement procedures.
   **RATIONALE:** *Medication must be administered so that peak action occurs during the burn dressing change.*

3. Wash your hands. You may need an assistant to position and hold the child and the burned extremity during care.

### EQUIPMENT AND SUPPLIES

- Basin
- Sterile normal saline solution
- Large supply of 4″ × 4″ gauze pads
- Forceps
- Scissors
- Sterile tongue blade
- Prescribed topical medication
- Tape
- Absorbent pad
- Clean and sterile gloves

### PROCEDURE

1. Place the absorbent pad under the area to be cleaned. Put on clean gloves. Soak the wound for about 10 minutes in normal saline solution, or apply a wet dressing to the area. Remove the dressing and then the gloves.
   **RATIONALE:** *This will soften the wound and make it easier to remove the old dressing.*

2. Using sterile gloves, wash the burn with the gauze pads and sterile normal saline to remove any medication and crusting. Use a firm, circular motion, moving from the inside to the outer edges. Bleeding may occur, but this is a sign of healing, healthy tissue. Rinse with normal saline solution. Pat dry with sterile gauze.

   RATIONALE: *The injured skin secretes serous fluid that forms a tough, leathery layer called eschar. This layer must be removed to promote healing.*

3. Some children are placed in a whirlpool bath to soften the eschar and increase circulation.

4. Remove (per physician's orders) any loose or dead skin around the burn's edges by gently lifting it with the forceps and snipping it. This is not painful to the child. Rinse and dry again.

   RATIONALE: *Debridement speeds the healing process.*

5. Place a thin layer of prescribed medication (about 0.125-inch thick) on the burn or gauze with fingers or a sterile tongue blade.

6. Place the medicated gauze on the burn and cover with a dry, sterile dressing.

7. Document the procedure, the condition of the burn area, the child's pain level, and the child's response to the procedure.

---

## SKILL 18–3  Suture and Staple Removal

Skin sutures and staples are used in repairing a wound to hold tissue and skin together. After a period of 1 to 2 weeks, skin healing is adequate and they need to be removed.

### *Suture Removal*

### PREPARATION

1. Verify the order.
2. Verify the identity of the child, and explain the procedure to the child and family.
3. Review the client's history to include date of repair and number of sutures placed.
4. Gather supplies.

### EQUIPMENT AND SUPPLIES

- Suture removal kit or sterile forceps and scissors
- Steri-Strips
- Gloves
- Wound-cleansing agent according to agency policy
- Clean and sterile gloves

### PROCEDURE

1. Perform hand hygiene and don clean gloves.
2. Remove any dressing covering the sutures. Remove clean gloves, perform hand hygiene, and don a sterile pair of gloves.
3. Assess the wound for healing. If the wound edges are gaping or if there are signs of infection, stop the procedure and consult the physician.

   RATIONALE: *If sutures are removed early, the wound is at risk to reopen. Some approximate adequate preliminary healing times are listed in Table 18–1.*

| TABLE 18–1 | Healing Times and Suture Removal Times Common for Various Body Parts |
|---|---|
| **Location of Sutures** | **Removal in Days** |
| Face | 5 |
| Chin | 5–6 |
| Scalp | 7 |
| Trunk | 10 |
| Arm/leg | 10 |
| Dorsum of hand | 10–14 |
| Palm | 10–14 |
| Sole | 10–14 |

4. Clean the site with a wound-cleansing agent, and gently pat dry with sterile gauze.

5. To remove sutures, using forceps, gently lift the suture knot away from the skin and cut one side of the suture close to the skin.

   RATIONALE: *One cut close to the skin avoids suture material that has been external to be pulled internally as it is removed. It also allows for all of the suture material to be removed.*

6. Slowly pull to remove the suture.

7. Remove every other suture. If the wound is healed and not pulling apart, remove the remaining sutures.

   RATIONALE: *Removing every other suture allows for further assessment of wound healing. If the wound is not adequately healed, there should be enough remaining sutures to support the wound during continued healing.*

8. Apply Steri-Strips to the suture line if needed.

   RATIONALE: *Steri-Strips provide additional support as needed.*

9. Remove gloves. Perform hand hygiene. Dispose of gloves and materials in an appropriate manner.

10. Instruct the client and family regarding further wound care.

11. Document time, the number of sutures removed, the condition of the wound, and how the client tolerated the procedure.

### Staple Removal

## PREPARATION

1. Verify the order.

2. Verify the identity of the child, and explain the procedure to the child and family.

3. Review the client's history to include date of repair and number of sutures placed.

4. Gather supplies.

## EQUIPMENT AND SUPPLIES

- Staple remover
- Steri-Strips
- Clean and sterile gloves
- Wound-cleansing agent according to agency policy

## PROCEDURE

1. Perform hand hygiene and don clean gloves.

2. Remove any dressing covering the staples; assess the dressing for drainage and assess the wound. Remove gloves, perform hand hygiene, and don sterile gloves.

3. Cleanse the wound according to agency policy.

4. To remove staples: Position a sterile staple remover under the staple to be removed. Squeeze the levers of the staple remover together. The staple will bend in the middle and the edges will pull out.

5. Remove every other staple. If the wound is healed, remove the remaining staples.

   RATIONALE: *Removing every other staple allows for further assessment of wound healing. If the wound is not adequately healed, there should be enough remaining staples to support the wound during continued healing.*

6. Apply Steri-Strips if needed.

   RATIONALE: *Steri-Strips provide additional support as needed.*

7. Remove gloves. Perform hand hygiene. Dispose of gloves and staples/materials in an appropriate manner.

8. Instruct the client and family regarding further wound care.

9. Document the time, the number of staples removed, the condition of the wound, and how the client tolerated the procedure.

# Casts

Children often have casts applied after surgery or to treat fractures. They may have white plaster casts that are generally heavy and sturdy. Alternatively, fiberglass casts are lighter and come in various colors, but generally do not last as long. Nurses may assist with cast application and are involved in immediate cast care after application. They commonly instruct the child and family on maintenance of the cast at home. The following procedure describes the nurse's role in care after cast application. See your textbook for further information about management of musculoskeletal treatments (Figure 18–1).

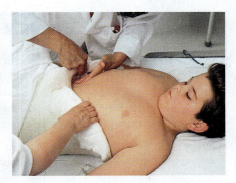

**Figure 18–1** *Nurses check the edges of the fresh cast for dryness and rough edges.*

## SKILL 18–4 Providing Cast Care

### PREPARATION

1. Consult the child's chart for a description of the injury or surgery.

### EQUIPMENT AND SUPPLIES

- Cast material (if assisting in application)
- Large basin with water (if assisting in application)
- Pillows with waterproof covering
- Absorbent pads and protectors
- Clean gloves

| **SAFETY ALERT** |
| --- |
| Neurovascular impairment under a cast is an emergency. If assessments indicate impaired circulatory or neurologic status, notify the physician immediately. Have a cast cutter at the bedside so the cast can quickly be removed if needed and the pressure relieved. |

### PROCEDURE

Following cast application:

1. Perform hand hygiene and don clean gloves.

2. Elevate a wet cast on pillows covered in plastic.
   RATIONALE: *Elevation decreases edema under the cast, which can restrict circulation.*

3. Use the palm of the hands when lifting a wet or damp cast.
   RATIONALE: *Fingertips can indent plaster and create pressure areas.*

4. Circle and note the date and time of any drainage on the cast.
   RATIONALE: *Some drainage is common after surgery. Monitoring its presence provides clues to the amount and type of fluid lost.*

5. Assess circulatory and neurologic status every 15 minutes immediately after surgery or cast placement, and then progress to every 30 minutes, 60 minutes, and 2 hours (see Skill 14–1 for further information about neurovascular assessment). Report abnormal findings or changes in condition. Include the following observations on the involved extremities:

   - Distal pulses
   - Color
   - Warmth
   - Sensation
   - Capillary refill
   - Edema
   - Movement
   - Pain, tingling
   
   RATIONALE: *Circulation and nerves under the cast can be injured if it is too tight.*

6. Use pain-control measures as needed and reassess pain. Report immediately worsening pain or pain that is not controlled by prescribed medication (see Chapter 8 in this manual).

7. Check the edges of the cast for roughness or crumbling. Pull the inner stockinette over the edge of the cast and tape once the cast has dried.
   RATIONALE: *These actions can prevent discomfort and skin breakdown.*

8. Keep the cast clean and dry. Cover it with a plastic bag during bathing or toileting.

9. Avoid use of lotions and powders under the cast.
   RATIONALE: *These products can cause skin irritation.*

| TABLE 18–2 | Instructions for Home Care of the Child With a Cast |
| --- | --- |

*Skin Care*

- Check the skin around the cast edges for irritation, rubbing, or blistering. The skin should be clean and dry.
- Cleanse the skin just under the cast edges and between the toes or fingers with a cotton-tipped applicator and rubbing alcohol. Avoid using lotions, oils, and powders near the cast as they may cause caking.
- Avoid poking sharp objects inside the cast as this may result in sores.

*Cast Care*

- Keep the cast dry. Protect plaster with a cast shoe, thick sock, or sling.
- Raise the casted arm or leg above heart level and rest it on pillows to prevent or reduce any swelling.
- Allow a new, wet cast to air-dry for 24 hours.
- Begin walking on a leg cast only when the physician gives permission.

*Be Alert for Possible Complications*

- Toes or fingers should be pink, not blue or white.
- Skin should be warm. The tips of the toes should blanch when pinched.

*Notify Your Healthcare Provider if Any of the Following Occur*

- Unusual odor beneath the cast
- Burning, tingling, or numbness in the casted arm or leg
- Drainage through the cast
- Swelling or inability to move the fingers or toes
- Fingers or toes that are blue or white
- Slippage of the cast
- Cracked, soft, or loose cast
- Sudden unexplained fever
- Unusual fussiness or irritability in an infant or child
- Pain that is not relieved by any comfort measures (e.g., repositioning or pain medication)

Source: Courtesy of Shriners Hospital for Children, Spokane, WA.

10. Keep shirts or other clothing over the top edges of casts on young children.
    RATIONALE: *This action helps to prevent the child from placing objects down into the cast, which can result in areas of discomfort or skin damage.*

11. Instruct the family about care of the cast at home and when to return for checks and removal of the cast (Table 18–2).

12. Document the cast application, how the child tolerated the procedure, the cast care provided, and the assessment of vascular and neurologic status.

# Crutches

Children may need crutches temporarily after surgery or injury of an extremity, or permanently to assist in ambulation. Crutches are generally supported under the axillae. For long-term use, they may be supported by attachment fitting over the forearms (Canadian crutches). Nurses assist children to set initial crutch height, reinforce instruction provided by a physical therapist about safety with crutches, ensure that children using crutches over time are evaluated as needed for correct fit, and monitor the skin that receives pressure from the crutches (Figure 18–2).

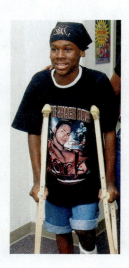

**Figure 18–2** *This young boy needs to use crutches to walk because he has a non–weight-bearing cast on his left lower leg.*

## SKILL 18–5  Setting Crutch Height

**PROCEDURE**

1. While the child is standing, the child's elbows should be slightly and comfortably flexed.

2. Place the tip of the crutches about 3 to 6 in. to the upper, outer border of the toes on each foot.

3. The upper pads on the crutches should now be lightly placed in the child's axillae.

   **RATIONALE:** *Crutches that are too high can put pressure on the brachial plexus, causing pain and injury. Crutches that are too low require that the child bend over to walk, and can injure or cause discomfort of the back and neck.*

4. The child should be taught safe crutch walking, a procedure generally taught by a physical therapist or other specialist.

# Braces

Braces are used to treat conditions temporarily (such as for scoliosis in a teenager), or may be used on a long-term basis (such as a child with cerebral palsy who needs leg braces for ambulation). The nurse helps the child accommodate to new braces and then periodically evaluates the fit of the braces and the condition of the skin. Brace wear is usually part of the home and community nursing role, so families are taught correct brace and skin assessment. See Table 18–3 for guidelines to teach families about brace wear.

| **TABLE 18–3** | Guidelines for Brace Wear |
|---|---|

- Braces should be as comfortable as possible, and the child should have adequate mobility while wearing the brace.
- Begin wearing the brace for periods of 1–2 hours and then progress to 2–4 hours.
- Check the skin at 1- to 2-hour intervals initially, then lengthening to every 4 hours once the skin has been clear for several days. If redness is apparent, leave the brace off and allow the skin to clear. If breakdown has occurred, the brace cannot be worn until healing is complete.
- Always have the child wear a clean white sock, T-shirt, or other thin white liner beneath the brace. Be sure the liner is wrinkle-free under the brace. Avoid using powders or lotions that can cause skin to break down. Toughen any sensitive areas by using alcohol wipes on that skin twice daily.
- Reapply the brace when the skin returns to its normal color.
- Return to the physician or orthotic specialist if discomfort or red areas persist, or if the brace needs adjustment or repair, or if the brace is outgrown.
- Check the brace daily for rough edges.

# Traction

Various types of traction are used to provide force on bones and muscles. See your textbook for descriptions of various types of traction. Skin or external traction is sometimes used, whereas skeletal or internal traction involves surgery to place pins into bones that are then attached to traction apparatus. The nurse sets up traction devices as ordered and often applies skin traction with prescribed weights. The nurse also maintains both skin and skeletal traction while monitoring the client's response and condition.

## SKILL 18–6  Applying and Monitoring Skin Traction

**PREPARATION**

1. Verify the identity of the child. Explain to the child and family the type of traction and what it will involve.

2. Gather equipment needed and review proper setup.

3. Check the weights to be certain they are the same as those ordered by the physician.

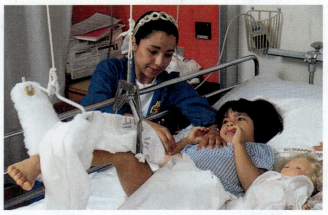

**Figure 18–3** *The child in traction needs close monitoring for alignment and proper traction application. Parents can often provide distraction and activities to help the child pass the time during their child's immobility.*

## EQUIPMENT AND SUPPLIES

- Poles, pulleys, rope, weight, pads
- Elastic wrap for skin traction

## PROCEDURE

1. Set up the prescribed type of traction with proper weights.
2. Apply skin traction as ordered to the particular extremity. Wrap the extremity and apply straps to freely movable prescribed weights.
3. Perform assessments every 30 minutes initially, and then advance to every 1 to 2 hours when stable. Include the following areas:
   - Proper position of traction
   - Proper body alignment
   - Neurovascular status of the extremity (see information on cast care earlier in this chapter and Skill 14–1 on neurovascular assessment)
   - Skin condition under and around the traction application
     - Skin on prominences exposed to the surface of the bed
     - Vital signs
     - Pain and psychologic status

   RATIONALE: *Traction can lead to skin breakdown or neurovascular impairment. Infections can result, especially with internal traction. Regular assessments help to identify problems early. Children may be pulled out of correct alignment by traction and movement in bed and may require frequent repositioning.*
4. Check the child's alignment in bed and reposition, as needed.
5. Remove traction according to agency policy, performing assessments and skin care. Reapply as directed in the medical orders.
6. Provide teaching and evaluation of the technique if the family will maintain traction at home (Figure 18–3).

---

## SKILL 18–7  Monitoring Skeletal Traction and Performing Pin Care

### PREPARATION

1. Verify orders for the type of traction and amount of weight as well as orders or agency policy regarding pin care.
2. Verify the identity of the child, and explain the procedure to the child and parents.
3. Gather supplies as needed for skin care.

### EQUIPMENT AND SUPPLIES

- Sterile gloves (two pairs)
- Sterile applicators
- Normal saline
- Gauze pads

### PROCEDURE

1. Identify that weights are correct and are freely movable. Ropes should be secure and not frayed.
2. Check the child's alignment in bed and reposition, as needed.
3. Perform an extremity check as described previously and in Skill 14–1, to include the following:
   - Neurovascular status of the extremity (see information on cast care earlier in this chapter)
     - Skin condition under and around the traction application
     - Presence and type of drainage
   - Skin on prominences exposed to the surface of the bed
   - Vital signs
   - Pain and psychologic status

*When Pin Care Is Needed, Perform the Following Steps*

1. Perform hand hygiene and don gloves. Remove old gauze from pin sites and assess the condition of the skin and the type of drainage.

2. Remove gloves, perform hand hygiene, open sterile containers so they are readily accessible, and don new gloves.

3. Using sterile technique, cleanse the area around the pins with normal saline or other ordered solution. Clean off dried drainage from pins.

   RATIONALE: *Pin care helps to maintain cleanliness and decrease microbial contamination at the insertion sites and minimizes the chance of infection.*

4. Reapply gauze or pin shields around pin sites.

5. Document assessment findings, the procedure, and the child's response.

## HOME AND COMMUNITY CARE CONSIDERATIONS

Children are increasingly being treated with traction at home. Be certain that the family understands how to set up and maintain the traction. Teach the observations to be made on the extremity involved. Siblings may change the weights or ropes, so close supervision may be needed by parents in some families. A home visit soon after traction begins is often made to evaluate the family's understanding and ability to carry out the regimen.

# Appendix A
# Physical Growth Charts

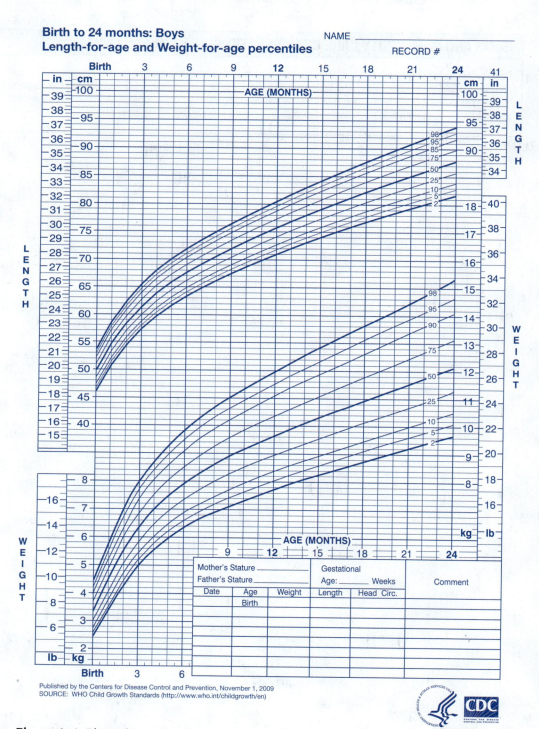

**Birth to 24 months: Boys**
**Length-for-age and Weight-for-age percentiles**

NAME _____

RECORD # _____

Published by the Centers for Disease Control and Prevention, November 1, 2009
SOURCE: WHO Child Growth Standards (http://www.who.int/childgrowth/en)

**Figure A–1** *Physical growth percentiles for length and weight—boys: birth to 24 months.*
Source: WHO Child Growth Standards, http://www.who.int/childgrowth/en.

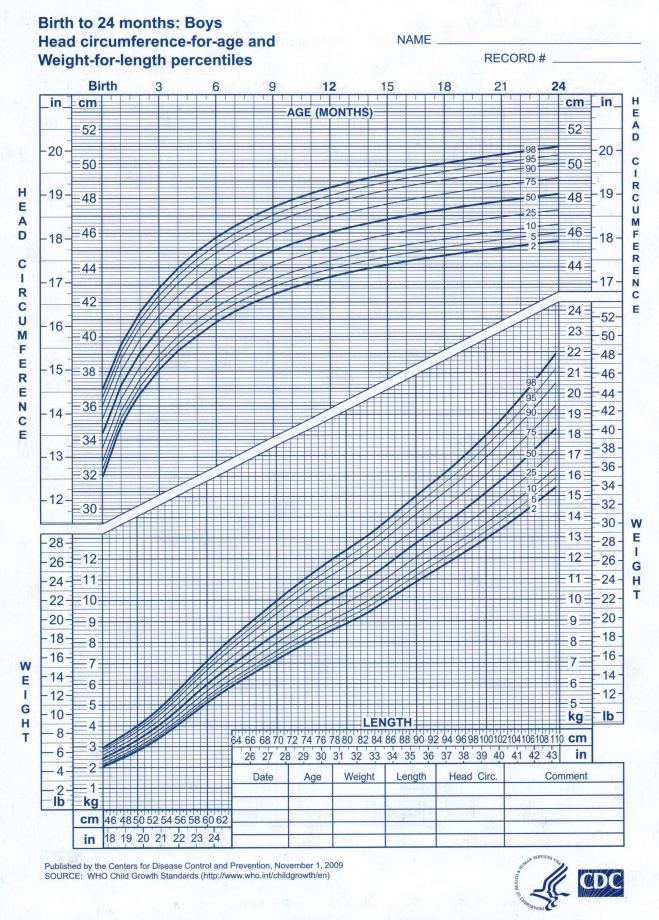

**Birth to 24 months: Boys
Head circumference-for-age and
Weight-for-length percentiles**

NAME _____

RECORD # _____

Published by the Centers for Disease Control and Prevention, November 1, 2009
SOURCE: WHO Child Growth Standards (http://www.who.int/childgrowth/en)

**Figure A–2** *Physical growth percentiles for head circumference, weight for length—boys: birth to 24 months.*
Source: WHO Child Growth Standards, http://www.who.int/childgrowth/en.

## Birth to 24 months: Girls
## Length-for-age and Weight-for-age percentiles

NAME _____

RECORD # _____

Published by the Centers for Disease Control and Prevention, November 1, 2009
SOURCE: WHO Child Growth Standards (http://www.who.int/childgrowth/en)

**Figure A–3** *Physical growth percentiles for length and weight—girls: birth to 24 months.*
Source: WHO Child Growth Standards, http://www.who.int/childgrowth/en.

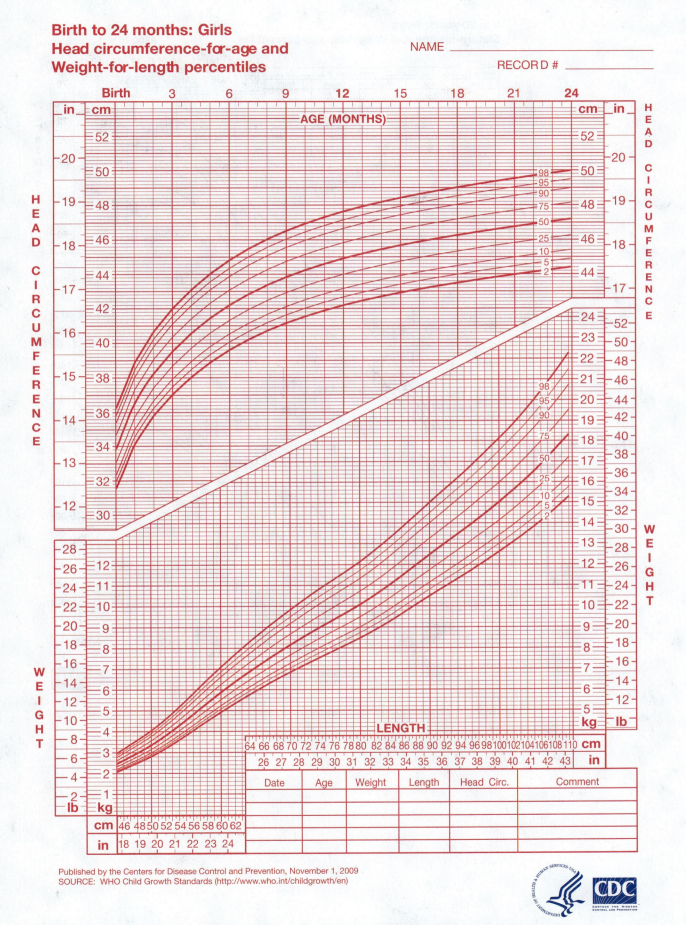

**Birth to 24 months: Girls**
**Head circumference-for-age and**
**Weight-for-length percentiles**

NAME _____

RECORD # _____

**Figure A–4** *Physical growth percentiles for head circumference, weight for length—girls: birth to 24 months.*
Source: WHO Child Growth Standards, http://www.who.int/childgrowth/en.

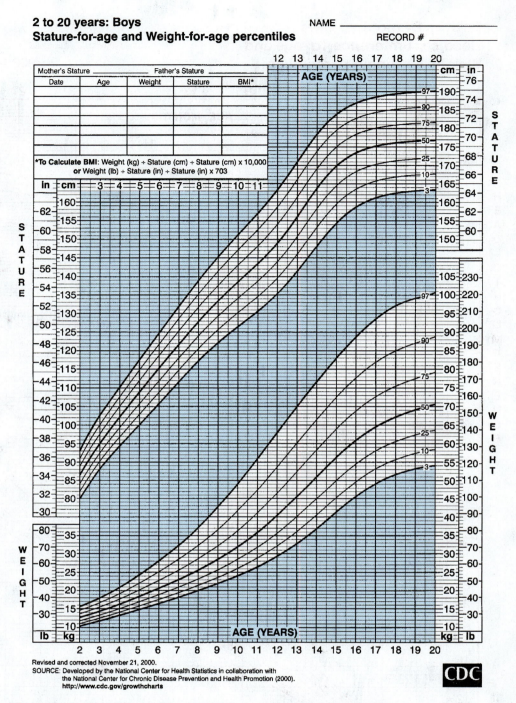

**Figure A–5** *Physical growth percentiles for stature and weight according to age—boys: 2 to 20 years.*
Source: CDC, 2001, http://www.cdc.gov/growthcharts.

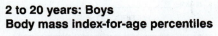

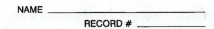

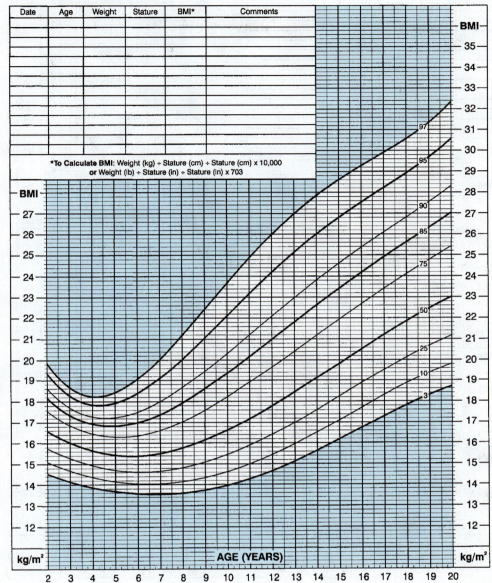

**Figure A–6**  *Physical growth percentiles for body mass index according to age—boys: 2 to 20 years.*
Source: CDC, 2001, http://www.cdc.gov/growthcharts.

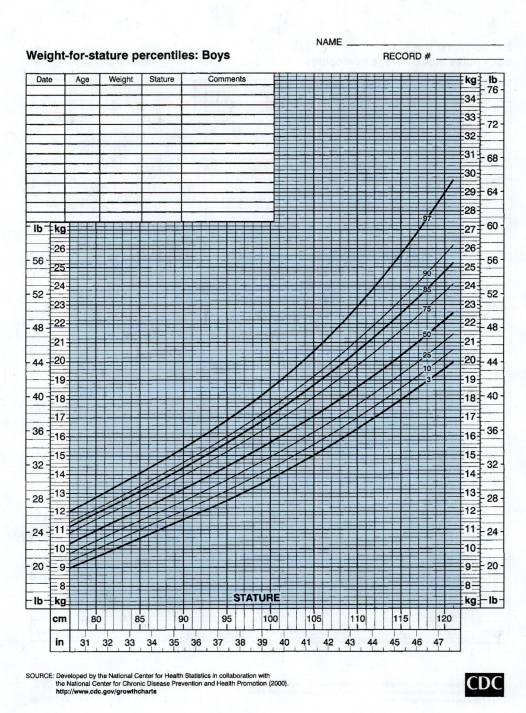

**Figure A-7** *Physical growth percentiles for weight for stature—boys: 2 to 20 years.*
Source: CDC, 2001, http://www.cdc.gov/growthcharts.

**2 to 20 years: Girls**
**Stature-for-age and Weight-for-age percentiles**

NAME _____

RECORD # _____

Revised and corrected November 21, 2000.
SOURCE: Developed by the National Center for Health Statistics in collaboration with
the National Center for Chronic Disease Prevention and Health Promotion (2000).
http://www.cdc.gov/growthcharts

**Figure A–8** *Physical growth percentiles for stature and weight according to age—girls: 2 to 20 years.*
Source: CDC, 2001, http://www.cdc.gov/growthcharts.

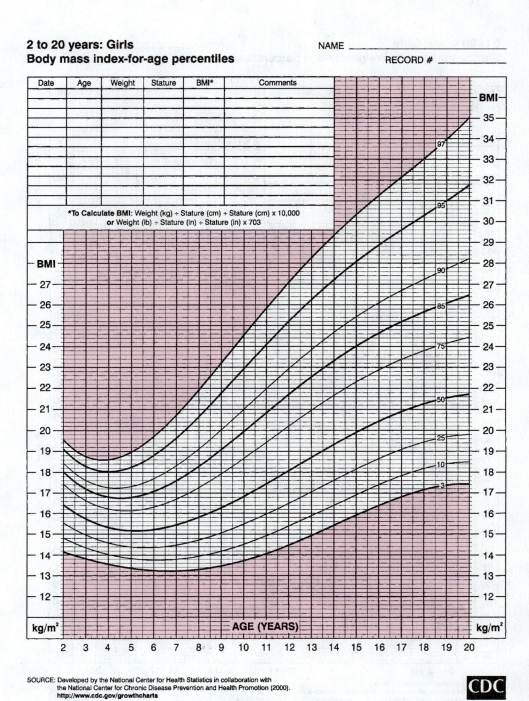

**Figure A–9**  *Physical growth percentiles for body mass index according to age—girls: 2 to 20 years.*
Source: CDC, 2001, http://www.cdc.gov/growthcharts.

**Weight-for-stature percentiles: Girls**

NAME _____

RECORD # _____

| Date | Age | Weight | Stature | Comments |
|------|-----|--------|---------|----------|
|      |     |        |         |          |
|      |     |        |         |          |
|      |     |        |         |          |
|      |     |        |         |          |
|      |     |        |         |          |

STATURE

cm  80  85  90  95  100  105  110  115  120

in  31  32  33  34  35  36  37  38  39  40  41  42  43  44  45  46  47

SOURCE: Developed by the National Center for Health Statistics in collaboration with
the National Center for Chronic Disease Prevention and Health Promotion (2000).
http://www.cdc.gov/growthcharts

CDC

**Figure A–10** *Physical growth percentiles for weight for stature—girls: 2 to 20 years.*
Source: CDC, 2001, http://www.cdc.gov/growthcharts.

# Blood Pressure Values by Age, Gender, and Height Percentiles

**Blood Pressure Levels for Boys by Age and Height Percentile. Use the child's height percentile for the age and gender from the standard growth charts found in Appendix A. A blood pressure value at 50th percentile for the child's age, gender, and height percentile is considered the midpoint of the normal range. A reading above the 95th percentile indicates hypertension.***

| Age (Year) | BP Percentile | Systolic BP (mmHg) Percentile of Height | | | | | | | Diastolic BP (mmHg) Percentile of Height | | | | | | |
|---|---|---|---|---|---|---|---|---|---|---|---|---|---|---|---|
| | | 5th | 10th | 25th | 50th | 75th | 90th | 95th | 5th | 10th | 25th | 50th | 75th | 90th | 95th |
| 1 | 50th | 80 | 81 | 83 | 85 | 87 | 88 | 89 | 34 | 35 | 36 | 37 | 38 | 39 | 39 |
| | 90th | 94 | 95 | 97 | 99 | 100 | 102 | 103 | 49 | 50 | 51 | 52 | 53 | 53 | 54 |
| | 95th | 98 | 99 | 101 | 103 | 104 | 106 | 106 | 54 | 54 | 55 | 56 | 57 | 58 | 58 |
| | 99th | 105 | 106 | 108 | 110 | 112 | 113 | 114 | 61 | 62 | 63 | 64 | 65 | 66 | 66 |
| 2 | 50th | 84 | 85 | 87 | 88 | 90 | 92 | 92 | 39 | 40 | 41 | 42 | 43 | 44 | 44 |
| | 90th | 97 | 99 | 100 | 102 | 104 | 105 | 106 | 54 | 55 | 56 | 57 | 58 | 58 | 59 |
| | 95th | 101 | 102 | 104 | 106 | 108 | 109 | 110 | 59 | 59 | 60 | 61 | 62 | 63 | 63 |
| | 99th | 109 | 110 | 111 | 113 | 115 | 117 | 117 | 66 | 67 | 68 | 69 | 70 | 71 | 71 |
| 3 | 50th | 86 | 87 | 89 | 91 | 93 | 94 | 95 | 44 | 44 | 45 | 46 | 47 | 48 | 48 |
| | 90th | 100 | 101 | 103 | 105 | 107 | 108 | 109 | 59 | 59 | 60 | 61 | 62 | 63 | 63 |
| | 95th | 104 | 105 | 107 | 109 | 110 | 112 | 113 | 63 | 63 | 64 | 65 | 66 | 67 | 67 |
| | 99th | 111 | 112 | 114 | 116 | 118 | 119 | 120 | 71 | 71 | 72 | 73 | 74 | 75 | 75 |
| 4 | 50th | 88 | 89 | 91 | 93 | 95 | 96 | 97 | 47 | 48 | 49 | 50 | 51 | 51 | 52 |
| | 90th | 102 | 103 | 105 | 107 | 109 | 110 | 111 | 62 | 63 | 64 | 65 | 66 | 66 | 67 |
| | 95th | 106 | 107 | 109 | 111 | 112 | 114 | 115 | 66 | 67 | 68 | 69 | 70 | 71 | 71 |
| | 99th | 113 | 114 | 116 | 118 | 120 | 121 | 122 | 74 | 75 | 76 | 77 | 78 | 78 | 79 |
| 5 | 50th | 90 | 91 | 93 | 95 | 96 | 98 | 98 | 50 | 51 | 52 | 53 | 54 | 55 | 55 |
| | 90th | 104 | 105 | 106 | 108 | 110 | 111 | 112 | 65 | 66 | 67 | 68 | 69 | 69 | 70 |
| | 95th | 108 | 109 | 110 | 112 | 114 | 115 | 116 | 69 | 70 | 71 | 72 | 73 | 74 | 74 |
| | 99th | 115 | 116 | 118 | 120 | 121 | 123 | 123 | 77 | 78 | 79 | 80 | 81 | 81 | 82 |
| 6 | 50th | 91 | 92 | 94 | 96 | 98 | 99 | 100 | 53 | 53 | 54 | 55 | 56 | 57 | 57 |
| | 90th | 105 | 106 | 108 | 110 | 111 | 113 | 113 | 68 | 68 | 69 | 70 | 71 | 72 | 72 |
| | 95th | 109 | 110 | 112 | 114 | 115 | 117 | 117 | 72 | 72 | 73 | 74 | 75 | 76 | 76 |
| | 99th | 116 | 117 | 119 | 121 | 123 | 124 | 125 | 80 | 80 | 81 | 82 | 83 | 84 | 84 |
| 7 | 50th | 92 | 94 | 95 | 97 | 99 | 100 | 101 | 55 | 55 | 56 | 57 | 58 | 59 | 59 |
| | 90th | 106 | 107 | 109 | 111 | 113 | 114 | 115 | 70 | 70 | 71 | 72 | 73 | 74 | 74 |
| | 95th | 110 | 111 | 113 | 115 | 117 | 118 | 119 | 74 | 74 | 75 | 76 | 77 | 78 | 78 |
| | 99th | 117 | 118 | 120 | 122 | 124 | 125 | 126 | 82 | 82 | 83 | 84 | 85 | 86 | 86 |
| 8 | 50th | 94 | 95 | 97 | 99 | 100 | 102 | 102 | 56 | 57 | 58 | 59 | 60 | 60 | 61 |
| | 90th | 107 | 109 | 110 | 112 | 114 | 115 | 116 | 71 | 72 | 72 | 73 | 74 | 75 | 76 |
| | 95th | 111 | 112 | 114 | 116 | 118 | 119 | 120 | 75 | 76 | 77 | 78 | 79 | 79 | 80 |
| | 99th | 119 | 120 | 122 | 123 | 125 | 127 | 127 | 83 | 84 | 85 | 86 | 87 | 87 | 88 |
| 9 | 50th | 95 | 96 | 98 | 100 | 102 | 103 | 104 | 57 | 58 | 59 | 60 | 61 | 61 | 62 |
| | 90th | 109 | 110 | 112 | 114 | 115 | 117 | 118 | 72 | 73 | 74 | 75 | 76 | 76 | 77 |
| | 95th | 113 | 114 | 116 | 118 | 119 | 121 | 121 | 76 | 77 | 78 | 79 | 80 | 81 | 81 |
| | 99th | 120 | 121 | 123 | 125 | 127 | 128 | 129 | 84 | 85 | 86 | 87 | 88 | 88 | 89 |

**Blood Pressure Levels for Boys by Age and Height Percentile. Use the child's height percentile for the age and gender from the standard growth charts found in Appendix A. A blood pressure value at 50th percentile for the child's age, gender, and height percentile is considered the midpoint of the normal range. A reading above the 95th percentile indicates hypertension.\*** (*continued*)

| Age (Year) | BP Percentile | Systolic BP (mmHg) Percentile of Height | | | | | | | Diastolic BP (mmHg) Percentile of Height | | | | | | |
|---|---|---|---|---|---|---|---|---|---|---|---|---|---|---|---|
| | | 5th | 10th | 25th | 50th | 75th | 90th | 95th | 5th | 10th | 25th | 50th | 75th | 90th | 95th |
| 10 | 50th | 97 | 98 | 100 | 102 | 103 | 105 | 106 | 58 | 59 | 60 | 61 | 61 | 62 | 63 |
| | 90th | 111 | 112 | 114 | 115 | 117 | 119 | 119 | 73 | 73 | 74 | 75 | 76 | 77 | 78 |
| | 95th | 115 | 116 | 117 | 119 | 121 | 122 | 123 | 77 | 78 | 79 | 80 | 81 | 81 | 82 |
| | 99th | 122 | 123 | 125 | 127 | 128 | 130 | 130 | 85 | 86 | 86 | 88 | 88 | 89 | 90 |
| 11 | 50th | 99 | 100 | 102 | 104 | 105 | 107 | 107 | 59 | 59 | 60 | 61 | 62 | 63 | 63 |
| | 90th | 113 | 114 | 115 | 117 | 119 | 120 | 121 | 74 | 74 | 75 | 76 | 77 | 78 | 78 |
| | 95th | 117 | 118 | 119 | 121 | 123 | 124 | 125 | 78 | 78 | 79 | 80 | 81 | 82 | 82 |
| | 99th | 124 | 125 | 127 | 129 | 130 | 132 | 132 | 86 | 86 | 87 | 88 | 89 | 90 | 90 |
| 12 | 50th | 101 | 102 | 104 | 106 | 108 | 109 | 110 | 59 | 60 | 61 | 62 | 63 | 63 | 64 |
| | 90th | 115 | 116 | 118 | 120 | 121 | 123 | 123 | 74 | 75 | 75 | 76 | 77 | 78 | 79 |
| | 95th | 119 | 120 | 122 | 123 | 125 | 127 | 127 | 78 | 79 | 80 | 81 | 82 | 82 | 83 |
| | 99th | 126 | 127 | 129 | 131 | 133 | 134 | 135 | 86 | 87 | 88 | 89 | 90 | 90 | 91 |
| 13 | 50th | 104 | 105 | 106 | 108 | 110 | 111 | 112 | 60 | 60 | 61 | 62 | 63 | 64 | 64 |
| | 90th | 117 | 118 | 120 | 122 | 124 | 125 | 126 | 75 | 75 | 76 | 77 | 78 | 79 | 79 |
| | 95th | 121 | 122 | 124 | 126 | 128 | 129 | 130 | 79 | 79 | 80 | 81 | 82 | 83 | 83 |
| | 99th | 128 | 130 | 131 | 133 | 135 | 136 | 137 | 87 | 87 | 88 | 89 | 90 | 91 | 91 |
| 14 | 50th | 106 | 107 | 109 | 111 | 113 | 114 | 115 | 60 | 61 | 62 | 63 | 64 | 65 | 65 |
| | 90th | 120 | 121 | 123 | 125 | 126 | 128 | 128 | 75 | 76 | 77 | 78 | 79 | 79 | 80 |
| | 95th | 124 | 125 | 127 | 128 | 130 | 132 | 132 | 80 | 80 | 81 | 82 | 83 | 84 | 84 |
| | 99th | 131 | 132 | 134 | 136 | 138 | 139 | 140 | 87 | 88 | 89 | 90 | 91 | 92 | 92 |
| 15 | 50th | 109 | 110 | 112 | 113 | 115 | 117 | 117 | 61 | 62 | 63 | 64 | 65 | 66 | 66 |
| | 90th | 122 | 124 | 125 | 127 | 129 | 130 | 131 | 76 | 77 | 78 | 79 | 80 | 80 | 81 |
| | 95th | 126 | 127 | 129 | 131 | 133 | 134 | 135 | 81 | 81 | 82 | 83 | 84 | 85 | 85 |
| | 99th | 134 | 135 | 136 | 138 | 140 | 142 | 142 | 88 | 89 | 90 | 91 | 92 | 93 | 93 |
| 16 | 50th | 111 | 112 | 114 | 116 | 118 | 119 | 120 | 63 | 63 | 64 | 65 | 66 | 67 | 67 |
| | 90th | 125 | 126 | 128 | 130 | 131 | 133 | 134 | 78 | 78 | 79 | 80 | 81 | 82 | 82 |
| | 95th | 129 | 130 | 132 | 134 | 135 | 137 | 137 | 82 | 83 | 83 | 84 | 85 | 86 | 87 |
| | 99th | 136 | 137 | 139 | 141 | 143 | 144 | 145 | 90 | 90 | 91 | 92 | 93 | 94 | 94 |
| 17 | 50th | 114 | 115 | 116 | 118 | 120 | 121 | 122 | 65 | 66 | 66 | 67 | 68 | 69 | 70 |
| | 90th | 127 | 128 | 130 | 132 | 134 | 135 | 136 | 80 | 80 | 81 | 82 | 83 | 84 | 84 |
| | 95th | 131 | 132 | 134 | 136 | 138 | 139 | 140 | 84 | 85 | 86 | 87 | 87 | 88 | 89 |
| | 99th | 139 | 140 | 141 | 143 | 145 | 146 | 147 | 92 | 93 | 93 | 94 | 95 | 96 | 97 |

BP, blood pressure

\*The 90th percentile is 1.28 SD, 95th percentile is 1.645 SD, and the 99th percentile is 2.326 SD over the mean.

National Heart, Lung, and Blood Institute. (2004). Blood pressure tables for children and adolescents from the fourth report on the diagnosis, evaluation, and treatment of high blood pressure in children and adolescents. *www.nhlbi.nih.gov/guidelines/hypertension/child_tbl.htm,* accessed 6/11/2004.

**Blood Pressure Levels for Girls by Age and Height Percentile.** Use the child's height percentile for the age and gender from the standard growth charts found in Appendix A. A blood pressure value at 50th percentile for the child's age, gender, and height percentile is considered the midpoint of the normal range. A reading above the 95th percentile indicates hypertension.*

| Age (Year) | BP Percentile | Systolic BP (mmHg) Percentile of Height | | | | | | | Diastolic BP (mmHg) Percentile of Height | | | | | | |
|---|---|---|---|---|---|---|---|---|---|---|---|---|---|---|---|
| | | 5th | 10th | 25th | 50th | 75th | 90th | 95th | 5th | 10th | 25th | 50th | 75th | 90th | 95th |
| 1 | 50th | 83 | 84 | 85 | 86 | 88 | 89 | 90 | 38 | 39 | 39 | 40 | 41 | 41 | 42 |
| | 90th | 97 | 97 | 98 | 100 | 101 | 102 | 103 | 52 | 53 | 53 | 54 | 55 | 55 | 56 |
| | 95th | 100 | 101 | 102 | 104 | 105 | 106 | 107 | 56 | 57 | 57 | 58 | 59 | 59 | 60 |
| | 99th | 108 | 108 | 109 | 111 | 112 | 113 | 114 | 64 | 64 | 65 | 65 | 66 | 67 | 67 |
| 2 | 50th | 85 | 85 | 87 | 88 | 89 | 91 | 91 | 43 | 44 | 44 | 45 | 46 | 46 | 47 |
| | 90th | 98 | 99 | 100 | 101 | 103 | 104 | 105 | 57 | 58 | 58 | 59 | 60 | 61 | 61 |
| | 95th | 102 | 103 | 104 | 105 | 107 | 108 | 109 | 61 | 62 | 62 | 63 | 64 | 65 | 65 |
| | 99th | 109 | 110 | 111 | 112 | 114 | 115 | 117 | 69 | 69 | 70 | 70 | 71 | 72 | 72 |
| 3 | 50th | 86 | 87 | 88 | 89 | 91 | 92 | 93 | 47 | 48 | 48 | 49 | 50 | 50 | 51 |
| | 90th | 100 | 100 | 102 | 103 | 104 | 106 | 106 | 61 | 62 | 62 | 63 | 64 | 64 | 65 |
| | 95th | 104 | 104 | 105 | 107 | 108 | 109 | 110 | 65 | 66 | 66 | 67 | 68 | 68 | 69 |
| | 99th | 111 | 111 | 113 | 114 | 115 | 116 | 117 | 73 | 73 | 74 | 74 | 75 | 76 | 76 |
| 4 | 50th | 88 | 88 | 90 | 91 | 92 | 94 | 94 | 50 | 50 | 51 | 52 | 52 | 53 | 54 |
| | 90th | 101 | 102 | 103 | 104 | 106 | 107 | 108 | 64 | 64 | 65 | 66 | 67 | 67 | 68 |
| | 95th | 105 | 106 | 107 | 108 | 110 | 111 | 112 | 68 | 68 | 69 | 70 | 71 | 71 | 72 |
| | 99th | 112 | 113 | 114 | 115 | 117 | 118 | 119 | 76 | 76 | 76 | 77 | 78 | 79 | 79 |
| 5 | 50th | 89 | 90 | 91 | 93 | 94 | 95 | 96 | 52 | 53 | 53 | 54 | 55 | 55 | 56 |
| | 90th | 103 | 103 | 105 | 106 | 107 | 109 | 109 | 66 | 67 | 67 | 68 | 69 | 69 | 70 |
| | 95th | 107 | 107 | 108 | 110 | 111 | 112 | 113 | 70 | 71 | 71 | 72 | 73 | 73 | 74 |
| | 99th | 114 | 114 | 116 | 117 | 118 | 120 | 120 | 78 | 78 | 79 | 79 | 80 | 81 | 81 |
| 6 | 50th | 91 | 92 | 93 | 94 | 96 | 97 | 98 | 54 | 54 | 55 | 56 | 56 | 57 | 58 |
| | 90th | 104 | 105 | 106 | 108 | 109 | 110 | 111 | 68 | 68 | 69 | 70 | 70 | 71 | 72 |
| | 95th | 108 | 109 | 110 | 111 | 113 | 114 | 115 | 72 | 72 | 73 | 74 | 74 | 75 | 76 |
| | 99th | 115 | 116 | 117 | 119 | 120 | 121 | 122 | 80 | 80 | 80 | 81 | 82 | 83 | 83 |
| 7 | 50th | 93 | 93 | 95 | 96 | 97 | 99 | 99 | 55 | 56 | 56 | 57 | 58 | 58 | 59 |
| | 90th | 106 | 107 | 108 | 109 | 111 | 112 | 113 | 69 | 70 | 70 | 71 | 72 | 72 | 73 |
| | 95th | 110 | 111 | 112 | 113 | 115 | 116 | 116 | 73 | 74 | 74 | 75 | 76 | 76 | 77 |
| | 99th | 117 | 118 | 119 | 120 | 122 | 123 | 124 | 81 | 81 | 82 | 82 | 83 | 84 | 84 |
| 8 | 50th | 95 | 95 | 96 | 98 | 99 | 100 | 101 | 57 | 57 | 57 | 58 | 59 | 60 | 60 |
| | 90th | 108 | 109 | 110 | 111 | 113 | 114 | 114 | 71 | 71 | 71 | 72 | 73 | 74 | 74 |
| | 95th | 112 | 112 | 114 | 115 | 116 | 118 | 118 | 75 | 75 | 75 | 76 | 77 | 78 | 78 |
| | 99th | 119 | 120 | 121 | 122 | 123 | 125 | 125 | 82 | 82 | 83 | 83 | 84 | 85 | 86 |
| 9 | 50th | 96 | 97 | 98 | 100 | 101 | 102 | 103 | 58 | 58 | 58 | 59 | 60 | 61 | 61 |
| | 90th | 110 | 110 | 112 | 113 | 114 | 116 | 116 | 72 | 72 | 72 | 73 | 74 | 75 | 75 |
| | 95th | 114 | 114 | 115 | 117 | 118 | 119 | 120 | 76 | 76 | 76 | 77 | 78 | 79 | 79 |
| | 99th | 121 | 121 | 123 | 124 | 125 | 127 | 127 | 83 | 83 | 84 | 84 | 85 | 86 | 87 |

**Blood Pressure Levels for Girls by Age and Height Percentile. Use the child's height percentile for the age and gender from the standard growth charts found in Appendix A. A blood pressure value at 50th percentile for the child's age, gender, and height percentile is considered the midpoint of the normal range. A reading above the 95th percentile indicates hypertension.*** *(continued)*

| Age (Year) | BP Percentile | Systolic BP (mmHg) Percentile of Height | | | | | | | Diastolic BP (mmHg) Percentile of Height | | | | | | |
|---|---|---|---|---|---|---|---|---|---|---|---|---|---|---|---|
| | | 5th | 10th | 25th | 50th | 75th | 90th | 95th | 5th | 10th | 25th | 50th | 75th | 90th | 95th |
| 10 | 50th | 98 | 99 | 100 | 102 | 103 | 104 | 105 | 59 | 59 | 59 | 60 | 61 | 62 | 62 |
| | 90th | 112 | 112 | 114 | 115 | 116 | 118 | 118 | 73 | 73 | 73 | 74 | 75 | 76 | 76 |
| | 95th | 116 | 116 | 117 | 119 | 120 | 121 | 122 | 77 | 77 | 77 | 78 | 79 | 80 | 80 |
| | 99th | 123 | 123 | 125 | 126 | 127 | 129 | 129 | 84 | 84 | 85 | 86 | 86 | 87 | 88 |
| 11 | 50th | 100 | 101 | 102 | 103 | 105 | 106 | 107 | 60 | 60 | 60 | 61 | 62 | 63 | 63 |
| | 90th | 114 | 114 | 116 | 117 | 118 | 119 | 120 | 74 | 74 | 74 | 75 | 76 | 77 | 77 |
| | 95th | 118 | 118 | 119 | 121 | 122 | 123 | 124 | 78 | 78 | 78 | 79 | 80 | 81 | 81 |
| | 99th | 125 | 125 | 126 | 128 | 129 | 130 | 131 | 85 | 85 | 86 | 87 | 87 | 88 | 89 |
| 12 | 50th | 102 | 103 | 104 | 105 | 107 | 108 | 109 | 61 | 61 | 61 | 62 | 63 | 64 | 64 |
| | 90th | 116 | 116 | 117 | 119 | 120 | 121 | 122 | 75 | 75 | 75 | 76 | 77 | 78 | 78 |
| | 95th | 119 | 120 | 121 | 123 | 124 | 125 | 126 | 79 | 79 | 79 | 80 | 81 | 82 | 82 |
| | 99th | 127 | 127 | 128 | 130 | 131 | 132 | 133 | 86 | 86 | 87 | 88 | 88 | 89 | 90 |
| 13 | 50th | 104 | 105 | 106 | 107 | 109 | 110 | 110 | 62 | 62 | 62 | 63 | 64 | 65 | 65 |
| | 90th | 117 | 118 | 119 | 121 | 122 | 123 | 124 | 76 | 76 | 76 | 77 | 78 | 79 | 79 |
| | 95th | 121 | 122 | 123 | 124 | 126 | 127 | 128 | 80 | 80 | 80 | 81 | 82 | 83 | 83 |
| | 99th | 128 | 129 | 130 | 132 | 133 | 134 | 135 | 87 | 87 | 88 | 89 | 89 | 90 | 91 |
| 14 | 50th | 106 | 106 | 107 | 109 | 110 | 111 | 112 | 63 | 63 | 63 | 64 | 65 | 66 | 66 |
| | 90th | 119 | 120 | 121 | 122 | 124 | 125 | 125 | 77 | 77 | 77 | 78 | 79 | 80 | 80 |
| | 95th | 123 | 123 | 125 | 126 | 127 | 129 | 129 | 81 | 81 | 81 | 82 | 83 | 84 | 84 |
| | 99th | 130 | 131 | 132 | 133 | 135 | 136 | 136 | 88 | 88 | 89 | 90 | 90 | 91 | 92 |
| 15 | 50th | 107 | 108 | 109 | 110 | 111 | 113 | 113 | 64 | 64 | 64 | 65 | 66 | 67 | 67 |
| | 90th | 120 | 121 | 122 | 123 | 125 | 126 | 127 | 78 | 78 | 78 | 79 | 80 | 81 | 81 |
| | 95th | 124 | 125 | 126 | 127 | 129 | 130 | 131 | 82 | 82 | 82 | 83 | 84 | 85 | 85 |
| | 99th | 131 | 132 | 133 | 134 | 136 | 137 | 138 | 89 | 89 | 90 | 91 | 91 | 92 | 93 |
| 16 | 50th | 108 | 108 | 110 | 111 | 112 | 114 | 114 | 64 | 64 | 65 | 66 | 66 | 67 | 68 |
| | 90th | 121 | 122 | 123 | 124 | 126 | 127 | 128 | 78 | 78 | 79 | 80 | 81 | 81 | 82 |
| | 95th | 125 | 126 | 127 | 128 | 130 | 131 | 132 | 82 | 82 | 83 | 84 | 85 | 85 | 86 |
| | 99th | 132 | 133 | 134 | 135 | 137 | 138 | 139 | 90 | 90 | 90 | 91 | 92 | 93 | 93 |
| 17 | 50th | 108 | 109 | 110 | 111 | 113 | 114 | 115 | 64 | 65 | 65 | 66 | 67 | 67 | 68 |
| | 90th | 122 | 122 | 123 | 125 | 126 | 127 | 128 | 78 | 79 | 79 | 80 | 81 | 81 | 82 |
| | 95th | 125 | 126 | 127 | 129 | 130 | 131 | 132 | 82 | 83 | 83 | 84 | 85 | 85 | 86 |
| | 99th | 133 | 133 | 134 | 136 | 137 | 138 | 139 | 90 | 90 | 91 | 91 | 92 | 93 | 93 |

BP, blood pressure

*The 90th percentile is 1.28 SD, 95th percentile is 1.645 SD, and the 99th percentile is 2.326 SD over the mean.

National Heart, Lung, and Blood Institute. (2004). Blood pressure tables for children and adolescents from the fourth report on the diagnosis, evaluation, and treatment of high blood pressure in children and adolescents. *www.nhlbi.nih.gov/guidelines/hypertension/child_tbl.htm,* accessed 6/11/2004.

# Appendix C
# Body Surface Area Nomogram

The proportion between height and weight in children is different from the proportion in adults. These differences are most manifest in newborns, infants, and young children. Therefore, dosages of drugs that have been established for adults cannot simply be reduced and correspondingly be safe for young children. Weight is used as a better method of calculating drug dosage in children and is used when medications have a dose of drug recommended in milligrams per kilogram (mg/kg).

However, weight alone is not always accurate as a method of calculating a drug dosage for a child. Another more accurate method is that of body surface area (BSA). BSA is a relationship of height to weight and is measured in square meters. BSA increases about 7 times from birth to adulthood, and is a good reflection of many physiologic processes significant in metabolizing, transporting, and eliminating drugs, such as metabolic rate, extracellular fluid and total fluid volumes, cardiac output, and glomerular filtration rate. BSA is calculated by the formula:

$$\text{Surface area (m}^2) = \sqrt{\frac{\text{height (cm)} \times \text{weight (kg)}}{3600}}$$

A nomogram, or graph, has been developed to calculate BSA quickly and accurately. The nomogram on the left can be used when a child has height and weight in proportion, or in the same percentile range. When the percentiles for height and weight differ, the nomogram on the right can be used. To calculate the BSA, draw a straight line from the height to the weight. The point at which this line intersects the surface area (SA) column is the BSA in square meters. Medications that are prescribed using the BSA are dosed in milligrams per meter squared (mg/m²).

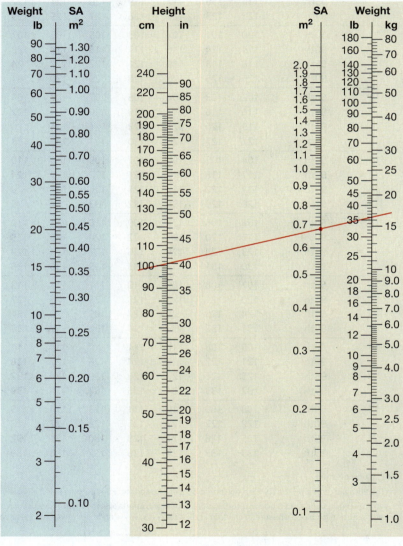

Nomogram for child with proportional height and weight

Nomogram for child with varied height and weight percentiles

# Appendix D
# Conversions and Equivalents

## TEMPERATURE CONVERSION

(Fahrenheit temperature − 32) × 5/9 = Centigrade temperature

(Centigrade temperature × 9/5) + 32 = Fahrenheit temperature

## SELECTED CONVERSION TO METRIC MEASURES

| Known Value | Multiply by | To Find |
|---|---|---|
| inches | 2.54 | centimeters |
| ounces | 28 | grams |
| pounds | 454 | grams |
| pounds | 0.45 | kilograms |

## SELECTED CONVERSION FROM METRIC MEASURES

| Known Value | Multiply by | To Find |
|---|---|---|
| centimeters | 0.4 | inches |
| grams | 0.035 | ounces |
| grams | 0.0022 | pounds |
| kilograms | 2.2 | pounds |

## Conversion of Pounds and Ounces to Grams

| Pounds \ Ounces | 0 | 1 | 2 | 3 | 4 | 5 | 6 | 7 | 8 | 9 | 10 | 11 | 12 | 13 | 14 | 15 |
|---|---|---|---|---|---|---|---|---|---|---|---|---|---|---|---|---|
| 0 | — | 28 | 57 | 85 | 113 | 142 | 170 | 198 | 227 | 255 | 283 | 312 | 340 | 369 | 397 | 425 |
| 1 | 454 | 482 | 510 | 539 | 567 | 595 | 624 | 652 | 680 | 709 | 737 | 765 | 794 | 822 | 850 | 879 |
| 2 | 907 | 936 | 964 | 992 | 1021 | 1049 | 1077 | 1106 | 1134 | 1162 | 1191 | 1219 | 1247 | 1276 | 1304 | 1332 |
| 3 | 1361 | 1389 | 1417 | 1446 | 1474 | 1503 | 1531 | 1559 | 1588 | 1616 | 1644 | 1673 | 1701 | 1729 | 1758 | 1786 |
| 4 | 1814 | 1843 | 1871 | 1899 | 1928 | 1956 | 1984 | 2013 | 2041 | 2070 | 2098 | 2126 | 2155 | 2183 | 2211 | 2240 |
| 5 | 2268 | 2296 | 2325 | 2353 | 2381 | 2410 | 2438 | 2466 | 2495 | 2523 | 2551 | 2580 | 2608 | 2637 | 2665 | 2693 |
| 6 | 2722 | 2750 | 2778 | 2807 | 2835 | 2863 | 2892 | 2920 | 2948 | 2977 | 3005 | 3033 | 3062 | 3090 | 3118 | 3147 |
| 7 | 3175 | 3203 | 3232 | 3260 | 3289 | 3317 | 3345 | 3374 | 3402 | 3430 | 3459 | 3487 | 3515 | 3544 | 3572 | 3600 |
| 8 | 3629 | 3657 | 3685 | 3714 | 3742 | 3770 | 3799 | 3827 | 3856 | 3884 | 3912 | 3941 | 3969 | 3997 | 4026 | 4054 |
| 9 | 4082 | 4111 | 4139 | 4167 | 4196 | 4224 | 4252 | 4281 | 4309 | 4337 | 4366 | 4394 | 4423 | 4451 | 4479 | 4508 |
| 10 | 4536 | 4564 | 4593 | 4621 | 4649 | 4678 | 4706 | 4734 | 4763 | 4791 | 4819 | 4848 | 4876 | 4904 | 4933 | 4961 |
| 11 | 4990 | 5018 | 5046 | 5075 | 5103 | 5131 | 5160 | 5188 | 5216 | 5245 | 5273 | 5301 | 5330 | 5358 | 5386 | 5415 |
| 12 | 5443 | 5471 | 5500 | 5528 | 5557 | 5585 | 5613 | 5642 | 5670 | 5698 | 5727 | 5755 | 5783 | 5812 | 5840 | 5868 |
| 13 | 5897 | 5925 | 5953 | 5982 | 6010 | 6038 | 6067 | 6095 | 6123 | 6152 | 6180 | 6209 | 6237 | 6265 | 6294 | 6322 |
| 14 | 6350 | 6379 | 6407 | 6435 | 6464 | 6492 | 6520 | 6549 | 6577 | 6605 | 6634 | 6662 | 6690 | 6719 | 6747 | 6776 |
| 15 | 6804 | 6832 | 6860 | 6889 | 6917 | 6945 | 6973 | 7002 | 7030 | 7059 | 7087 | 7115 | 7144 | 7172 | 7201 | 7228 |
| 16 | 7257 | 7286 | 7313 | 7342 | 7371 | 7399 | 7427 | 7456 | 7484 | 7512 | 7541 | 7569 | 7597 | 7626 | 7654 | 7682 |
| 17 | 7711 | 7739 | 7768 | 7796 | 7824 | 7853 | 7881 | 7909 | 7938 | 7966 | 7994 | 8023 | 8051 | 8079 | 8108 | 8136 |
| 18 | 8165 | 8192 | 8221 | 8249 | 8278 | 8306 | 8335 | 8363 | 8391 | 8420 | 8448 | 8476 | 8504 | 8533 | 8561 | 8590 |
| 19 | 8618 | 8646 | 8675 | 8703 | 8731 | 8760 | 8788 | 8816 | 8845 | 8873 | 8902 | 8930 | 8958 | 8987 | 9015 | 9043 |
| 20 | 9072 | 9100 | 9128 | 9157 | 9185 | 9213 | 9242 | 9270 | 9298 | 9327 | 9355 | 9383 | 9412 | 9440 | 9469 | 9497 |
| 21 | 9525 | 9554 | 9582 | 9610 | 9639 | 9667 | 9695 | 9724 | 9752 | 9780 | 9809 | 9837 | 9865 | 9894 | 9922 | 9950 |
| 22 | 9979 | 10007 | 10036 | 10064 | 10092 | 10120 | 10149 | 10177 | 10206 | 10234 | 10262 | 10291 | 10319 | 10347 | 10376 | 10404 |

Ounces

Pounds

# Appendix E
# Diagnostic Procedures

Consider the growth and developmental level of the child when preparing the child for a procedure, and support the child during and after the procedure. See your textbook for preparing a child for procedures. Parents need to complete a signed consent after making sure they have an understanding of the procedure, results, and risk factors. When possible, allow the parents to remain with the child during the procedure.

| Procedure, Description, and Purpose | Nursing Management |
| --- | --- |
| **ACTH (adrenocorticotropic hormone) stimulation test**<br><br>A drug, metyrapone, is administered to block the production of cortisol. In persons with pituitary insufficiency, the ACTH level does not increase as expected. | ■ Phenytoin and estrogen compounds interfere with the test results.<br>■ Contact the laboratory for timing of the blood specimens to be collected. |
| **ACTH (adrenocorticotropic hormone) suppression test**<br><br>Dexamethosone, a potent corticosteroid, is administered to suppress the pituitary and ACTH production. In cases of Cushing syndrome, high levels of serum cortisol continue to be produced. | ■ Administer dexamethosone in the dose and at the time prescribed.<br>■ Contact the laboratory for timing of the blood specimens to be collected. A plastic tube is used rather than glass. Urine may also be collected to test level of cortisol. |
| **Arteriography/angiogram**<br><br>A contrast dye is injected intravenously to allow visualization of blood vessels. Useful in evaluating patency of blood vessels and blood flow to parts of the body and in identifying abnormal vasculature. | ■ Obtain history of hypersensitivity to iodine, seafood, or radiographic contrast dye. Antihistamines and/or steroids may be prescribed if allergy is suspected.<br>■ Administer sedation as prescribed and follow assessment guidelines to monitor the child during and after the procedure; assess for vasovagal and allergic reactions.<br>■ Tell the child to expect a warm, flushing feeling that could last a few minutes. |
| **Arthrogram**<br><br>After a local anesthetic, a needle is inserted into a joint (e.g., knee or shoulder). Samples of joint fluid may be aspirated, and then air or contrast medium is injected into the joint cavity. The joint is moved to spread the dye. Radiographs are taken with the joint in various positions to detect injuries to cartilage or ligaments, and to visualize the joint capsule. | ■ Prepare the child and family for the procedure.<br>■ Local anesthesia is often used with general anesthesia for very young children. Support the child when the local anesthetic is inserted.<br>■ Rest, ice on the joint, elevation, and an analgesic may be needed for discomfort after the procedure. |
| **Barium or contrast enema**<br><br>Barium or barium and air are administered via a tube through the rectum to the colon. The large intestine is visualized to detect any abnormalities. Fluoroscopy is used to monitor the process and radiographs are taken. | ■ Give parents preprocedure instructions regarding diet, laxatives, and/or enemas so the colon is clear.<br>■ Prepare the child and parents for the procedure and to expect the sensation of fluid entering the rectum. Tell the child of the need not to have a bowel movement until told it is okay to do so.<br>■ Ensure that the child holds still while the radiographs are taken. |

*(continued)*

| Procedure, Description, and Purpose | Nursing Management |
|---|---|
| **Biopsy**<br><br>Removal and examination of tissue from the body organs or skin to detect malignancies or the presence of disease.<br><br>Biopsies can be obtained in several ways:<br><br>■ Surgical excision at tissue site<br>■ Needle aspiration at tissue site, with or without ultrasound<br>■ Needle insertion into skin<br>■ Brush method, scraping cells and tissue with stiff bristles as is done with a Pap smear<br>■ Punch, using an instrument to excise a small area of tissue | ■ Prepare necessary instruments and specimen containers. Assist with preparation of biopsy site.<br>■ Monitor the child receiving sedation and analgesia according to protocol.<br>■ Ensure that the child remains still during the procedure.<br>■ Apply dressing, if appropriate, to the site after the procedure.<br>■ Label specimens accurately and arrange for specimen transport as recommended.<br>■ Teach family to care for wound and to monitor site for infection. |
| **Bone marrow aspiration**<br><br>Marrow is removed from pelvic or iliac crest bones through a large-gauge needle with a syringe used for aspiration. The test is diagnostic for leukemia, metastatic tumors, and some anemias, and it tests for response to treatment. Marrow may also be harvested for transplant. | ■ The child is usually given anesthesia, or sedation and analgesia. Follow monitoring guidelines during and after the procedure.<br>■ The site is prepped with a cleansing agent according to agency protocol.<br>■ Positioning is determined by the site used, e.g., side-lying for the iliac crest.<br>■ After the procedure, maintain the child on bed rest for at least 1 hour.<br>■ Mild analgesics are provided for pain at the harvest site. |
| **Bronchoscopy**<br><br>A flexible fiberoptic bronchoscope is used to visualize the trachea and bronchi to identify and extract foreign objects in the airway, or for a biopsy. | ■ Maintain NPO status preprocedure according to agency guidelines.<br>■ The child will often be sedated for the procedure; if the child is not sedated, a local anesthetic spray will be used prior to passing the bronchoscope. Monitor the child according to agency guidelines.<br>■ Monitor vital signs per protocol postprocedure. Resume oral feedings as prescribed. |
| **Cardiac catheterization**<br><br>A radiopaque catheter is passed through a large vein or artery in an arm or leg to the heart. It is then threaded to the heart chambers or coronary arteries, or both, guided by fluoroscopy. The procedure enables precise measurement of oxygen saturation within the heart's chambers and great arteries and pressure gradients in the pulmonary vessels or heart chambers. This helps assess for:<br><br>■ Congenital heart defects<br>■ Cardiac valvular disease<br>■ Coronary artery disease<br>■ Evaluation of artificial valves<br><br>Other purposes of cardiac catheterization include heart muscle biopsy, tissue sampling for heart transplant rejection, or radiofrequency ablation for a heart rhythm disturbance. | ■ Preparation includes discontinuation of anticoagulant therapy a week prior to the test and no food or fluid 6–8 hours preprocedure (may be a shorter interval for infants). Have the child void.<br>■ Prepare the child for the equipment to be used and sensations that will be felt.<br>■ Obtain history of hypersensitivity to iodine, seafood, or radiographic contrast dye. Antihistamines and/or steroids may be ordered if allergy is suspected. Assess for allergic reaction during procedure.<br>■ An IV is started for sedation administration, and to provide access for emergency drugs if needed.<br>■ ECG leads are applied to the chest to monitor heart activity. Baseline vital signs and extremity circulation and pulses are assessed and documented. Vital signs, heart rhythm, as well as the pulse strength and neurovascular assessment of the affected extremity are monitored according to agency protocol.<br>■ See your textbook for nursing management after the procedure. |

*(continued)*

| *Procedure, Description, and Purpose* | *Nursing Management* |
|---|---|
| **Computed tomography (CT)**<br><br>The CT scan is a radiographic procedure that examines body sections from 360 degrees, producing cross-section images that build into a two-dimensional image of any body structure. It may be performed with or without contrast dye. Multislice CT is performed with a greater number of images obtained simultaneously for a more rapid procedure so that moving organs are not blurred.<br><br>CT is used to screen for head, liver, abdominal, and renal lesions; tumors; edema; abscesses; bone destruction; and to locate foreign objects in soft tissue, such as the eye. | ■ If contrast dye is required, the infant or child may be NPO. It must be performed 4 days after any other barium studies of abdomen.<br>■ If contrast dye is to be used, obtain a history about any hypersensitivity to iodine, seafood, or radiographic contrast dye. If allergy is suspected, antihistamines and/or steroids may be ordered prior to procedure. Assess for allergic reaction during procedure.<br>■ Prepare child for the procedure by describing the equipment, noises, and other expected sensations, and how the child can help during the procedure by not moving.<br>■ If sedation is ordered for infants and small children to keep them still, monitor them according to protocol.<br>■ If contrast dye is used, encourage fluids after the procedure. |
| **Cultures**<br><br>Cultures are taken to isolate and identify microorganisms causing infection, and often to identify the specific antibiotics to which the organisms are sensitive.<br><br>Cultures commonly used with children include: blood, throat, sputum, stool, wound, urine, and cerebrospinal fluid. | ■ Collect culture specimens before administering new antimicrobials to prevent false results. List any antimicrobials given on laboratory slip.<br>■ Send all specimens immediately to the laboratory, or refrigerate the specimen.<br>■ Use strict aseptic technique to handle the specimen. Keep lids on sterile specimen containers. |
| **Cystoscopy**<br><br>A flexible fiberoptic scope is inserted through the urethra into the bladder to inspect the interior urethra and bladder for inflammation, tumors, stones, or structural abnormalities. The procedure may be done simultaneously with a voiding cystourethrogram (see below). | ■ Keep infants and children NPO prior to the study if sedation will be used.<br>■ Administer sedation and/or analgesia as prescribed and monitor the child according to protocol.<br>■ Encourage fluids after the procedure to detect problems with voiding.<br>■ Inform the child and parents that dysuria and frequency may occur for a short time following the procedure. |
| **Dual-energy x-ray absorptiometry (DEXA)**<br><br>DEXA is a radiographic procedure emitting two photon energy beams used to measure bone mineral density in children at risk for glucocorticoid-induced osteoporosis. | ■ Identify factors increasing a child's risk for osteoporosis or skeletal problems.<br>■ Explain the procedure and equipment to be used to the child and parents.<br>■ Inform the child of the need to not move, and let the child know the test does not cause pain. |
| **Echocardiography**<br><br>An ultrasound study of the heart used to identify the heart size, structure, pattern of movement, hemodynamics, valvular disease, blood flow, and blood flow disturbances. The ultrasound probe (transducer) is held over the chest (transthoracic) or inserted through the esophagus (transesophageal) to send an ultrasound beam to the tissues. The reflected sound waves are then transformed into scans, graphs, or sounds (Doppler). | ■ Explain the procedure to the parents and child. Inform the child of the need to hold still for the procedure.<br>■ Inform the child that patches and a gel will be applied to the skin and a transducer will move over the area with some pressure, but that the test should cause no pain. |

*(continued)*

| *Procedure, Description, and Purpose* | *Nursing Management* |
|---|---|
| **Electrocardiography (ECG or EKG) and ambulatory electrocardiography**<br><br>An (ECG) records the electrical impulses of the heart via electrodes and a galvanometer (ECG machine). Eight electrodes are placed on the chest and an electrode is placed on each extremity. The lead selector is turned to read the 12 standard leads. A Holter monitor may be attached to capture ambulatory ECG readings over a 24-hour period.<br><br>An ECG is used to detect cardiac arrhythmias, identify electrolyte imbalances, or to monitor ECG changes during an exercise or stress test. | ▪ Obtain list of current medications and when they were last taken.<br>▪ Inform the child that patches will be applied to the chest, arms, and legs. Then wires will then be attached to the patches. Tell the child that the test causes no pain.<br>▪ Ask the child to hold still for a brief time. A pacifier or bottle may help the infant be still.<br>▪ Encourage the child with a Holter monitor to engage in usual activities, but no swimming or bathing in a tub or shower is allowed until electrodes are removed.<br>▪ Ask the parents of the child wearing a Holter monitor to keep a diary of any events or emotional stress that cause symptoms. A daily schedule of sleep, eating, exercise, and other activities may be requested. |
| **Electroencephalogram (EEG)**<br><br>Approximately 20 electrodes are applied to the scalp to record cerebral cortex electrical activity over 1–2 hours. In some cases, an EEG is performed when the child is asleep. An EEG is used to identify the potential for seizures, to determine brain death, and to detect other abnormalities such as a tumor, abscess, or intracranial hemorrhage. | ▪ Inform the parents and child about all medications and other substance (e.g., cola, tea, or coffee) to withhold for 24 to 48 hours.<br>▪ Ensure that the hair is clean and dry, and that no hair products (e.g., oil, gel, spray) have been applied.<br>▪ Do not permit infants or children to nap before the test.<br>▪ Explain that the procedure is not painful as electrodes are applied.<br>▪ Explain that washing the child's hair will remove the electrode gel. |
| **Electromyography (EMG)**<br><br>Needle electrodes are inserted into skeletal muscles, and muscle activity is measured during rest, voluntary activity, and electrical stimulation.<br><br>The test is useful in assisting with diagnosis of muscular dystrophy and to differentiate muscle diseases and lower motor neuron neuropathies such as those caused by hypothyroidism or diabetes. | ▪ Be alert to medications (muscle relaxants, anticholinergics, and cholinergics) or caffeine use that could affect EMG results, and whether they should be withheld.<br>▪ Inform the child that there may be slight pain when the needle electrodes are inserted. Support the child with age-appropriate relaxation techniques or distraction techniques. If pain persists, inform technician. Pain may cause false reports.<br>▪ Administer analgesic as needed for residual pain. |
| **Esophagogastroduodenoscopy/esophagastroscopy**<br><br>A flexible fiberoptic endoscope is used to visualize the internal structures of the esophagus, stomach, and duodenum. This procedure is also used to collect cytology specimens and to confirm gastrointestinal pathology (e.g., tumors, ulcerations, bleeding). | ▪ Keep the child NPO prior to the procedure.<br>▪ Administer sedation as prescribed and monitor the child during and postprocedure according to protocol.<br>▪ Inform children that they may be asked to swallow and may feel some pressure when the endoscope is inserted.<br>▪ Resume oral feedings as prescribed. Explain that some burping may occur that helps remove air inserted to visualize the GI tract. |
| **Evoked potential**<br><br>A child who is awake is monitored by electrodes measuring brain (e.g., electroencephalogram) and related muscle activity. The baseline of electrical activity obtained is then used during later surgery, such as a spinal fusion for scoliosis, in order to monitor innervation to muscle groups and avoid injury to the spinal cord during the surgical procedure. | ▪ Prepare the child for the procedure, including the size of equipment, sounds, and time it will take.<br>▪ Assist the child to relax with quiet music during the test. |

*(continued)*

| Procedure, Description, and Purpose | Nursing Management |
|---|---|
| **Exercise testing**<br><br>A test performed with a treadmill or stationary bicycle to evaluate exercise tolerance. ECG leads, a blood pressure cuff, and sometimes an oxygen consumption monitor are attached. Acceleration and pitch of the treadmill or bicycle are increased at intervals until the client is fatigued, symptomatic, or a predetermined endpoint is reached.<br><br>An ECG recording with a controlled activity increase helps to identify significant cardiac compensation or inadequate cardiac output. | ■ Prepare the adolescent for the test, what to expect, and that the test can be stopped at any time.<br>■ Instruct the adolescent to report vertigo, extreme shortness of breath, chest pain, and excessive fatigue.<br>■ Ensure that the adolescent understands that the test is of greater value when the exercise continues until the predetermined stopping level is reached.<br>■ Take baseline vital sign measurements prior to the exercise and throughout according to agency guidelines. |
| **GI series**<br><br>Upper GI and small bowel series are fluoroscopic and radiographic examinations of the esophagus, stomach, and small intestine as ingested oral barium or water-soluble contrast agent passes through the digestive tract.<br><br>This series identifies: ulcers; gastroesophageal reflux; polyps, tumors, or hiatal hernias in the GI tract; pyloric stenosis; or foreign bodies, varices, or strictures. | ■ Keep child NPO after midnight or for a number of hours according to agency guidelines. A low-residue diet may be ordered for the night before the test.<br>■ Withhold medications as ordered.<br>■ Record vital signs; note epigastric pain or discomfort.<br>■ Inform child that all of the liquid must be swallowed, but that the test will not cause pain or discomfort.<br>■ Inform the child that the room will be dark and the table on which the child is lying may be tilted.<br>■ Inform parents that the stool will be light colored after the test. |
| **Hyperoxitest**<br><br>Arterial blood is collected before and at least 10 minutes after giving the infant 100% oxygen to see how the child's $Po_2$ level responds to the oxygen. Differences between the arterial blood gas levels when an infant has central cyanosis help to distinguish between cardiac disease and pulmonary disease (Park, 2014). | ■ Follow guidelines for arterial blood collection from the upper right side of the body.<br>■ Administer oxygen through a plastic hood for at least 10 minutes to replace all alveolar air with oxygen. |
| **Intraesophageal pH probe monitoring**<br><br>A probe is placed in the distal esophagus for 24 hours to detect pH changes below 4. The pH is measured and recorded every 4–8 seconds. The test determines how frequently stomach acid enters the esophagus and how long it stays there. It is used to diagnose gastroesophageal reflux disease and for evaluating atypical symptoms such as apnea, stridor, or cough. | ■ Inform the family of medications that must be withheld before and during the test (e.g., antacids, $H_2$ inhibitors, proton pump inhibitors).<br>■ Prevent infant or child from inadvertent removal of probe. Use soft mittens on the child's hands if necessary.<br>■ Monitor and record pH measurements per protocol.<br>■ Instruct parents to keep a diary of the child's activities while probe is in place, e.g., feeding or sleeping. |
| **Intravenous pyelogram**<br><br>A contrast dye is administered by IV and excreted by the urinary system. A series of radiographs are taken at various intervals over an hour to evaluate the entire urinary system, including the kidney cortex, kidney pelvis, ureters, and bladder. A postvoid radiograph is taken to see how well the bladder empties. The test is used to diagnose structural defects and tumors in the urinary system. | ■ Assess for potential allergy to the contrast dye. An antihistamine or corticosteroid may be given to children with a potential allergy. Monitor the child carefully for an allergic reaction.<br>■ Obtain a serum creatinine and BUN prior to the test to assess renal function.<br>■ Follow orders for an NPO or clear liquid diet prior to the study and cleansing enema the morning of the test.<br>■ Encourage fluids after the procedure to flush out the contrast media, and monitor urinary output. |

*(continued)*

| *Procedure, Description, and Purpose* | *Nursing Management* |
|---|---|
| **Lumbar puncture**<br><br>A lumbar puncture is performed at the L3–L4 or L4–L5 level to obtain a specimen of cerebrospinal fluid (CSF) and to measure the CSF pressure. CSF is cultured and analyzed for glucose and protein content, and the number of lymphocytes present. | ■ Obtain a blood glucose level prior to the test for comparison with the CSF glucose level.<br>■ Hold the infant or child in knee–chest position and keep the child still during the procedure.<br>■ Label the tubes of CSF obtained by numeric sequence.<br>■ Assess breathing and any changes in neurologic function during the test.<br>■ Administer analgesics as ordered for headache. |
| **Magnetic resonance imaging (MRI)**<br><br>A radiographic examination that uses a large magnet to produce a magnetic field and radio waves to produce detailed images without ionizing radiation. The MRI scanner is a large, doughnut-shaped cylinder and the child lies on a table in the cylinder. An intravenous contrast dye is often used. An MRI provides detailed images of internal organ structure, blood flow patterns, and abnormalities in soft tissues. | ■ Prepare the child for loud sounds, the size of the equipment, and the tunnel. Cardiorespiratory leads are often placed on the chest when contrast dye is used.<br>■ Assess the child for potential allergy to the contrast dye. An antihistamine or corticosteroid may be ordered if the child is at risk for allergy. Monitor the child for allergy during the procedure.<br>■ Carefully check for and remove all metal objects from the body. Only preapproved medical equipment can be in the room.<br>■ Sedation may be needed to keep the infant or child still. Headphones with music may help older children to cooperate. Monitor the child according to agency guidelines. Commonly, the examiner can talk with the child via a speaker system to provide information and reassurance. |
| **Nuclear scan or radionuclide imaging**<br><br>A radionuclide (an unstable radioisotope that decays or disintegrates, emitting radiation) is given by mouth or IV, which concentrates in certain parts of the body. Scintillation (gamma) camera detectors are used to create a two-dimensional image of an organ in gray tones or color that is sent to a computer. The scans may be taken in several minutes, hours, or 24 hours later.<br><br>The test may identify a functional (rather than a structural) problem in the bone, brain, gastrointestinal tract, or kidney, or a thyroid scan may diagnose hyperthyroidism or hypothyroidism. | ■ Explain the procedure to the parents and child. Inform them that the amount of radiation received from radionuclide imaging is usually less than that received from a radiograph, and that there will be no discomfort.<br>■ The child may be NPO for several hours before the initial scan.<br>■ The nurse should wear two pairs of disposable gloves when in direct contact with the child's wastes for several hours. Follow agency guidelines for handling waste products.<br>■ Inform the child and family that radionuclide is excreted from the body in 6–24 hours. Ask the child and family to flush the toilet 3 times after voiding. Ask parents to schedule the test when airline travel is not planned for several days as the radioactive substance may set off security scanners. |
| **Polysomnography (sleep study)**<br><br>Electrodes are attached to the head and chest, and a pulse oximeter is used. Recordings of brain activity, eye movement, apnea episodes, oxygen desaturation, and sleep disturbances are taken during sleep over an 8-hour period. The test is used to identify apnea during sleep and to determine the cause of sleep disorders. | ■ Instruct family to keep sleep log 1 to 2 weeks prior to sleep studies, including notes about snoring and sleepiness during the day. Review the sleep log.<br>■ Instruct client/family to avoid caffeine products, sedatives, and naps for 1 to 2 days prior to testing.<br>■ Obtain a history related to medications, head injury, headache, and seizures. Caffeine and sedatives may be withheld.<br>■ Explain the procedure to the parents and child.<br>■ Monitor vital signs and observe for respiratory distress during the test. |

*(continued)*

| Procedure, Description, and Purpose | Nursing Management |
|---|---|
| **Positron emission tomography (PET) scan and single photon emission computed tomography (SPECT)**<br><br>PET alone or in combination with CT uses an intravenous radioisotope to measure emission of positive electrons in body organs, such as the brain or heart, or detect tumors and metastases. PET is effective in evaluating cerebral blood flow and myocardial perfusion as well as detecting recurrent cancer. SPECT is used to measure blood perfusion in the brain, evaluating central nervous system disorders. | ▪ Inform the child and family if food and fluids must be withheld.<br>▪ Prepare the child for the procedure in order to reduce anxiety.<br>▪ Start two IVs, one for the radioisotope and the other for serial blood gases.<br>▪ Monitor vital signs.<br>▪ Assess for potential allergies to the radioisotope medium. |
| **Pulmonary function tests (spirometry)**<br><br>The client breathes into a spirometer connected to a computer, and the results are analyzed. The vital capacity (maximum amount of air that can be expired after a normal inspiration) and forced expiratory volume (FEV), the percentage of air expired at 1, 2, and 3 seconds, can be calculated.<br><br>Pulmonary function tests are used to assess pulmonary function and to identify the severity of obstructive airway disease. | ▪ Obtain a list of any bronchodilators and steroids the child is taking.<br>▪ Record child's age, gender, height, weight, and vital signs.<br>▪ Assess for signs and symptoms of respiratory distress.<br>▪ Explain the purpose of the tests and procedures.<br>▪ Help the child to practice breathing patterns required for the test.<br>▪ Take two readings, average the values, and compare to expected values for age, gender, and height. |
| **Pulse oximetry**<br><br>Pulse oximetry provides an estimate of the hemoglobin saturated by oxygen, measured percutaneously ($SpO_2$). It serves as an alternate to the direct measurement of $PaO_2$ ($SaO_2$) through arterial blood gas analysis. | ▪ Explain that the sensor needs to be over a finger or nailbed.<br>▪ Monitor the skin under the sensor regularly if it is kept in place for a constant measurement. |
| **Radiograph (x-ray)**<br><br>The most common form of imaging, radiographs use electromagnetic radiation to obtain images of body structures on film for diagnostic purposes.<br><br>Radiographs are commonly used to detect abnormalities in the size, structure, and shape of bone and body structures, or to detect abnormalities of the chest, such as air trapping in the alveoli (hyperinflation), consolidation of lung tissue (pneumonia), or lung collapse. | ▪ Determine if any other radiographic procedures have been performed recently, as the contrast dye used may distort radiographic images.<br>▪ Explain the procedure to the parents and child and the need for a lead apron. Explain that one or more films will be taken in about 5–10 minutes. Explain that modern equipment decreases radiation exposure.<br>▪ Prepare the child. Have the child practice holding still and holding a breath in preparation for the test. |
| **Sweat chloride test**<br><br>Gel pads containing pilocarpine are placed on the child's arms. A small electrode is attached to the pads to stimulate sweating until enough sweat is collected. The arms are covered with plastic. Sweat is collected and analyzed for the concentration of chloride and osmolality. The test is used to diagnose cystic fibrosis. | ▪ Explain the purpose of the test to the parents and child.<br>▪ Explain the need for the child to keep the plastic covering over the lower arms in place for the duration of test (about 30 minutes). |
| **Tympanogram**<br><br>The procedure provides an estimate of middle ear pressure and an indirect measure of tympanic membrane movement. This helps identify the presence of fluid accumulation in the middle ear. | ▪ Explain the procedure to the parents and child. A parent should hold the young child still.<br>▪ Insert the earpiece with the probe into the auditory canal until the canal is sealed tightly.<br>▪ Use the machine according to the manufacturer's instructions.<br>▪ Repeat the test in the other ear. |

*(continued)*

| *Procedure, Description, and Purpose* | *Nursing Management* |
|---|---|
| **Ultrasound**<br><br>An ultrasound probe (transducer) is held over the skin or body cavity to transmit ultrasound waves to the tissues and receives deflected sound waves as they bounce off various body structures. The computer transforms the deflected sound waves into two-dimensional electronic scans or audible sounds (Doppler). Ultrasound is usually a noninvasive procedure used to detect tissue abnormalities. | ■ Explain the procedure to the parents and child. Inform them that the procedure is painless, and there is no exposure to radiation.<br>■ Maintain NPO status preprocedure for abdominal studies.<br>■ Confirm the child has not received any tests that will interfere with results (e.g., upper GI series).<br>■ Instruct child to remain still during the procedure. |
| **Voiding cystourethrogram or radionuclide cystography**<br><br>A cystoscopy procedure is combined with a radionucleotide scan to examine bladder structure and function, urethral anatomy, and bladder masses. The test may detect vesicoureteral reflux. | ■ Assess for potential allergies to radioisotope medium.<br>■ Explain catheterization to the child and that the bladder will be filled.<br>■ Provide coaching strategies for parents accompanying the child to help the child cooperate and cope during the test.<br>■ Encourage fluids after the procedure to flush out the contrast media. |

Source: Data from Corbett, J. V., & Banks, A. D. (2013). *Laboratory tests and diagnostic procedures with nursing diagnosis* (8th ed.). Upper Saddle River, NJ: Pearson; Kee, J. L. (2014). *Laboratory and diagnostic tests with nursing implications* (9th ed.). Upper Saddle River, NJ: Pearson; Park, M. (2014). *Pediatric cardiology for practitioners* (6th ed., pp. 207–208). Philadelphia, PA: Elsevier Saunders; Bindler, R. C., & Ball, J. W. (2012). *Clinical skills manual for principles of pediatric nursing: Caring for children* (5th ed.). Upper Saddle River, NJ: Pearson; U.S. National Library of Medicine. (2012). *Esophageal pH monitoring.* Retrieved from http://www.nlm.nih.gov/medlineplus/ency/article/003401.htm

# Citations and General References

Allison, J., & George, M. (2014). Using preoperative assessment and patient instruction to improve patient safety. *AORN Journal, 99*(3), 364–375.

American Academy of Allergy, Asthma, and Immunology (AAAAI). (2014). *Peak flow meter*. Retrieved from http://www.aaaai.org/conditions-and-treatments/library/at-a-glance/peak-flow-meter.aspx

American Academy of Pediatrics (AAP). (2009). *Guidelines for care of children in the emergency department*. Retrieved from http://aappolicy.aappublications.org/cgi/reprint/pediatrics;124/4/1233.pdf

American Academy of Pediatrics (AAP). (2013). Transporting children with special healthcare needs. *Pediatrics, 104*, 988–992; reaffirmed *132*, e281.

American Academy of Pediatrics (AAP) & American Heart Association (AHA). (2011). *Textbook of neonatal resuscitation* (6th ed.). Elk Grove Village, IL: AAP; Dallas, TX: AHA.

American Academy of Pediatrics (AAP) Committee on Drugs. (2015). Metric units and the preferred dosing of orally administered liquid medications. *Pediatrics, 135*(4), 784–787.

American Academy of Pediatrics (AAP) Committee on Fetus and Newborn, & American College of Obstetricians and Gynecologists (ACOG) Committee on Obstetrics. (2012). *Guidelines for perinatal care* (7th ed.). Evanston, IL: Author.

American Academy of Pediatrics (AAP) Section on Ophthalmology and Committee on Practice and Ambulatory Medicine, American Academy of Ophthalmology, American Association for Pediatric Ophthalmology and Strabismus, & American Association of Certified Orthoptists. (2012). Instrument-based pediatric vision screening policy statement, *Pediatrics, 130*(5), 983–986.

American Academy of Pediatrics (AAP) Task Force on Circumcision. (2012). Circumcision policy statement. *Pediatrics, 130*, 585–586.

American Association for Pediatric Ophthalmology and Strabismus. (2014). *Vision screening recommendations*. Retrieved from http://www.aapos.org/terms/conditions/131

American Association of Critical Care Nurses. (2010). *Verification of feeding tube placement (blindly inserted)*. Retrieved from http://www.aacn.org/WD/Practice/Docs/PracticeAlerts/Verification_of_Feeding_Tube_Placement_05-2005.pdf

American Association of Neuroscience Nurses (AANN). (2011). Care of the patient undergoing intracranial pressure monitoring/external ventricular drainage or lumbar drainage. In *AANN Clinical Practice Guideline Series*. Glenview, IL: Author.

Association of Women's, Health, Obstetrics and Neonatal Nurses (AWHONN). (2013). *Neonatal skin care: Evidence based clinical practice guideline* (3rd ed.). Washington, DC: Author.

Atkins, D. L., Berger, S., Duff, J. P., Gonzales, J. C., Hunt, E. A., Joyner, B. L., … Schexnayder, S. M. (2015). Part 11: Pediatric basic life support and cardiopulmonary resuscitation quality: 2015 American Heart Association guidelines update for cardiopulmonary resuscitation and emergency cardiovascular care. *Circulation, 132*(18, Suppl. 2), S519–S525.

Berman, A., Snyder, S., & Jackson, C. (2009). *Skills in clinical nursing* (6th ed.). Upper Saddle River, NJ: Pearson Prentice Hall.

Bethel, J. (2012). Emergency care of children and adults with head injury. *Nursing Standard, 26*(43), 49–56.

Bhutani, V. K., Committee on Fetus and Newborn, & American Academy of Pediatrics. (2011). Phototherapy to prevent severe neonatal hyperbilirubinemia in the newborn infant 35 or more weeks of gestation. *Pediatrics, 128*, e1046–e1052.

Bindler, R. C., & Ball, J. W. (2012). *Clinical skills manual for principles of pediatric nursing: Caring for children* (5th ed.). Upper Saddle River, NJ: Pearson.

Bindler, R. M., & Howry, L. B. (2005). *Pediatric drug guide and nursing implications*. Upper Saddle River, NJ: Prentice Hall Health.

Blackburn, S. T. (2013). *Maternal, fetal, & neonatal physiology: A clinical perspective* (4th ed.). Maryland Heights, MO: Elsevier Saunders.

Boroughs, D. S., & Dogherty, J. (2011). *Evidence-based pediatric secretion management: How do you measure up?* Retrieved from http://ce.nurse.com/ce619/evidence-based-pediatric-secretion-management/

Burchell, P. L., & Powers, K. A. (2011). Focus on central venous pressure monitoring. *Nursing 2011, 41*(12), 39–43.

Casey, G. (2013). Too much pressure on the brain. *Kai Tiaki Nursing New Zealand, 19*(3), 20–24.

Centers for Disease Control and Prevention (CDC). (2011). *Guidelines for the prevention of intravascular device-related infections, 2011*. Retrieved from http://www.cdc.gov/hicpac/pdf/guidelines/bsi-guidelines-2011.pdf

Centers for Disease Control and Prevention (CDC). (2014a). *Infection prevention and control recommendations for hospitalized patients under investigation (PUIs) for Ebola virus disease (EVD) in U.S. hospitals*. Retrieved from http://www.cdc.gov/vhf/ebola/healthcare-us/hospitals/infection-control.html

Centers for Disease Control and Prevention (CDC). (2014b). *Hand hygiene basics*. Retrieved from http://www.cdc.gov/handhygiene/Basics.html

Centers for Disease Control and Prevention (CDC). (2015a). *Epidemiology and prevention of vaccine-preventable disease* (13th ed.). Washington, DC: Author.

Centers for Disease Control and Prevention (CDC). (2015b). *Vaccines and immunizations*. Retrieved from http://www.cdc .gov/vaccines/recs/vac-admin/default.htm

Chameides, L., Samson, R. A., Schexnayder, S. M., & Hazinski, M. F. (2011). *Pediatric advanced life support*. Dallas, TX: American Heart Association.

Chan, E. D., Chan, M. M., & Chan, M. M. (2013). Pulse oximetry: Understanding its basic principles facilitates appreciation of its limitations. *Respiratory Medicine, 107*, 789–799.

Chan, E. Y., Ng, I. H., Tan, S. L., Jabin, K., Lee, L. N., & Ang, C. C. (2012). Nasogastric feeding practices: A survey using clinical scenarios. *International Journal of Nursing Studies, 49*, 310–319.

Chau, J. P. C., Lee, D. T. F., & Lo, S. H. S. (2012). A systematic review of methods of eye irrigation for adults and children with ocular chemical burns. *Worldviews on Evidence-Based Nursing, Third Quarter 2012*, 129–138.

Chin-Sang, S. (2015). Emergency management, In B. Engorn, & J. Flerlage (Eds.), *The Harriet Lane handbook* (20th ed., pp. 3–16). Philadelphia, PA: Elsevier Saunders.

Chung, J., & Morgan, S. H. (2013). Neonatal hearing screening. In M. G. MacDonald, J. Ramasethu, & K. Rais-Bahrami. *Atlas of procedures in neonatology* (5th ed., pp. 385–388). Philadelphia, PA: Wolters Kluwer.

Clores, L. (2014). *How to measure CVP (central venous pressure)*. Retrieved from http://nursingcrib.com/nursing-notes-reviewer/fundamentals-of-nursing/how-to-measure-cvp-central-venous-pressure/

Coin, I., & Scott, P. (2014). Alternatives to restraining children for clinical procedures. *Nursing Children and Young People, 26*(2), 22–27.

Coleman, D. L., & Rosoff, D. M. (2013). The legal authority of mature minors to general medical treatment. *Pediatrics, 131*, 786–793.

Corbett, J. V., & Banks, A. D. (2013). *Laboratory tests and diagnostic procedures with nursing diagnosis* (8th ed.). Upper Saddle River, NJ: Pearson.

Correa, J. A., Fallon, S. C., Murphy, K. M., Victorian, V. A., Bisset, G. S., Vasudevan, S. A., … Lee, T. C. (2014). Resource utilization after gastrostomy tube placement: Defining areas of improvement for future quality improvement projects. *Journal of Pediatric Surgery, 49*, 1598–1601.

Cystic Fibrosis Foundation. (2012). *Airway clearance techniques*. Retrieved from http://www.cff.org/treatments/Therapies/Respiratory/AirwayClearance/

Daniels, S. R. (2012). Diagnosis and management of hypertension in children and adolescents, *Pediatric Annals, 41*(7), 1–10.

Dumont, C., & Nesselrodt, D. (2012). Preventing central line-associated bloodstream infections. *Nursing 2012, June*, 41–46.

Emergency Nurses Association. (2012). *Provider manual: Emergency nursing pediatric course* (4th ed.). Des Plains, IL: Author.

Engorn, B., & Flerlage, J. (2015). *The Harriet Lane handbook* (20th ed.). St. Louis: Elsevier Mosby.

Flynn, J. T., Pierce, C. B., Miller, E. R., Charleston, J., Samuels, J. A., Kupferman, J., … the Chronic Kidney Disease in Children Study Group. (2012). Reliability of resting blood pressure measurement and classification using an oscillometric device in children with chronic kidney disease. *Journal of Pediatrics, 160*(3), 434–440.

Foresman-Capuzzi, J. (2009). More big help from little tools. *Journal of Emergency Nursing, 35*(3), 260–262.

Gasim, G. I., Musa, I. R., Abdien, M. T., & Adam, I. (2013). Accuracy of tympanic temperature measurement using an infrared tympanic membrane thermometer. *BMC Research Notes, 6*, 194–199.

Glomella, T. L. (2013). *Neonatology: Management, procedure, on-call problems, disease, and drugs* (7th ed.). New York, NY: Lange Medical Books/McGraw-Hill.

Gomez, R. J., Barrowman, N., Elia, S., Manias, E., Royle, J., & Harrison, D. (2013). Establishing intra- and inter-rater agreement of the Faces, Legs, Activity, Cry, Consolability scale for evaluating pain in toddlers during immunization. *Pain Research & Management, 18*(6), e124–e128.

Goossens, G. A. (2015). Flushing and locking of venous catheters: Available evidence and evidence deficit. *Nursing Research Practice*. doi: 10.1155/2015/985686

Greenway, K. (2014). Rituals in nursing: Intramuscular injections. *Journal of Clinical Nursing, 23*, 3583–3588.

Guido, G. W. (2010). *Legal & ethical issues in nursing* (5th ed.). Upper Saddle River, NJ: Prentice Hall Health.

Hadaway, L. (2012). Needleless connectors for IV catheters. *American Journal of Nursing, 112*(11), 31–44.

Hall, R. T., Domenico, H. J., Self, W. H., & Hain, P. D. (2013). Reducing the blood culture contamination rate in a pediatric emergency department and subsequent cost savings. *Pediatrics, 131*(1), e292–e297.

Hannah, E., & John, R. M. (2013). Everything the nurse practitioner should know about pediatric feeding tubes. *Journal of the American Association of Nurse Practitioners, 25*, 567–577.

Harrington, J. W., Logan, S., Harwell, C., Gardner, J., Swingle, J., McGuire, E., & Santos, R. (2012). Effective analgesia using physical interventions for infant immunizations. *Pediatrics, 129*(5), 815–822.

Heidari Gorji, M. A., Rezaei, F., Jafari, H., & Yazdani Cherati, J. (2015). Comparison of the effects of heparin and 0.9% sodium chloride solutions in maintenance of patency of central venous catheters. *Anesthesia and Pain Medicine, 5*, e22595.

Hered, R. W. (2011). Effective vision screening of young children in the pediatric office. *Pediatric Annals, 40*(2), 76–82.

James, H. E. (1986). Neurologic evaluation and support in the child with acute brain insult. *Pediatric Annals, 15*(1), 16–22.

Johns Hopkins Medicine. (2012). *Peak flow measurement*. Retrieved from http://www.hopkinsmedicine.org/healthlibrary/test_procedures/pulmonary/peak_flow_measurement_92,P07755/

Johnstone, L., Spence, D., & Koziol-McClain, J. (2010). Oral hygiene care in the pediatric intensive care unit: Practice recommendations. *Pediatric Nursing, 36*(2), 85–96.

Joint Commission. (2015a). *Universal protocol*. Retrieved from http://www.jointcommission.org/standards_information/up.aspx

Joint Commission. (2015b). *State operations manual.* Retrieved from http://www.cms.gov/Regulations-and-Guidance/Guidance/Manuals/downloads/som107ap_a_hospitals.pdf

Kee, J. L. (2014). *Laboratory and diagnostic tests with nursing implications* (9th ed.). Upper Saddle River, NJ: Pearson.

Ladewig, P. W., London, M. L., & Davidson, M. R. (2014). *Contemporary maternal-newborn care* (8th ed.). Upper Saddle River, NJ: Prentice Hall.

Lawrence, J., Alcock, D., McGrath, P., Kay, J., MacMurray, S. B., & Dulberg, C. (1993). The development of a tool to assess neonatal pain. *Neonatal Network, 12*(6), 59–66.

Merkel, S. I., Voepel-Lewis, T., Shayevitz, J. R., & Malviya, S. (1997). The FLACC: A behavioral scale for scoring postoperative pain in young children. *Pediatric Nursing, 23*(3), 293–297.

National Institute for Occupational Safety and Health (NIOSH). (2014). *Latex allergy: A prevention guide.* Retrieved from http://www.cdc.gov/niosh/docs/98-113/

O'Farrelly, C., & Hennessy, E. (2013). Brief report: A comparison of saliva collection methods with preschool children: The perspectives of children, parents, and childcare practitioners. *Journal of Pediatric Nursing, 28*(3), 292–295.

Office of the National Coordinator for Health Information Technology. (2015). *Guide to privacy and security of electronic health information.* Retrieved from http://www.healthit.gov/sites/default/files/pdf/privacy/privacy-and-security-guide.pdf

O'Grady, N. P., Alexander, M., Burns, L. A., Dellinger, E. P., Garland, J., Heard, S., … Healthcare Infection Control Practices Advisory Committee (HICPAC). (2011). *Guidelines for the prevention of intravascular catheter-related infections, 2011.* Bethesda, MD: U.S. Department of Health and Human Services.

O'Neill, J. l., Bull, M. J., & Sobus, K. (2011). Issues and approaches to safely transporting children with special healthcare needs. *Journal of Pediatric Rehabilitation Medicine, 4,* 279–288.

Padon, A. A., & Baren, J. M. (2011). Achieving a decision-making triad in adolescent sexual health care. *Adolescent Medicine State of the Art Reviews, 22*(2), 183–194.

Park, M. (2014). *Pediatric cardiology for practitioners* (6th ed., pp. 207–208). Philadelphia, PA: Elsevier Saunders.

Parker, L. C. (2012). Top 10 care essentials for ventilator patients. *American Nurse Today, 7*(3), 13–16.

Salimetrics. (2012). *Saliva collection and handling advice* (3rd ed.). State College, PA: Author.

Sarnaik, A. P., Clark, J. A., & Sarnaik, A. A. (2016). Respiratory distress and failure. In R. M. Kleigman, B. F. Stanton, J. W. St. Geme, & N. F. Schor, *Nelson textbook of pediatrics* (20th ed., pp. 529–545). Philadelphia, PA: Elsevier.

Schrauf, C. M. (2012). Monitoring blood pressure: Do method and body location matter? *Nephrology Nursing Journal, 39*(6), 502–505, 512.

Schweitzer, M., Aucoin, J., Docherty, S. L., Rice, H. E., Thompson, J., & Sullivan, D. T. (2014). Evaluation of a discharge education protocol for pediatric patients with gastrostomy tubes. *Journal of Pediatric Health Care, 28*(5), 420–428.

SGNA Practice Committee. (2008). Guideline for preventing sensitivity and allergic reactions to natural rubber latex in the workplace. *Gastroenterology Nursing, 31*(3), 239–246.

Siegel, J. D., Rhinehart, E., Jackson, M., Chiarello, L., & the IHC Infection Control Practices Advisory Committee. (2007). *2007 guidelines for isolation precautions: Preventing transmission of infectious agents in health care settings.* Retrieved from http://www.cdc.gov/hicpac/2007IP/2007isolationPrecautions.html

Simons, S. R. (2012). Bedside assessment of enteral tube placement: Aligning practice with evidence. *American Journal of Nursing, 112*(2), 40–46.

Sisson, H. (2015). Aspirating during the intramuscular injection procedure: A systematic literature review. *Journal of Clinical Nursing.* doi:10.1111.jocn.12824

Smith, J., Alcock, G., & Usher, K. (2013). Temperature measurement in the preterm and term infant: A review of the literature. *Neonatal Network, 31*(1), 16–25.

Sona, C., Prentice, D., & Schallom, L. (2012). National survey of central venous catheter flushing in the intensive care unit. *Critical Care Nurse, 32,* e12–e19.

Stine, C. A., Flook, D. M., & Vincze, D. L. (2012). Rectal versus axillary temperatures: Is there a significant difference in infants less than 1 year of age? *Journal of Pediatric Nursing, 27,* 265–270.

Taddio, A., Hogan, M. E., Moyer, P., Girgis, A., Gerges, S., Wang, L., & Ipp, M. (2011). Evaluation of the reliability, validity and practicality of 3 measures of acute pain in infants undergoing immunization injections. *Vaccine, 29,* 1390–1394.

Teasdale, G., & Jennett, B. (1974). Assessment of coma and impaired consciousness. *Lancet, 2,* 81–84.

Teasdale, G., Allan, D., Brennan, P., McElhinney, E., & Mackinnon, L. (2014). Forty years on: Updating the Glasgow Coma Scale. *Nursing Times, 110*(42), 12–16.

Teasdale, G., Maas, A., Lecky, F., Manley, G., Stocchetti, N., & Murray, G. (2014). The Glasgow Coma Scale at 40 years: Standing the test of time. *Lancet Neurology, 13*(8), 844–854.

Tho, P. C., Mordiffi, S., Ang, E., & Chen, H. (2011). Implementation of the evidence review on best practice for confirming the correct placement of nasogastric tube in patients in an acute care hospital. *International Journal of Evidence Based Healthcare, 9,* 51–60.

Unguru, Y. (2011). Making sense of adolescent decision-making: Challenge and reality. *Adolescent Medicine State of the Art Research, 22*(2), 195–206.

U.S. Department of Health and Human Services. (2015). *Safety and effectiveness of health care antiseptics.* Retrieved from http://www.gpo.gov/fdsys/pkg/FR-2015-05-01/pdf/2015-10174.pdf

U.S. National Library of Medicine. (2012). *Esophageal pH monitoring.* Retrieved from http://www.nlm.nih.gov/medlineplus/ency/article/003401.htm

WebMD. (2012). *Asthma and the peak flow meter*. Retrieved from http://www.webmd.com/asthma/guide/peak-flow-meter

White, M. L., Crawley, J., Rennie, E. A., & Lewandowski, L. A. (2011). Examining the effectiveness of 2 solutions used to flush capped pediatric peripheral intravenous catheters. *Journal of Infusion Nursing, 34*(4), 260–270.

Wong, D. L., & Baker, C. M. (1988). Pain in children: Comparison of assessment scales. *Pediatric Nursing, 14*, 9–16.

Woolley, S. (2011). The limits of parental responsibility regarding medical treatment decisions. *Archives of Disease in the Child, 96*(11), 1060–1065.

World Health Organization (WHO). (2014). *Good hand hygiene by health workers protects patients from drug resistant infections.* Retrieved from http://www.who.int/mediacentre/news/releases/2014/hand-hygiene/en/

Worrall, K. (2004). Use of the Glasgow Coma Scale in infants. *Paediatric Nursing, 16*(4), 45–47.

Yin, H. S., Dreyer, B. P., Ugboaja, D. C., Sanchez, D. C., Paul, I. M., Horeira, H. A., … Mendelsohn, A. L. (2014). Unit of measurement used and parent medication dosing errors. *Pediatrics, 134*, e354–e361.

Yönt, G. H., Korhanb, E. A., & Dizer, B. (2014). The effect of nail polish on pulse oximetry readings. *Intensive and Critical Care Medicine, 30*, 111–115.

# Index

Note: Page numbers followed by f indicate figures; those followed by t indicate tables.